Stilianos E. Kountakis · Metin Önerci (Eds.)

Rhinologic and Sleep Apnea Surgical Techniques

Stilianos E. Kountakis · Metin Önerci (Eds.)

Rhinologic and Sleep Apnea Surgical Techniques

With 480 Figures and 32 Tables

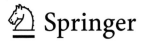

Springer

Stilanos E. Kountakis, MD
Medical College of Georgia
Department of Otolaryngology
Head and Neck Surgery
1120 Fifteeth Street
30912-4060 Augusta
USA

Metin Önerci, MD
Hacettepe University
Faculty of Medicine
Department of Otorhinolaryngology
06100 Ankara
Turkey

Library of Congress Control Number: 2006939423

ISBN 978-3-540-34019-5 Springer Berlin Heidelberg New York

Springer is a part of Springer Science+Business Media
springer.com
© Springer-Verlag Berlin Heidelberg 2007

Editor: Marion Philipp, Heidelberg, Germany
Desk Editor: Irmela Bohn, Heidelberg, Germany
Production: LE-TeX, Jelonek, Schmidt & Vöckler GbR, Leipzig, Germany
Cover design: Frido Steinen-Broo, EStudio, Calamar, Spain
Reproduction and typesetting: Satz-Druck-Service (SDS), Leimen, Germany

Printed on acid-free paper 24/3180/YL   5 4 3 2 1 0

Dedication

To my father Emmanuel.
To the memory of my mother Eftihia – to you I owe what I am and there has never been
a day in my life without missing you.
To my beautiful wife Eleni and children Eftihia, Emmanuel and Nikoleta
for their love and support.

Stilianos E. Kountakis

To my nurturing and supporting parents.
To my loving wife, Semra, and my daughters, Özlem and Zeynep,
for their support and accepting a part-time father.
To my colleagues who inspire me to learn and to my students who inspire me to teach.

Metin Önerci

Preface

The fields of rhinology and sleep apnea surgery have rapidly advanced with new instrumentation and surgical techniques. Surgeons in these fields stay abreast by attending scientific meetings, by participating in hands-on laboratory workshops and by reading the literature. This surgical book fills the void of a single concise surgical-atlas-like book that contains precise description of the surgical techniques used in rhinology and sleep apnea surgery. We have invited internationally recognized faculty with extensive experience to author the chapters. These authors share their wisdom on each topic through diagrammatic and illustrated chapters with the purpose of providing the basis for the successful management of the surgical rhinologic and sleep apnea patient.

The chapters are grouped into a rhinologic and a sleep apnea section and are arranged in a logical fashion so that the reader first learns basic techniques followed by more advanced and revision surgery. In addition to the illustrated surgical descriptions, surgical chapters contain information about the workup of the abnormality that is described followed by indications of surgery and tips and pearls to avoid complications. All authors share their secrets that lead to successful and uncomplicated surgical outcomes. Almost all surgical techniques in the field of rhinology and sleep apnea surgery are addressed, including the latest on balloon dilatation of sinus ostia or, more precisely, endoscopic balloon sinusotomy.

In addition to illustrated surgical descriptions, the DVD version of the book contains video files of actual procedures performed by the authors. So the readers have a 360° learning experience by first reading the chapter text and visualizing the illustrations, and then reinforcing their learning experience by reviewing the actual video of the procedures. The result is a comprehensive volume of surgical information in the form of a 360° learning experience that can be used by all practicing and in-training otolaryngologists as a reference source and to augment their surgical education.

Stilianos E. Kountakis MD
Metin Önerci MD

Contents

List of Contributors

Marcelo Antunes
Department of Otolaryngology
University of Pennsylvania
5th Floor, Ravdin Building
3400 Spruce Street, Philadelphia
PA 19104-4283
USA

Raghu S. Athre
Department of Otolaryngology –
Head and Neck Surgery
University of Texas Southwestern Medical Center
5323 Harry Hines Blvd., Dallas
TX 75235-9035
USA
E-mail: raghu@athre.com

Alexander Baisch
Department of Otorhinolaryngology –
Head and Neck Surgery
University Hospital Mannheim
Theodor-Kutzer-Ufer, 68167 Mannheim
Germany
E-mail: alexander.baisch@hno.ma.uni-heidelberg.de

Pete S. Batra
Department of Otolaryngology
Cleveland Clinic Foundation
Desk A71, 9500 Euclid Avenue,
Cleveland, OH 44195
USA
E-mail: batrap@ccf.org

Adam M. Becker
Department of Otolaryngology –
Head and Neck Surgery
Medical College of Georgia
1120 15th Street, Augusta, GA 30912-4060
USA
E-mail: abecker@mcg.edu

Bernard Bertrand
Department of Otolaryngology
and Head and Neck Surgery
University UCL Hospital of Mont-Godinne
Avenue Therasse 1, 330 Yvoir
Belgium
E-mail: bernard.bertrand@orlo.ucl.ac.be

Benjamin Bleier
Department of Otolaryngology –
Head and Neck Surgery
Hospital University of Pennsylvania
5th Floor, Ravdin Building
3400 Spruce Street, Philadelphia, PA 19104
USA
E-mail: benjamin.bleier@uphs.upenn.edu

Jean M. Bruch
Department of Otolaryngology
Massachusetts Eye and Ear Infirmary
243 Charles Street, Boston, MA 02114
USA

Nicolas Y. Busaba
Department of Otolaryngology –
Head and Neck Surgery
Massachusetts Eye and Ear Infirmary
243 Charles Street, Boston, MA 02114
USA
E-mail: nicolas_busaba@meei.harvard.edu

Roy R. Casiano
Department of Otolaryngology
Leonard Miller School of Medicine
University of Miami
Suite 4025, 1475 N.W. 12th Avenue
Miami, FL 33136-1002
USA
E-mail: rcasiano@med.miami.edu

Thomas T. Le
Department of Otorhinolaryngology,
University of Maryland Medical System,
Suite 500, 16 South Eutaw Street, Baltimore
MD 21201
USA

Richard A. Lebowitz
Department of Otolaryngology
New York University Medical Center
Suite 3C, 530 1st Avenue, New York
NY 10016-6402
USA
E-mail: richard.lebowitz@nyumc.org

Kasey K. Li
University Sleep Disorders and Research Center
Stanford University, Suite 105
1900 University Ave
East Palo Alto
CA 94303-2212
USA
E-mail: drli@drkaseyli.com

Francis T.K. Ling
Department of Otolaryngology –
Head and Neck Surgery
Medical College of Georgia
1120 15th Street, Augusta
GA 30912-4060
USA
E-mail: fling@mail.mcg.edu

Robert H. Maisel
Department of Otolaryngology
University of Minnesota
Hennepin County Medical Center
701 Park Avenue, Minneapolis
MN 55415
USA
E-mail: maise001@umn.edu

Steven Mariën
Department of Otorhinolaryngology
General Hospital Middelheim, Lindendreef 1
2020 Antwerp
Belgium
E-mail: stevenmarien@yahoo.com

Bradley F. Marple
Department of Otolaryngology –
Head and Neck Surgery
University of Texas Southwestern
Medical Center, 5323 Harry Hines Blvd., Dallas
TX 75235-9035
USA
E-mail: bradley.marple@utsouthwestern.edu

Christopher T. Melroy
Georgia Nasal & Sinus Institute
Suite 112, 4750 Waters Avenue, Savannah
GA 31404-6220
USA

Tanya K. Meyer
Department of Otorhinolaryngology
University of Maryland Medical System
Suite 500, 16 South Eutaw Street, Baltimore
MD 21201
USA

Amir Minovi
Department for ENT Diseases
Head, Neck and Facial Plastic Surgery
Hospital of Fulda, Pacelliallee 4, 36043 Fulda
Germany
E-mail: minovi@web.de

Chairat Neruntarat
Department of Otolaryngology
Faculty of Medicine, Srinakharinwirot University
Vajira Hospital, 681 Sam saen Road
Bangkok 10300
Thailand
E-mail: xyratana@yahoo.com

Oguz Ögretmenoglu
Department of Otorhinolaryngology –
Head and Neck Surgery
University of Hacettepe
06100 Sıhhıye, Ankara
Turkey

Metin Önerci
Department of Otorhinolaryngology –
Head and Neck Surgery
University of Hacettepe, 06100 Sıhhıye, Ankara
Turkey
E-mail: metin@tr.net

James N. Palmer
Department of Otolaryngology –
Head and Neck Surgery, Hospital
University of Pennsylvania
5th Floor, Ravdin Building, 3400 Spruce Street
Philadelphia, PA 19104
USA
E-mail: james.palmer@uphs.upenn.edu

Kenny P. Pang
Department of Otolaryngology
Tan Tock Seng Hospital, 11 Jalan Tan Tock Seng
Singapore 308433
Republic of Singapore
E-mail: kennypang@hotmail.com

Wolfgang Pirsig
ENT Department, University Hospital Ulm
Mozartstrasse 22/1, 89075 Ulm
Germany
E-mail: wolfgang.pirsig@extern.uni-ulm.de

Hassan H. Ramadan
Department of Otolaryngology
West Virginia University, PO Box 9200, Morgantown
WV 26506-9200
USA
E-mail: hramadan@hsc.wvu.edu

Marc Remacle
Department of ORL and Head and Neck Surgery
University UCL Hospital of Mont-Godinne
Avenue Therasse 1
5530 Yvoir, Belgium
E-mail: remacle@orlo.ucl.ac.be

Daniel Rodenstein
Department of Pneumology
Université Catholique de Louvain
Cliniques Universitaires Saint Luc
Avenue Hippocrate 10, 1200 Brussels
Belgium

Philippe Rombaux
Department of Otorhinolaryngology
Université Catholique de Louvain
Cliniques Universitaires Saint Luc
Avenue Hippocrate 10, 200 Brussels,
Belgium
E-mail: philippe.rombaux@orlo.ucl.ac.be

Zoukaa B. Sargi
Department of Otolaryngology
Leonard Miller School of Medicine
University of Miami, UMHC Suite 4025, 1475 NW
12th Avenue, Miami, FL 33136-1002
USA
E-mail: zsargi@um-jmh.org

Rodney J. Schlosser
Department of Otolaryngology
Medical University of South Carolina
Suite 1130, 135 Rutledge Ave., Charleston
SC 29425
USA
E-mail: schlossr@musc.edu

Paul Schalch
Suite 1107, 30 N. Michigan Ave.
Chicago, IL 60602-3747
USA
E-mail: paulschalch@yahoo.com

Joseph M. Scianna
Department of Otolaryngology
Loyola University, 2160 South 1st Avenue
Maywood, IL 60153-3304
USA

Joachim Schmeck
ENT Department, St. Lucas Andreas Hospital
Jan Tooropstraat 164, 1061 AE Amsterdam
The Netherlands

Bert Schmelzer
Department of Otorhinolaryngology
General Hospital Middelheim
Lindendreef 1, 2020 Antwerp
Belgium
E-mail: bert.schmelzer@belgacom.net

Brent A. Senior
Department of Otolaryngology –
Head and Neck Surgery
The University of North Carolina at Chapel Hill
G0412 Neurosciences Hospital, CB 7070
Chapel Hill, NC 27599
USA
E-mail: brent_senior@med.unc.edu

Michael J. Sillers
Alabama Nasal and Sinus Center, Suite 301
7191 Cahaba Valley Road, Birmingham
AL 35242
USA
E-mail: michaelsillers@charter.net

Ioannis G. Skoulas
Member of Greek Partiament
Allending Physician at Venizetion Hospital
Heraklion, Crete/ G. Katehaki St 26 Heraklion
Crete 71500
Greece

Timothy L. Smith
Department of Otolaryngology/
Head and Neck Surgery
Oregon Sinus Center
Oregon Health & Science University
PV-01, 3181 S.W. Sam Jackson Park Rd., Portland
OR 97239
USA
E-mail: smithtim@ohsu.edu

James A. Stankiewicz
Department of Otolaryngology
Loyola University
2160 South 1st Avenue, Maywood
IL 60153-3304, USA
E-mail: jstank@lumc.edu

dictates an endless combination of anatomic variations that force the rhinologist to evaluate each side of the face as a completely independent anatomic, functional and surgical entity.

Recent significant advances in computed tomography (CT), especially the introduction of multidetector helical scanning and the routine availability of computer workstations, have made demonstration of this complex anatomy easier and more useful to rhinologic surgical planning. This improvement in imaging clarity and multiplanar demonstration of sinus complex anatomy is now of even more clinical relevance in view of the extensive developments in powered instruments, better endoscopic devices and surgical navigation with CT cross-registration.

Functional Concepts

The sinonasal embryologic development during the first trimester is characterized by the emergence of more than six ethmoturbinals, which progressively coalesce and differentiate into the final anatomy of the lateral nasal wall [9].

The ethmoturbinals give rise to the following structures:

- The most superior remnant of the first ethmoturbinal becomes the agger nasi mound.
- The remnant of the descending portion of the first ethmoturbinal becomes the uncinate process.
- The basal lamella of the second ethmoturbinal pneumatizes and gives rise to the bulla ethmoidalis.
- The basal lamella of the third ethmoturbinal becomes the basal lamella of the middle turbinate.

The nasal mucosa invaginates at specific points in the lateral nasal wall forming nasal pits that develop into the anlages of maxillary, frontal sinuses and ethmoid cells [2]. The mesenchyme resorbs around the invagination of the nasal pits, allowing progressive development of the sinus cavity. The embryologic point at which the initial invagination occurs becomes the future sinus ostium. Cilia develop and orient towards this ostium, allowing mucus to flow towards and through the ostium. The efficiency of the mucociliary drainage is then dictated and impacted by the patency, tortuosity and/or frank narrowing of the resulting drainage pathways, which are progressively modified by the sequential ongoing pneumatization process occurring during the patient's life. Typically the ethmoid cells and the maxillary antra are pneuma-

tized at birth, with the maxillary antra progressively expanding into mature sinuses as the maxilla matures and the teeth erupt. The frontal sinus develops and expands in late childhood to early adolescence, and continues to grow into adulthood. The rate of sinus growth is modified by the efficiency of ventilation and mucociliary drainage dictated by the patency of the sinus ostium and the corresponding drainage pathways. The frontal sinus drainage pathway is the most complex of all sinus outflow tracts, impacted by its anatomic relationships with the agger nasi, anterior ethmoid cells and pattern of vertical insertion of the uncinate process [3, 4]. The frontal sinus mucociliary output joins the outflow from the anterior ethmoid and maxillary sinuses at the ostiomeatal complex, with the mucociliary transport continuing posteriorly over the attachment of the inferior turbinate, through the choanna and towards the nasopharynx anterior to the torus tubarius. Similarly, the mucociliary transport output of the posterior ethmoid and sphenoid sinuses emerges into the sphenoethmoid recess at the level of the superior meatus to be transported downwards towards the nasopharynx posterior to the torus tubarius.

Sinus Imaging Evaluation

The evaluation of the paranasal sinuses for functional endoscopic sinus surgery is traditionally performed with continuous coronal and axial 3-mm CT slices to provide orthogonal sinus anatomy planes [6, 7]. Recent CT scanner advances with the introduction of multidetector helical designs and faster computers with larger processing capacities now allow single-plane thin-section high-resolution databases to be acquired and postprocessed to depict the sinus anatomy in any planar projection, with high definition of the underlying anatomy. This multiplanar capability has mostly impacted the evaluation of all sinus drainage pathways, since perpendicular reconstructions of the frontal recess, ostiomeatal complex and sphenoethmoid recess can now be easily obtained from a single-plane image acquisition.

Typical high-resolution multidetector scanning is performed in the axial plane (Fig. 1.1a) following the long axis of the hard palate, using low milliampere technique, a small field of view (18–20 cm) and 1.25-mm collimation, with data back-processed in 0.65-mm thickness in a bone algorithm and displayed in mucosal (window of 2,000, level of –200) and bone (3,500/800) detail. Most centers use this pattern of data acquisition for three-dimensional computer-assisted surgical navigation. Interactive processing and evaluation of the data is then performed on the CT workstation to define a coronal plane perpendic-

Fig. 1.1. High-resolution sinus navigation CT protocol. **a** Lateral scout view showing the typical prescription of axial thin-section slices. **b** An axial image at the level of the nasal cavity helps prescribe the coronal reformatted images. **c** The sagittal reformatted images are more accurately prescribed from the coronal reformatted images

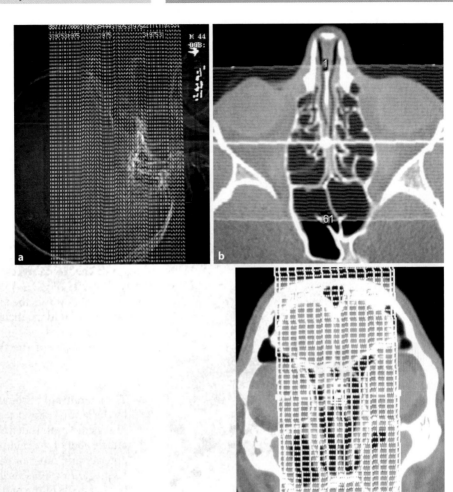

ular to the hard palate for the ostiomeatal complex (Fig. 1.1b) and a sagittal plane perpendicular to the hard palate for the frontal recess (Fig. 1.1c). The axial plane perpendicular to the rostrum of the sphenoid sinus allows for adequate evaluation of the sphenoethmoid recess.

Frontal Sinus Drainage Pathway

The frontal sinus grows and expands within the diploic space of the frontal bone from the frontal sinus ostium medial and superior to the orbital plates, enclosed anteriorly by the cortical bone of the anterior frontal sinus wall and posteriorly by the cortical bone of the skull base and the posterior frontal sinus wall (which is also the anterior wall of the anterior cranial fossa). Each frontal sinus grows independently, with its rate of growth, final volume and configuration dictated by its ventilation, drainage and the corresponding growth (or lack of it) of the competing surrounding sinuses and skull base.

Frontal Sinus Ostium

The frontal sinus narrows down inferiorly and medially into a funnel-shaped transition point, which is defined as the frontal sinus ostium (Fig. 1.2a–c), extending between the anterior and posterior frontal sinus walls at the skull base level. This point is typically demarcated along its anterior wall by the variably shaped bone ridge of the nasofrontal buttress, frequently called the "nasal beak" (Fig. 1.2d). The frontal sinus ostium is oriented nearly perpendicular to the posterior wall of the sinus at the level of the anterior skull base [3].

Anterior Ethmoid Artery

The anterior ethmoid artery is a terminal branch of the ophthalmic artery that crosses the lamina papyracea along the posterior wall of the frontal recess to supply the dura of the olfactory fossa and the anterior

1

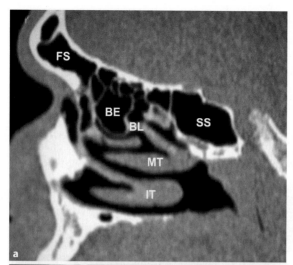

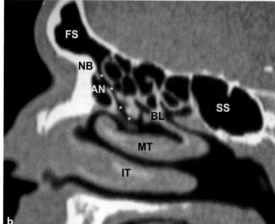

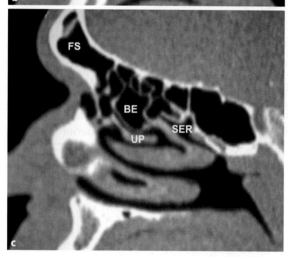

Fig. 1.2. The frontal sinus ostium: sagittal sequential refor-matted images from midline to lateral showing the many im-portant anatomic landmarks. Axial (a), coronal (b) and sag-ittal (c) images at the level of the frontal sinus (FS) illustrate the frontal sinus ostium. *Asterisks* ethmoid infundibulum, *AE* anterior ethmoid, *AN* agger nasi cells, *BE* bulla ethmoidalis, *BL* basal lamella of the middle turbinate (*MT*), *IT* inferior tur-binate, *NB* nasal beak, *PE* posterior ethmoid, *UP* uncinate pro-cess, *SER* sphenoethmoid recess, *SS* sphenoid sinus

falx cerebri. It is a constant vascular landmark of the posterior wall of the frontal recess, crossing through the anterior ethmoid canal, which can be frequently dehiscent, posing a risk of vascular injury when ex-ploration of the frontal recess is surgically necessary (Fig. 1.3b).

Frontal Recess, Agger Nasi and Uncinate Process

The Anatomic Terminology Group defined the fron-tal recess as "the most anterior and superior part of the anterior ethmoid complex from where the fron-tal bone becomes pneumatized, resulting in a frontal sinus" [9]. The frontal recess frequently looks like an inverted funnel (Fig. 1.3a) on sagittal images, open-ing superiorly towards the frontal sinus ostium, with its anatomic boundary dictated by the walls of sur-rounding structures.

The boundaries of the frontal recess are as fol-lows:

- The lateral wall of the frontal recess is defined by the lamina papyracea of the orbit.
- The medial wall is defined by the vertical attachment of the middle turbinate (its most anterior and superior part).
- Its posterior wall is variable, depending on the basal lamella of the bulla ethmoidalis reaching (or not) the skull base, or if it is dehiscent al-lowing communication with the suprabullar recess, or if it is hyperpneumatized anteriorly, producing a secondary narrowing of the fron tal recess from forward deformity of its poste-rior wall [2].

The agger nasi cells and the uncinate process dictate the floor and the pattern of drainage of the frontal recess. The frontal recess can be narrowed from an-terior-inferior direction by hyperpneumatized agger nasi cells. Furthermore, the frontal recess inferior drainage is dictated by the insertion of the vertical attachment of the uncinate process, a sagittally ori-ented hooklike bony leaflet (Fig. 1.4a). Whenever the uncinate process attaches to the skull base or the su-perior-anterior portion of the middle turbinate, the frontal recess will drain directly into the superior end of the ethmoid infundibulum (Fig. 1.4b). If the uncinate process attaches laterally into the lamina papyracea of the orbit, the frontal recess will open directly into the superior aspect of the middle me-atus and the ethmoid infundibulum will end blindly into the recessus terminalis.

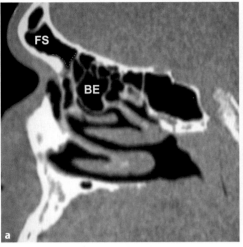
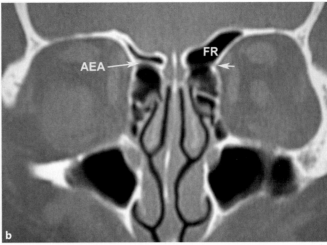

Fig. 1.3. The frontal recess. **a** Sagittal reformatted image at the frontal recess showing the frontal sinus ostium as a funnel shaped outflow tract (*dashed line*). **b** Coronal image showing the right anterior ethmoid artery (*AEA*) coursing through its bony canal (*long arrow*). The left anterior ethmoid artery is dehiscent (*short arrow*) just below the frontal recess

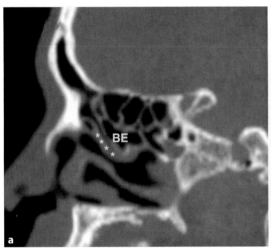
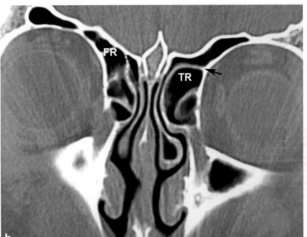

Fig. 1.4. The uncinate process. In the sagittal image (**a**) the uncinate process (*asterisks*) is shown as a curved bony projection that extends towards the frontal recess. It defines the anterior margin of the ethmoid infundibulum. The bulla ethmoidalis (*BE*) defines the posterior wall of the ethmoid infundibulum. In the coronal image (**b**) the left uncinate process attaches to the lamina papyracea (*arrow*), with the frontal recess (*FR*) opening directly to the middle meatus, and the left ethmoid infundibulum ending in a blind end or "terminal recess" (*TR*). The right uncinate process attaches to the skull base (*dotted line*), with the right frontal recess emptying into the right ethmoidal infundibulum

Ethmoid Infundibulum

The ethmoid infundibulum is a true three-dimensional space and is defined (Fig. 1.5a):

- Laterally by the lamina papyracea
- Anteromedially by the uncinate process
- Posteriorly by the bulla ethmoidalis

It opens medially into the middle meatus across the hiatus semilunaris inferioris, a cleftlike opening between the free posterior margin of the uncinate process and the corresponding anterior face of the bulla ethmoidalis (Fig. 1.5b). This is the functional common pathway of mucociliary drainage for the anterior ethmoid, agger nasi and maxillary sinus mucus. The frontal sinus mucus also drains in this direction when the frontal recess opens to the top of the ethmoid infundibulum.

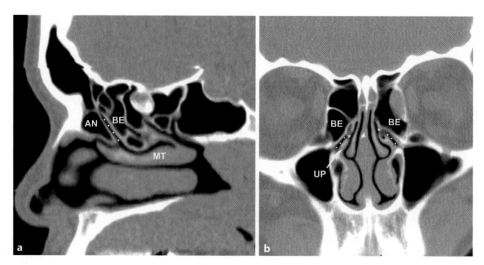

Fig. 1.5. The ostiomeatal complex. Notice on the sagittal image (**a**) the cleftlike ethmoid infundibulum (*dotted line*), bordered anteriorly by a pneumatized agger nasi cell (*AN*) and posteriorly by the bulla ethmoidalis (*BE*). The middle turbinate (*MT*) is seen below. In the coronal image (**b**) the ethmoid infundibulum (*dotted line*) lies between the uncinate process(*UP*) and the bulla ethmoidalis (*BE*), opening into the middle meatus across the hiatus semilunaris inferior (*asterisks*). Notice the deep olfactory fossa (Keros type III)

Anatomic Variants of the Frontal Recess

Several important anatomic variants impact on the anatomy of the frontal recess and the anterior skull base. Familiarity with these anatomic variants is required for safe anterior skull base and frontal recess surgical considerations.

Frontal Cells

The frontal cells are uncommon anatomic variants of anterior ethmoid pneumatization that impinge upon the frontal recess and typically extend within the lumen of the frontal sinus ostium above the level of the agger nasi cells (Fig. 1.6).

The different types of frontal cells as described by Bent are as follows [1, 9]:

- Type I frontal cells are described as a single frontal recess cell above the agger nasi cell (Fig. 1.6a).
- Type II frontal cells are a tier of cells above the agger nasi cell, projecting within the frontal recess.
- A type III frontal cell is defined as a single massive cell arising above the agger nasi, pneumatizing cephalad into the frontal sinus (Fig. 1.6b).
- A type IV frontal cell is a single isolated cell within the frontal sinus acting as a "sinus within a sinus," frequently difficult to visualize owing to its thin walls (Fig. 1.6c).

All frontal cells can be clinically significant if they become primarily infected or if they stenose the frontal sinus ostium, leading to mucus recirculation and secondary frontal sinusitis.

Supraorbital Ethmoid Cells

This is when the anterior ethmoid sinus pneumatizes the orbital plate of the frontal bone posterior to the frontal recess and lateral to the frontal sinus (Fig. 1.7), frequently developing from the suprabullar recess [2]. The degree of pneumatization of the supraorbital ethmoid cells can reach the anterior margin of the orbital plate and mimic a frontal sinus. We can best trace the supraorbital ethmoid cell towards the anterior ethmoid sinus on axial CT images, which allows us to recognize this variant better

Depth of Olfactory Fossa

The orbital plate of the frontal bone slopes downwards medially to constitute the roof of the ethmoid labyrinth (foveola ethmoidalis), ending medially at the lateral border of the olfactory fossa (Fig. 1.8). This configuration makes the olfactory fossa the lowermost point in the floor of the anterior cranial fossa,

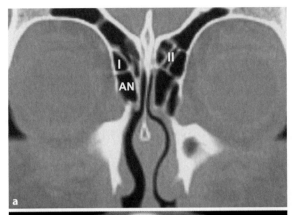

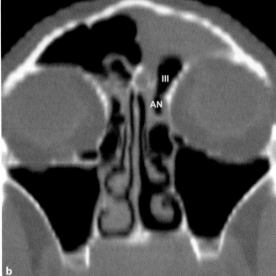

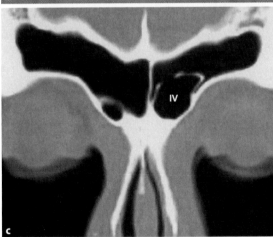

Fig. 1.6. Frontal cells. Frontal cells are rare air cells above the agger nasi (*AN*) that impinge upon the frontal recess and frontal sinus. Type *I* is a single cell above the agger nasi, while type *II* is a tier arrangement above the agger nasi (**a**). Type *III* is a single large frontal cell projecting into the frontal sinus lumen (**b**). Type *IV* is a large cell completely contained in the frontal sinus ("sinus within a sinus") (**c**)

frequently projecting between the pneumatized air cells of both ethmoid labyrinths [9]. The depth of the olfactory fossa into the nasal cavity is dictated by the height of the lateral lamella of the cribriform plate, a very thin sagittally oriented bone, continuous with the vertical attachment of the middle turbinate, defining the lateral wall of the olfactory fossa.

Keros [5] described the anatomic variations of the ethmoid roof and the olfactory fossa, classifying it in three surgically important types:

1. Type I has a short lateral lamella, resulting in a shallow olfactory fossa of only 1–3 mm in depth in relation to the medial end of the ethmoid roof.
2. Type II has a longer lateral lamella, resulting in an olfactory fossa depth of 4–7 mm.
3. Type III has a much longer lateral lamella (8–16 mm), with the cribriform plate projecting deep within the nasal cavity well below the roof of the ethmoid labyrinth.

The type III configuration represents a high-risk area for lateral lamella iatrogenic surgical perforation in ethmoid endoscopic surgical procedures. Occasionally there may be asymmetric depth of the olfactory fossa from side to side, which must be recognized and considered prior to surgery.

Ostiomeatal Complex

The ostiomeatal complex is the common pathway of drainage of the anterior paranasal sinuses, acting as the functional unit that controls and modulates the mucociliary drainage from the frontal sinus, anterior ethmoid sinus and maxillary sinus.

The ostiomeatal complex comprises a combination of structures:

- Uncinate process
- Ethmoid bulla
- Middle turbinate
- Spaces between these structures (ethmoid infundibulum, hiatus semilunaris and middle meatus) (Fig. 1.5).

The efficiency of drainage is dictated by the patency or closure of these spaces in response to the nasal cycle of alternating phases of mucosal engorgement and mucosal thinning, typically on cycles of 4–6 h. Whenever the ostiomeatal complex spaces are further narrowed by anatomic variants, mucosal polyps, inflamed mucosa, scars or synechiae, the resulting decreased drainage capacity of the system will result in backpressure accumulation of mucous

1

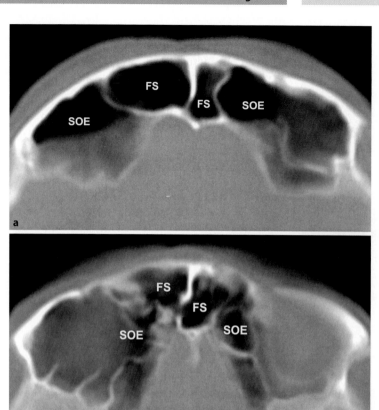

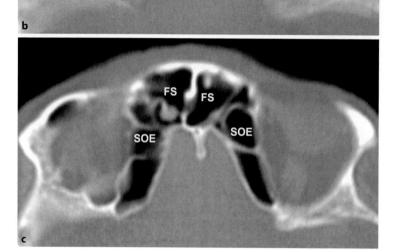

Fig 1.7. Supraorbital ethmoid cells. In the sequential axial images the supraorbital ethmoid cells (*SOE*) expand and pneumatize anteriorly the orbital plate of the frontal bone, not to be confused with the frontal sinus (*FS*)

secretions within the corresponding sinus spaces, increasing the likelihood of secondary bacterial colonization of the previously sterile sinus secretions by backflow of nasal cavity bacteria into the obstructed sinus spaces.

Structures and Spaces

The ethmoid infundibulum is the key element to understand the anatomy and physiology of the ostiome-atal complex (Fig. 1.5a). The ethmoid infundibulum is a sickle-shaped sagittally oriented three-dimensional space extending from the agger nasi/frontal recess region towards the middle meatus, running downwards and posteriorly between the lamina papyracea of the ipsilateral orbit laterally and the uncinate process medially. This resulting V-shaped drainage channel collects the mucociliary output of the frontal sinus, agger nasi cells, anterior ethmoid cells and maxillary sinus. The maxillary sinus mucous secretions are transported by mucociliary clearance towards its natural ostium, located along the superior aspect of the maxil-

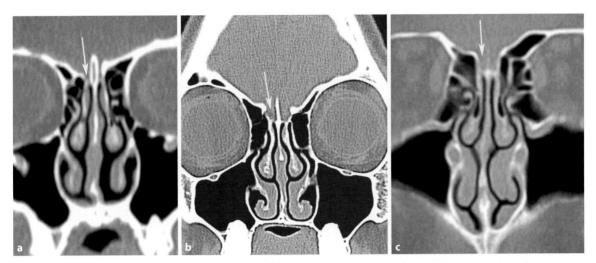

Fig. 1.8. Depth of the olfactory fossa. The length of the lateral lamella of the cribriform plate determines the depth of the olfactory fossa (*arrows*), categorized by Keros in type I (**a** 1–3-mm deep), type II (**b** 4–7-mm deep) and type III (**c** 8–16-mm deep)

lary sinus medial wall, opening into the junction of the middle and posterior third of the ethmoid infundibulum, which in turn opens medially into the middle meatus to direct the mucociliary transport secretions towards the choanna and nasopharynx.

The space connecting the ethmoid infundibulum and the middle meatus is the hiatus semilunaris inferioris, a two-dimensional cleft between the free edge of the uncinate process and the leading anterior ethmoid air cell in the middle meatus, the ethmoid bulla (Fig. 1.5b).

The uncinate process projects from the maxilla, easily recognized as a bony leaflet oriented upwards from the base of the inferior turbinate and the posterior margin of the nasolacrimal duct bony buttress. Its free edge defines the hiatus semilunaris inferioris and constitutes the medial wall of the ethmoid infundibulum.

The ethmoid bulla is the dominant ethmoid air cell projecting into the middle meatus, arising medially from the lamina papyracea of the orbit. Its attachment or bulla lamella can insert upwards into the skull base and the undersurface of the basal lamella of the middle turbinate, or into the lamina papyracea laterally. When it attaches to the lamina papyracea, the ethmoid bulla will create a narrow space between its roof and the basal lamella of the middle turbinate, recognized as the sinus lateralis, which can on occasion extend superiorly towards the frontal recess above the roof of the ethmoid bulla. The opening of the sinus lateralis towards the middle meatus is known as the hiatus semilunaris superioris.

The middle turbinate is a process of the ethmoid bone that defines the functional space of the middle meatus underneath it. Its basal lamella is attached vertically in the sagittal plane into the lateral lamella of the cribriform plate (Fig. 1.9). It continues posteriorly in a coronal orientation along the lamina papyra-

cea and ends in an axial plane along the lateral nasal wall towards the choanna. This three-planar pattern of attachment is of paramount importance for the stability of the middle turbinate. This is most obvious after endoscopic surgical procedures, since surgical fracture of any of these planar attachments increases the likelihood of turbinate lateralization and secondary ostiomeatal complex postsurgical scarring and obstruction. In addition, the basal lamella of the middle turbinate represents the anatomic, embryologic and functional boundary between the anterior and posterior ethmoid sinuses. Any sinus spaces anterior to the basal lamella of the middle turbinate will drain towards the ostiomeatal complex, while any sinus spaces posterior to this structure will drain towards the sphenoethmoid recess.

Anatomic Variants of the Ostiomeatal Complex

- *Paradoxical middle turbinate*: inverted configuration of the middle turbinate, which curves towards the lateral nasal wall at the level of the ostiomeatal complex. It decreases the caliber of the middle meatus and may impair mucociliary drainage (Fig. 1.10a).
- *Concha bullosa*: pneumatization of the middle turbinate from its vertical attachment to its bulbous portion. By decreasing middle meatal caliber, it may become an obstructing lesion on the active phase of the nasal cycle. It may pneumatize from the anterior or the posterior ethmoid air cells (Fig. 1.10b).

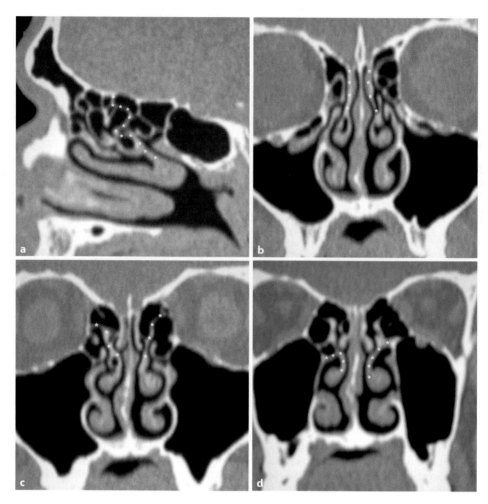

Fig. 1.9. Middle turbinate anatomy. The sagittal image (**a**) shows the complex deformity of the basal lamella of the middle turbinate (*asterisks*) deflected by the asymmetric competing growth of the anterior and posterior ethmoid cells. Sequential coronal images show the basal lamella of the middle turbinate in the sagittal plane (**b**) at the olfactory fossa, the coronal plane (**c**) at the lamina papyracea and the axial plane (**d**) at the posterior nasal cavity

- *Pneumatized uncinate process*: may decrease the hiatus semilunaris caliber (Fig. 1.10c).
- *Posterior fontanelle*: occasional defect in the lateral nasal wall behind the ethmoid infundibulum that freely communicates the maxillary sinus and the middle meatus (Fig. 1.10d). No mucociliary transit occurs through this space. Its presence must be recognized to avoid confusing it with the natural ostium of the maxillary sinus, which can result in failed middle meatal antrostomy.

Sphenoethmoid Recess

Structures and Spaces

The sphenoethmoid recess is a vertically oriented posterior nasal cavity–nasopharynx channel defined anteriorly by the posterior border of the superior turbinate and posteriorly by the anterior wall of the sphenoid sinus (Fig. 1.11a). It is easily recognizable on axial images as a narrow space between the posterior nasal septum medially and the superior turbinate laterally, right in front of the anterior wall of the sphenoid sinus and its natural ostium (Fig. 1.11b). It is the common pathway for mucociliary drainage from posterior ethmoid air cells and the sphenoid sinus.

Fig. 1.10. Anatomic variants of the ostiomeatal complex. **a** Bilateral paradoxical turn of the middle turbinates (*dots*). **b** A typical pneumatized middle turbinate or concha bullosa (*CB*). Notice the uncinectomy at the natural ostium of the right maxillary sinus (*MS*). **c** Bilateral pneumatized uncinate processes (*asterisks*). **d** A wide right maxillary sinus posterior fontanelle (*arrow*), which may mimic a maxillary sinus ostium by endoscopy. *CB* concha bullosa, *MS* maxillary sinus

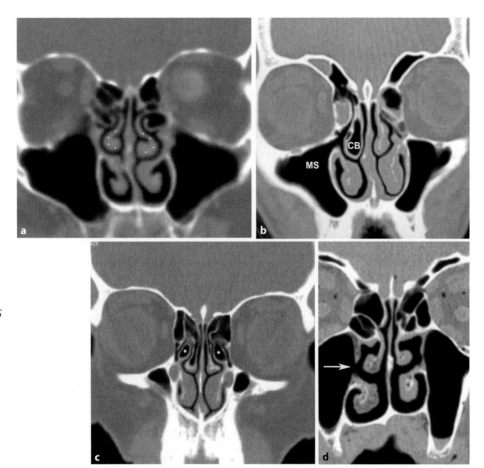

Fig. 1.11. Sphenoethmoid recess. **a** The vertical orientation of the sphenoethmoid recess on sagittal images (*asterisks*). **b** The diverging orientation of each sphenoethmoid recess (*asterisks*) as each gets closer to the corresponding sphenoid sinus ostium (*arrow*)

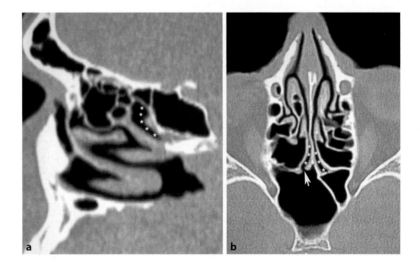

Posterior Ethmoid Sinus

The posterior ethmoid air cells comprise all the ethmoid sinus spaces that lie posterosuperior to the basal lamella of the middle turbinate, draining through the superior meatus into the sphenoethmoid recess (Fig. 1.11b). The posterior ethmoid sinus comprises a variable number of air cells, typically fewer in number and larger in size than the anterior ethmoid sinus cells. It is typically pneumatized at birth.

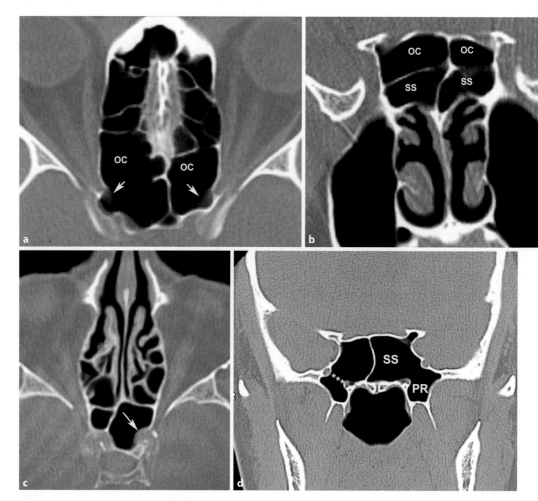

Fig. 1.12. Anatomic variants of the sphenoethmoid recess. **a** The expanded posterior ethmoid pneumatization constituting bilateral Onodi cells (*OC*), extending to the border of the optic nerves (*arrows*). **b** Coronal image showing the classic "two-story" appearance of the Onodi cells riding on top of the sphenoid sinuses (*SS*). **c** Axial image illustrating a dehiscent left internal carotid artery (*arrow*) in the left sphenoid sinus. **d** Coronal image showing bilateral pterygoid recesses (*PR*) from the sphenoid sinuses defined lateral to a line between the foramen rotundum and the vidian canal (*asterisks*). Notice a dehiscent left optic nerve in the pneumatized left clinoid process

Sphenoid Sinus

The sphenoid sinus develops from the sphenoethmoid recess as a small air cell that progressively pneumatizes the body of the sphenoid bone, growing continuously from childhood to adulthood. Its pneumatization volume, configuration and position of the intersinus septum are dynamically dictated by its ventilation, drainage and competition for space with its contralateral sphenoid sinus. This dynamic competition dictates the extreme variability in sphenoid sinus configuration experienced clinically (Fig. 1.11b).

Anatomic Variants of the Sphenoethmoid Recess Region

- Onodi cells are hyperpneumatized posterior ethmoid air cells that grow posteriorly on the planum sphenoidale above the sphenoid sinuses, typically towards the clinoid processes. Onodi cells frequently have associated dehiscence of the optic nerves whenever the clinoid process is pneumatized. It is a surgical danger zone as a potential site for iatrogenic endoscopic optic nerve injury or intracranial penetration (Fig. 1.12a, b).
- Dehiscent internal carotid arteries can occur whenever there is hyperpneumatization of the

sphenoid sinus, with the dehiscent internal carotid artery projecting submucosally along the lateral superior border of the posterior wall of the sphenoid sinus (Fig. 1.12c).

■ The pterygoid recess of the sphenoid sinus is defined by the sphenoid sinus pneumatization laterally into the pterygoid plate across a virtual line defined between the vidian canal and the foramen rotundum (Fig. 1.12d).

Conclusion

The paranasal sinus drainage pathways and their surrounding structures must be evaluated in an integrated fashion, emphasizing the interrelation between sinus anatomy and function. The dynamic competition of each aerated sinus space with the neighboring sinuses and anatomic structures dictates its high variability and complexity, requiring detailed CT examinations to map the anatomy and determine targets for functional surgery prior to any surgical intervention. An intimate knowledge of its anatomy and a clear understanding of its physiology and anatomic variants are required for safe and effective surgical management of paranasal sinus drainage pathway problems.

References

1. Bent JP, Cuilty-Siller C, Kuhn FH (1994) The frontal ell as a cause of frontal sinus obstruction. 8(4):185–191 \ CEnote{Please provide the name of the journal}
2. Bolger WE, Mawn CB (2001) Analysis of the suprabullar and retrobullar recesses for endoscopic sinus surgery. Ann Oto Rhinol Laryngol 110:3–14
3. Daniels DL, Mafee MF, Smith MM, et al (2003) The frontal sinus drainage pathway and related structures. AJNR Am J Neuroradiol 24:1618–1626
4. Kayalioglu G, Oyar O, Govsa F (2000) Nasal cavity and paranasal sinus bony variations: a computed tomographic study. Rhinology 38(3):108–113
5. Keros P (1965) Uber die praktische bedeutung der niveauunterschiede der lamina cribosa des ethmoids. Laryngol Rhinol Otol (Stuttgart) 41:808–813
6. Melhelm ER, Oliverio PJ, Benson ML, et al (1996) Optimal CT evaluation for functional endoscopic sinus surgery. AJNR Am J Neuroradiol 17:181–188
7. Perez P, Sabate J, Carmona A et al (2000) Anatomical variations in the human paranasal sinus region studied by CT. J Anat 197(Pt 2):221–227
8. Stammberger HR (1991) Functional endoscopic sinus surgery. BC Decker, Philadelphia
9. Stammberger HR, Kennedy DW, Bolger WE, et al (1995) Paranasal sinuses: anatomic terminology and nomenclature. Ann Rhinol Otol Laryngol (Suppl) 167:7–16

Chapter 2

Surgical Anatomy of the Paranasal Sinuses

Zoukaa B. Sargi, Roy R. Casiano

2

Core Messages

■ There are learned anatomical landmarks that can help surgeons perform safe endoscopic sinus surgery.

■ All sinuses are lined by a respiratory pseudostratified epithelium, which is directly attached to bone and is referred to as mucoperiosteum The middle meatus is the area that is most commonly involved in the pathophysiology of chronic rhinosinusitis.

■ The sphenoethmoid recess drains the posterior ethmoid and sphenoid sinuses and is referred to as the "posterior ostiomeatal complex.

■ The tail of the superior turbinate constitutes a very important surgical landmark in the sphenoethmoid recess as it points medially toward the natural ostium of the sphenoid sinus.

■ Removing the uncinate process is the first step of most endoscopic sinus surgeries.

■ The posterior fontanelle can have an opening to the maxillary sinus, the accessory ostium, that could be mistaken for the natural ostium during surgery if an incomplete uncinectomy is performed.

■ The most common anatomical variation in the maxillary sinus is the infraorbital ethmoid cell or Haller cell.

■ During endoscopic sinus surgery, supraorbital ethmoid cells can be mistaken for the frontal sinus by inexperienced surgeons.

■ The sphenoethmoid (or Onodi) cell is intimately related to the optic nerve.

■ Many factors contribute to make the frontal sinus infundibulum one of the most challenging areas to access in endoscopic sinus surgery.

Contents

Introduction

Understanding the anatomy of the paranasal sinuses is probably the most important prerequisite for endoscopic sinus surgery (ESS). As a matter of fact, most feared complications of ESS are the result of an uncontrolled maneuvering beyond the boundaries of the sinuses, mainly into the orbit or through the base of the skull. Even with the most experienced surgeons, these complications are still encountered, facilitated by some preexisting anatomical variants or pathological modifications caused by the underlying disease. Many constant landmarks have been described by different authors since ESS was first introduced in the late 1970s. These anatomical landmarks let beginners achieve a good spatial orientation when navigating within the sinuses, and help them perform the most complete sinus surgery while minimizing the risk to the patient. However, there is a definite learning curve that can make one divide ESS into increasing levels of difficulty in surgical skills, starting with the simple nasal endoscopy and ending with the most advanced frontal sinus procedures. In addition to the understanding of the anatomy, a thorough knowledge of the embryology, pathology and imaging of the sinuses is also very important for a comprehensive management of sinuses problems, but these topics are beyond the scope of this chapter.

2

Introduction to the Anatomy of the Paranasal Sinuses

The literature on the anatomy and physiology of the sinuses extends back to Galen (AD 130–201) who referred to the "porosity" of the bones of the head. Leonardo Da Vinci (1452–1519), whose classical sections of the head illustrate the maxillary antrum and the frontal sinus, apparently recognized the existence of these cavities as separate functional entities. He referred to the maxillary sinus as "the cavity of the bone which supports the cheek." Highmore (1651) was the first to give a detailed description of the maxillary antrum (antrum of Highmore) [2]. However, it was only in the late nineteenth century that the first detailed and systematic anatomical and pathological descriptions of the paranasal sinuses were published by Zuckerkandl. These descriptions became even more valuable as they could be applied directly to patients and their problems. The invention of the X-ray technique did not add much to the anatomical knowledge of the sinuses, and computed tomography (CT), available since the mid-1970s, made again the relationship between the largest sinuses and the ethmoids very clear, applying the knowledge that had been developed more that 100 years ago. Comparisons of CT with the drawings of Onodi, Grunwald and Zuckerkandl demonstrate the incredible accuracy of these pioneers' knowledge [17].

The paranasal sinuses form a complex unit of four paired air-filled cavities at the entrance of the upper airway. They start developing from ridges and furrows in the lateral nasal wall as early as the eighth week of embryogenesis, and they continue their pneumatization until early adulthood [4]. Each one is named after the skull bone in which it is located [8, 19]. However, during the development of a sinus, pneumatization may involve adjacent bones, as is the case for the ethmoid sinus developing into the frontal, maxillary or sphenoid bone, and for the maxillary sinus extending into the zygomatic bone.

All sinuses are lined by a respiratory pseudostratified epithelium, composed of four major types of cells:

1. Ciliated columnar cells
2. Nonciliated columnar cells
3. Goblet type mucous cells
4. Basal cells

This mucosa is directly attached to bone and is referred to as mucoperiosteum. Although it is somewhat thinner, the mucoperiosteum of the sinuses is continuous with that of the nasal cavity through the various ostia of the sinuses [8]. The ostium is a natural opening through which the sinus cavity drains into the airway, either directly into the nasal cavity (i.e., sphenoid ostium), or indirectly by means of more complex anatomical structures (i.e., frontal recess). The most important progress offered by the concept of functional ESS compared with older surgical approaches to the paranasal sinuses is the acknowledgement of the essential role of the sinus ostia and mucosa in the surgical management of inflammatory disease of the paranasal sinuses. By achieving an adequate drainage around the natural ostium, the mucosal disease and subsequent symptoms could become reversible in many cases.

The Nasal Cavity

The nasal cavity is the first cavity encountered by the surgeon during ESS. Its lateral and posterior-superior walls contain the openings for the paranasal sinuses, and its posterior-inferior wall leads to the nasopharynx through the choana. The identification of the choana and its relations to the posterior nasal septum and the eustachian tube opening (torus tubarius) in the nasopharynx is very important at the beginning of every ESS (Fig. 2.1). When polyps obstruct the nasal airway in its inferomedial part, reestablishing the patency of the nasal cavity should be performed first to allow for a good visualization of the choana at any time and provide a drainage route for the blood into the nasopharynx [5].

The turbinates, or conchae, are constant ridges of the lateral nasal wall. The inferior turbinate is a separate structure deriving embryologically from the maxilloturbinal. It inserts anteriorly on the maxilla and posteriorly on the palatine bone. The other turbinates, also called ethmoid turbinates, develop from the ethmoturbinals into a common structure or conchal lamina described by Mouret in 1922. This bony plate is attached all along the junction between the ethmoid roof and the cribriform plate. All the ethmoid turbinates originate from this bony lamina: one middle turbinate and one superior turbinate that are constant, and occasionally a supreme turbinate [3].

The lateral part of the nasal cavity is thus subdivided by the turbinates into four meati (Fig. 2.2). The inferior meatus is the space between the lateral side of the inferior turbinate and the medial wall of the maxillary sinus. It contains the distal opening of the nasolacrimal duct, covered by a mucosal valve (Hasner's valve). The middle meatus is the space lateral to the middle turbinate, and is often functionally referred to as the ostiomeatal complex [18]. It contains the drainage pathways for the anterior ethmoids, the maxillary and the frontal sinuses. The middle meatus is the area that is most commonly involved in the pathophysiology of chronic rhinosinusitis.

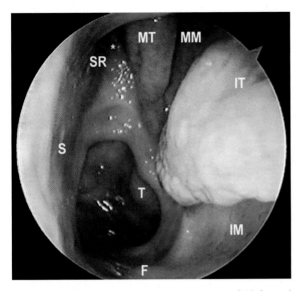

Fig. 2.1. Endoscopic view of the posterior part of a left nasal cavity showing the choana and the torus (*T*). Turning clockwise around the choana, the following structures and spaces can be recognized: the sphenoethmoid recess (*SR*), the tail of the superior turbinate (*asterisk*), the tail of the middle turbinate (*MT*), the middle meatus (*MM*), the tail of the inferior turbinate (*IT*), the inferior meatus (*IM*), the floor of the nose (*F*) and the nasal septum (*S*). Keeping this orientation in mind becomes more important when one or more of these structures are distorted or hidden by the disease

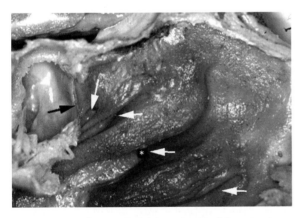

Fig. 2.2. Sagittal view of a left lateral wall of the nose showing the four turbinates. The *white arrows* point to the four meati. Note the accessory ostium of the maxillary sinus in the posterior fontanelle (marked by an *asterisk*). The *black arrow* points to the anterior wall of the sphenoid sinus. The middle, superior and supreme turbinates represent the third, fourth and fifth embryological lamellae. The first and second lamellae (uncinate and bulla) are hidden by the middle turbinate on this view

The middle meatus hosts from anterior to posterior the:

■ Agger nasi cells
■ Uncinate process
■ Hiatus semilunaris
■ Ethmoid bulla
■ Sinus lateralis
■ Posterior fontanelle

These structures will be detailed in the following paragraphs. The superior meatus is the lateral space between the superior and the middle turbinates. It drains the posterior ethmoid cells. The supreme meatus is the area above the superior turbinate, which drains the most posterior ethmoid cells.

The superior part of the nasal cavity is divided into the olfactory cleft anteriorly and the sphenoethmoid recess posteriorly. The olfactory cleft is located under the olfactory fossa between the insertion of the middle turbinate and the nasal septum. It lies just inferior to the cribriform plate. Keros (1965) described three types of olfactory fossa depending on how low the level of the cribriform plate is with relation to the roof of the ethmoids, this level being determined by the width of the lateral lamella of the cribriform plate which articulates with the roof of the ethmoids (Fig. 2.3).

The Keros classification is as follows:

■ Type 1 corresponds to an olfactory fossa 1–3-mm deep in relationship to the roof of the ethmoids.
■ Type 2 is 4–7-mm deep.
■ Type 3 refers to a depth of 8 mm and above [18].

Recognizing the relationship between the cribriform plate, the fovea ethmoidalis and the insertions of the middle and superior turbinates is very important to avoid an inadvertent breaking into the anterior skull base, especially in the anterior ethmoid where the junction between the conchal lamina and the ethmoid roof is the least-resistant zone [10]. Posterior to the olfactory cleft, and as the roof of the nasal cavity becomes more inferior, the sphenoethmoid recess lies between the tail of the superior turbinate and the posterior-superior septum, just above the choana (Fig. 2.1) [18]. This recess drains the sphenoid sinus and the posterior ethmoids via the superior and supreme meati. Functionally, this area is referred to as the "posterior" ostiomeatal complex, in contrast to the "anterior" ostiomeatal complex in the middle meatus. The tail of the superior turbinate constitutes a very important surgical landmark in the sphenoeth-

2

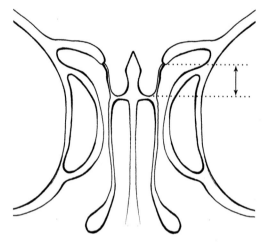

Fig. 2.3. Coronal view of the olfactory clefts and fossae, in a plane transecting the ethmoid bullae. The *arrow* measures the length of the lateral lamella of the cribriform plate, defining the type of olfactory fossa according to Keros. Note the insertion of the basal lamella of the middle turbinate on the cribriform plate, as well as the relatively thicker fovea ethmoidalis lateral to the cribriform plate. The intracranial bony spur that continues the septum corresponds to the crista galli. In most of the cases, the cribriform plate is symmetrical, however, an asymmetric skull base is an anatomical variant that should be recognized on a preoperative CT scan

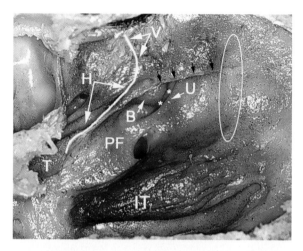

Fig. 2.4. Sagittal view of the left lateral wall of the nose after a partial middle turbinectomy exposing the contents of the middle meatus: The *black arrows* point to the resection margin anteriorly, and the *white line* draws the vertical (*V*) portion and the horizontal (*H*) portion of the basal lamella of the middle turbinate. The sagittal most anterior part of the basal lamella inserts on the anterior skull base marked in methylene blue. The uncinate process (*U*) and the ethmoid bulla (*B*) border the hiatus semilunaris marked by *asterisks*. Also note the prominence of the lacrimal bone (*circled*), the posterior fontanelle (*PF*) with the accessory ostium of the maxillary sinus, and the tail (*T*) of the middle turbinate

moid recess as it points medially toward the natural ostium of the sphenoid sinus [16].

The Uncinate Process and the Maxillary Sinus

The uncinate process is a very important surgical landmark in the lateral nasal wall for endonasal sinus surgery. Although considered part of the ethmoid labyrinth since it derives from the descending portion of the first ethmoturbinal, the uncinate process is typically discussed when addressing the maxillary sinus because of its intimate relationship with the maxillary ostium. The uncinate process is a crescent-shaped bony structure that typically projects from posteroinferior (at the palatine bone and inferior turbinate) to anterosuperior where it runs along the lateral nasal wall attaching to the ethmoid crest of the maxilla, the lacrimal bone, the skull base or the lamina papyracea. Its anterior-inferior margin has no bony attachments, and posteriorly it attaches to the ethmoid process of the inferior turbinate (Fig. 2.4) [4]. Its anterior convex part forms the anterior boundary of the (anterior) ostiomeatal complex, where the maxillary, anterior ethmoid and frontal sinuses drain. It endoscopically hides the hiatus semilunaris, which could

fairly be represented by the space between the uncinate and the ethmoid bulla. The uncinate process can be displaced medially by polypoid disease or laterally against the orbit as in maxillary sinus hypoplasia. Removing the uncinate process is the first step of most endoscopic sinus surgeries. When performing this, one must keep in mind the anterior insertion of the uncinate process in order to avoid injuries to the medial orbital wall (lamina papyracea). This step usually reveals the natural ostium of the maxillary sinus. The superior border of the maxillary sinus ostium identifies the level of the orbital floor.

The maxillary sinus is the largest and most constant of the paranasal sinuses. It is the first sinus to develop in utero. After birth, it undergoes two periods of rapid growth, between birth and 3 years of life, then between ages 7 and 18 years. The maxillary sinus has a pyramidal shape with an anterior wall corresponding to the facial surface of the maxilla. Its posterior bony wall separates it from the pterygomaxillary fossa medially and from the infratemporal fossa laterally. Its medial wall does not contain any bone; it is formed by the middle meatus mucosa, a layer of connective tissue and the sinus mucosa [19]. This is best recognized at the level of the posterior fontanelle which corresponds to the area between the tails of the middle and inferior turbinates, behind the hiatus semilunaris and under the ethmoid bulla. The posterior fontanelle can have an opening to the maxillary sinus, the accessory ostium, which could be mistaken for the natural ostium during ESS if an incomplete uncinectomy is performed (Fig. 2.4). A smaller anterior fontanelle is located between the anterior part of the uncinate superiorly and the insertion of the inferior turbinate inferiorly. The floor of the maxillary sinus is formed by the alveolar process of the maxillary bone and the hard palate. It lies at the same level of the floor of the nose in children, and 5–10 mm under the floor of the nose in adults [19]. The roof of the maxillary sinus corresponds to the floor of the orbit, and frequently shows a posteroanterior bony canal for the distal part of the second branch of the trigeminal nerve. The most common anatomical variation in the maxillary sinus is the infraorbital ethmoid cell, or Haller cell; Haller cells are pneumatized ethmoid cells that project along the floor of the orbit, arising most often from the anterior ethmoids [11, 14]. They can in some cases compromise the patency of the maxillary sinus infundibulum, and in other cases can be involved in the chronic polypoid disease, which will mandate opening them. In addition to this, removing the infraorbital ethmoid cell will allow an accurate identification of the floor of the orbit and the posterior wall of the maxillary sinus, which represent reliable surgical landmarks in the presence of advanced disease or distortion of the middle meatal anatomy.

The Ethmoid Labyrinth

Located lateral to the olfactory cleft and fossa, between the lateral nasal wall and the medial orbital wall, the ethmoid sinus is the most compartmentalized paranasal sinus. At birth, only a few cells are pneumatized, but in adulthood their number can go beyond 15 cells. The frontal bone in its posterior extension covers the roof of the ethmoid sinus, forming the so-called fovea, or foveolae ethmoidales [18]. The anterior and posterior ethmoid arteries, terminal branches of the internal carotid artery via the ophthalmic artery, run along the roof of the ethmoid from lateral to medial. The width of the ethmoid increases from anterior to posterior because of the conelike structure of the orbit.

The ethmoid sinus is referred to as the ethmoid labyrinth because of the complexity of its anatomy, due to the honeycomb-like appearance of its air cells with intricate passageways and blind alleys. Rhinologists have tried to simplify its difficult anatomy by considering the sinus as a series of five obliquely oriented parallel lamellae. These derive from the ridges in the lateral nasal wall of the fetus called ethmoturbinals [4, 15]. The lamellae are relatively constant

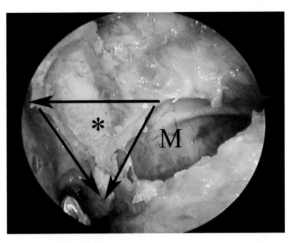

Fig. 2.5. Triangular zone of safe entry (*asterisk*) into the inferior-posterior ethmoid air cells through the basal lamella of the middle turbinate. The *base of the triangle* corresponds to a horizontal line drawn from the medial floor of the orbit (posteriorly) to the nasal septum. The *other two lines* correspond to the cut edge of the middle turbinate lamella and the vertical ridge (cut edge of the posterior fontanelle) of the middle meatal maxillary sinusotomy (*M*)

and easy to recognize intraoperatively. The first and most anterior lamella corresponds to the uncinate process, which embryologically represents the basal lamella of the first ethmoturbinal. The second lamella is the ethmoid bulla, or bulla ethmoidalis as first referred to by Zuckerkandl, the largest and most constant anterior ethmoid cell [14]. It has a round shape with thin walls, extending from the lamina papyracea laterally and bulging into the middle meatus medially (Fig. 2.3). Rarely, when nonpneumatized, a bony projection from the lamina papyracea results and is referred to as the torus lateralis. The most important lamella is the third one, the ground or basal lamella of the middle turbinate, not only defining the anatomical separation between the anterior and the posterior ethmoid cells, but also creating a bony septation that dictates the drainage pattern of the ethmoid cells into the middle meatus (for the anterior ethmoid cells) and the superior and supreme meati (for the posterior ethmoid cells). It thus represents the surgical posterior limit for an anterior ethmoidectomy. Its S-shaped insertion with a sagittal anterior third and a vertical middle third gives the middle turbinate its mechanical stability, and its posterior horizontal part at the level of the tail of the middle turbinate represents the most straightforward way for entry into the posterior ethmoids (Figs. 2.4, 2.5). The fourth lamella is the basal lamella of the superior turbinate and the fifth is the basal lamella of the supreme turbinate [4, 15].

Besides the bony lamellae, particular groups of ethmoid cells have been identified, and recognizing them helps understanding the pathophysiology and spread

2

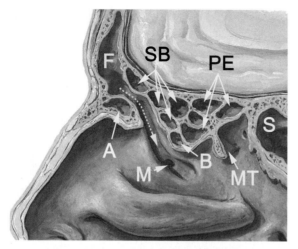

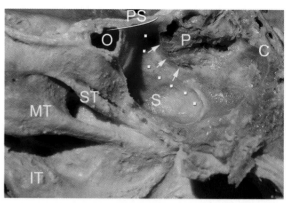

Fig. 2.6. Parasagittal view of a right frontal recess. The agger nasi (*A*) and suprabullar (*SB*) cells are, respectively, the anterior and posterior boundaries of the frontal recess (*dotted arrow*). The anterior portion of the middle turbinate, missing on this view, represents its medial limit. Note the frontal sinus (*F*), the ethmoid bulla (*B*), the posterior ethmoid cells (*PE*) and their relation to the tail of the middle turbinate (*MT*), the sphenoid sinus (*S*) and the natural ostium of the maxillary sinus (*M*).

Fig. 2.7. Sagittal view of a right lateral wall of the nose showing the sphenoid sinus and the pituitary gland (*P*). The *arrows* point to the sphenoid side of the floor of the sella turcica, separating the planum sphenoidale (*PS*) anteriorly from the clivus (*C*) posteriorly. The right carotid artery prominence is marked with a *dotted line*. A right Onodi cell (*O*) hides the optic nerve prominence, and the direction of the right optic nerve is represented by a *plain line*. Note the relationship of the tail of the superior turbinate (*ST*) with the ostium of the sphenoid sinus

of sinus disease, as well as performing the most complete ethmoid surgery with the least surgical complications. The agger nasi cells are the most anterior ethmoid cells, and are endoscopically visualized as a prominence anterior to the insertion of the middle turbinate. From Latin, *agger* means mound or eminence, and agger nasi refers to the pneumatized superior remnant of the first ethmoturbinal which persists as a mound anterior and superior to the insertion of the middle turbinate. Rarely, the pneumatization can extend inferiorly to involve the anterosuperior part of the uncinate process, which as described previously derives from the descending portion of the first ethmoturbinal. The agger nasi pneumatization can also have a significant impact on the uncinate process insertion, as well as on the patency of the frontal recess (Fig. 2.6) [15, 18]. Accurate identification of the agger nasi is the key to the surgical access to the frontal recess [20].

The middle turbinate can sometimes be pneumatized, resulting in a concha bullosa with a pneumatization usually originating from the frontal recess or the agger nasi. The concha bullosa is a normal variant that in itself does not require surgery; however, extensive pneumatization may narrow the ostiomeatal complex and contribute to sinus disease [9]. Conchal cells are ethmoid air cells that invade the middle turbinate in its anterior aspect, whereas interlamellar cells, originally described by Grunwald, arise from pneumatization of the vertical lamella of the middle turbinate from the superior meatus [18].

The supraorbital ethmoid cells (also referred to as suprabullar cells) are anterior ethmoid cells that arise immediately behind the frontal recess and extend over the orbit through pneumatization of the orbital plate of the frontal bone. They can compromise posteriorly the frontal sinus drainage, in a similar way as the agger nasi anteriorly (Fig. 2.6). During ESS, supraorbital cells can be mistaken for the frontal sinus by inexperienced surgeons. Transillumination of these cells with a telescope reveals the light in the inner canthal area, rather than the supraorbital area when the frontal sinus is transilluminated [14].

The sphenoethmoid cells, or Onodi cells, are another important group of ethmoid cells, with reference to Adolf Onodi from Budapest who studied the relationship of the ethmoid and the optic nerve [11, 17]. In this case, the posterior ethmoid cells extend superiorly or laterally to the sphenoid sinus, and the pneumatization can reach the posterior clinoid process. The sphenoethmoid cell is intimately related to the optic nerve, whether the latter is prominent or not in its lateral wall (Fig. 2.7). Also, if large enough, the carotid artery can bulge through its posterior wall. Thus, attempts to open the sphenoid through a sphenoethmoid cell can result in serious damage to the optic nerve or the carotid artery. Theese important structures are usually related to the lateral wall of the sphenoid sinus; however, accurate identification of these structures and possibly Onodi cells on a preoperative CT scan is the best way to avoid such severe complications.

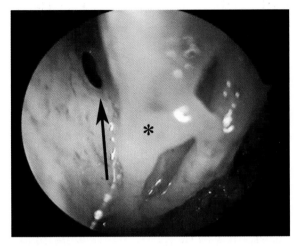

Fig. 2.8. Tail of the superior turbinate as a sphenoid ostium. The sphenoid ostium is found superomedial (*arrow*) to the tail of the superior turbinate (*asterisk*)

The Sphenoid Sinus

The sphenoid sinuses are located at the skull base at the junction of the anterior and middle cerebral fossae. Their growth starts between the third and fourth months of fetal development, as an invagination of the nasal mucosa into the posterior portion of the cartilaginous nasal capsule. Between birth and 3 years of age, the sphenoid is primarily a pit in the sphenoethmoid recess. Pneumatization of the sphenoid bone starts at age three, extends toward the sella turcica by age seven, and reaches its final form in the the mid-teens [15, 19]. The two sinuses generally develop asymmetrically, separated by the intersinus bony septum. In some cases, because of this asymmetry, the intersinus septum goes off the midline and can have a posterior insertion on the bony carotid canal, in the lateral wall of the sphenoid [16]. For this reason, care must be taken when removing the septum in these cases, as a brisk avulsion may result in carotid rupture. Pneumatization of the sphenoids can invade the anterior and the posterior clinoid processes as well as the posterior part of the nasal septum, the Vomer. The sphenoid sinus drains through a single ostium into the sphenoethmoid recess: this ostium is classically situated 7 cm from the base of the columella at an angle of 30° with the floor of the nose in a parasagittal plane, and this usually corresponds to a location halfway up the anterior wall of the sinus. Endoscopically, the posteroinferior end of the superior turbinate points superiorly and medially toward the ostium and thus represents a very important landmark to identify it (Fig. 2.8). When polypoid changes are present distorting the normal anatomy, the ostium can be located adjacent to the nasal septum, at the level of the posterior orbital floor seen through the middle meatal sinusot-

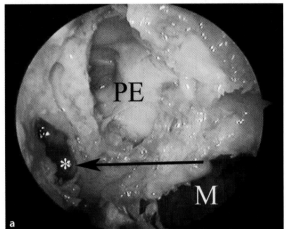

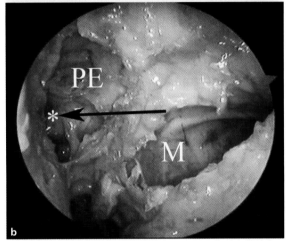

Fig. 2.9. **a** Anatomic landmarks for a sphenoid sinusotomy. In advanced disease the sphenoid (*asterisk*) is safely entered at the level of the posterior orbital floor (*arrow*), approximately 7 cm from the anterior columella, and adjacent to the nasal septum. This also corresponds to the level of the sphenoid natural ostium. **b** Completed sphenoidotomy. Endoscopically, most of the posterior ethmoid cavity (*PE*) is located superior to a line drawn at the level of the posterior orbital floor. By contrast, the sphenoid sinus (*asterisk*) and the maxillary sinus (*M*) are below this line

omy, usually within 10–12 mm from the superior arch of the choana, and approximately 7 cm from the columella [5, 12] (Fig. 2.9).

The superior wall of the sphenoid sinus usually represents the floor of the sella turcica (Fig. 2.7).

Depending on the extent of pneumatization, the sphenoid sinus can be classified into three types:

1. *Conchal*: the area below the sella is a solid block of bone without pneumatization.
2. *Presellar*: the sphenoid is pneumatized to the level of the frontal plane of the sella and not beyond.
3. *Sellar*: the most common type, where pneumatization extends into the body of the sphenoid beyond

the floor of the sella, reaching sometimes the clivus [6, 16].

The lateral wall of the sphenoid sinus can show various prominences, the most important being the carotid canal and the optic canal: the internal carotid artery is the most medial structure in the cavernous sinus, and rests against the lateral surface of the sphenoid bone. Its prominence within the sphenoid varies from a focal bulge to a serpigenous elevation marking the full course of the intracavernous portion of the carotid artery from posteroinferior to posterosuperior (Fig. 2.10). In some cases, even without advanced sinus disease, dehiscence in the bony margin can be present, and this should be particularly looked for on the CT scan [16].

The optic canal is found in the posterosuperior angle between the lateral, posterior and superior walls of the sinus, horizontally crossing the carotid canal from lateral to medial (Fig. 2.10). Pneumatization of the sphenoid above and below the optic canal can result, respectively, in a supraoptic recess and an infraoptic recess (the opticocarotid recess). The infraoptic recess lies between the optic nerve superiorly and the carotid canal inferiorly, and can sometimes pneumatize the anterior clinoid process [15].

The canals of two other nerves can be encountered in the lateral wall of the sphenoid sinus, below the level of the carotid canal:

- The second branch of the trigeminal nerve superiorly through the foramen roduntum
- The vidian nerve in the pterygoid canal inferiorly (Fig. 2.10).

In some cases, these nerves are easily identified on a coronal CT scan defining the superior and the inferior borders of the entry into the so-called lateral recess in an extensively pneumatized sphenoid sinus.

The Frontal Sinus

The frontal sinus is intimately related to the anterior ethmoid in both its embryology and its anatomy. It has been suggested that the frontal sinus develops from an upward extension of the anterior ethmoid cells into the most inferior aspect of the frontal bone between its two tables. However, Stammberger considers that the frontal sinus develops from the frontal recess, which is embryologically the superior continuation of the groove between the first ethmoturbinal (agger nasi and uncinate process) and the second ethmoturbinal (bulla ethmoidalis). At birth, the fron-

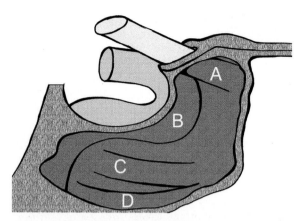

Fig. 2.10. Simplified drawing of a lateral wall of the left sphenoid sinus. The optic canal (*A*) runs from anterolateral to posteromedial in the most superior aspect of the lateral wall. The carotid prominence (*B*) is usually seen at the junction of the posterior and lateral walls. Note the supraoptic recess (*above A*) and the infraoptic or opticocarotid recess (*between A and B*). The canals for the second branch of the trigeminal nerve (*C*) and the vidian nerve (*D*) can sometimes be endoscopically identified, and define the superior and inferior boundaries for the lateral recess (*between C and D*) in a very pneumatized sphenoid

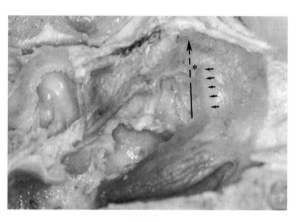

Fig. 2.11. Frontal sinus orientation. The correct trajectory into the frontal sinus is along a line (*dotted line*) parallel to the convexity of the nasolacrimal apparatus (*small arrows*), starting at the maxillary natural ostium area, and extending several millimeters behind the anterior attachment of the middle turbinate (*asterisk*)

tal sinus is a small blind pouch often indistinguishable from the anterior ethmoid cells. Starting around 2 years of age, pneumatization of the frontal sinus will become significant in early adolescence, and complete in the late teens. The right and left frontal sinuses develop independently, and are often asymmetrical: As with the sphenoid sinus, it is not uncommon to find one "dominant" frontal sinus, one or two hypoplastic frontal sinuses, one aplastic frontal sinus, and more rarely bilaterally aplastic sinuses [7].

The frontal sinus lies within the frontal bone between a thick anterior table and a relatively thin posterior table, separating the sinus from the frontal lobe of the brain posteriorly. It has classically been described as a pyramid: its medial wall corresponds to a bony septum, the intersinus septum, which can sometimes be pneumatized, forming an intersinus cell. The floor of the frontal sinus corresponds to the anterior roof of the orbit, and the thin bone at this level, in a similar way as the posterior table, can be eroded by a mucocele [7].

The frontal sinus drainage pathway has an hourglass shape, and opens in the nose at the level of the frontal recess (Fig. 2.6). The narrowest point of this tract is called the frontal infundibulum or ostium, and is located at the most inferomedial aspect of the sinus.

The frontal ostium is bounded by:

- The roof of the agger nasi anteroinferiorly
- The roof of the bulla ethmoidalis or suprabullar cells posteriorly
- The lamina papyracea laterally
- The lamella of the middle turbinate anteriorly

If the bulla ethmoidalis does not have an anterior insertion on the skull base, the frontal recess communicates with the suprabullar recess [20], and depending on the anterior insertion of the uncinate process, the frontal recess will drain medial or anterior to the uncinate (when it inserts on the lamina papyracea) and lateral or posterior to the uncinate into the anterior ethmoid (when the uncinate inserts on the skull base or on the middle turbinate) [13].

Besides the different anterior ethmoid cell groups that could be related to the frontal infundibulum, other cells can originate from the frontal recess and, when present, are called the frontal infundibular cells.

Bent and Kuhn classified the frontal cells into four types:

1. Type 1 is a single air cell above the agger nasi.
2. Type 2 is a group of small cells above the agger nasi but below the orbital roof.
3. Type 3 is a single cell extending from the agger nasi into the frontal sinus.
4. Type 4 is an isolated cell within the frontal sinus not contiguous with the agger nasi [1].

Many factors contribute to make the frontal sinus infundibulum one of the most challenging areas to access in ESS: the small diameter, the anterior location

and orientation within the frontal bone, as well as the anatomical relationship with the orbit, the skull base and the different groups of cells make the endoscopic anatomy very difficult to understand. The keys to achieving a good and safe visualization of the frontal sinus are opening the agger nasi cells and palpating with a probe to identify the posterior wall of the frontal sinus away and in front of the anterior ethmoid artery. The roof of the suprabullar and agger nasi cells should be down-fractured and removed carefully to visualize the infundibulum (Fig. 2.6). The trajectory for entry into the frontal infundibulum should be in the direction of a line drawn parallel to the convexity of the lacrimal bone, a few millimeters behind the anterior attachment of the middle turbinate, starting at the coronal plane of the natural ostium of the maxillary sinus [5] (Fig. 2.11).

Conclusion

The anatomy of the paranasal sinuses, despite its obvious complexity, can be comprehensively understood by subdividing the sinuses into different groups similar in their embryology and function. Even with the most sophisticated radiological techniques and surgical navigation tools, the safety of endoscopic sinus surgery still depends to a great extent on the surgeon's knowledge and experience. The preoperative imaging, mandatory before any ESS, helps the surgeon to recognize anatomical and pathological variants, in order to reduce the risk of complications while achieving an adequate surgery.

References

1. Bent J, Kuhn FA, Cuilty C (1994) The frontal cell in frontal recess obstruction. Am J Rhinol 8:185–91.
2. Blanton PL, Biggs NL (1969) Eighteen hundred years of controversy: the paranasal sinuses. Am J Anat 124(2):135–47.
3. Bodino C, Jankowski R, Grignon B et al (2004) Surgical anatomy of the turbinal wall of the ethmoidal labyrinth. Rhinology 42(2):73–80.
4. Bolger WE, Anatomy of the Paranasal Sinuses. In: Kennedy DW, Bolger WE, Zinreich J (2001) Diseases of the sinuses, Diagnosis and management. B.C. Decker.
5. Casiano RR (2001) A stepwise surgical technique using the medial orbital floor as the keylandmark in performing endoscopic sinus surgery. Laryngoscope 111(6):964–74.
6. Chan R, Astor FC, Younis RT, Embryology and Anatomy of the Nose and Paranasal Sinuses. In: Younis RT (2006) Pediatric Sinusitis ans Sinus Surgery. Taylor & Francis.

2

7. Duque CS, Casiano RR, Surgical Anatomy and Embryology of the Frontal Sinus. In: Kountakis S, Senior BA, Draf W (2005) The Frontal Sinus. Springer.

8. Graney DO, Rice DH, Paranasal sinuses anatomy. In: Cummings CW, Fredrickson JM, Harker LA et al (1998) Otolaryngology Head and Neck Surgery. Mosby, 3rd edn.

9. Joe JK, Ho SY, Yanagisawa E (2000) Documentation of variations in sinonasal anatomy by intraoperative nasal endoscopy. Laryngoscope 110(2):229–35.

10. Kainz J, Stammberger H (1988) [The roof of the anterior ethmoid: a locus minoris resistentiae in the skull base]. Laryngol Rhinol Otol (Stuttg) 67(4):142–9.

11. Kantarci M, Karasen RM, Alper F et al (2004) Remarkable anatomic variations in paranasal sinus region and their clinical importance. Eur J Radiol 50(3):296–302.

12. Kim HU, Kim SS, Kand SS et al (2001) Surgical anatomy of the natural ostium of the sphenoid sinus. Laryngosope 111(9):1599–1602.

13. Lee D, Brody R, Har-El G (1997) Frontal sinus outflow anatomy. Am J Rhinol 11(4):283–5.

14. Polavaram R, Devaiah AK, Sakai O et al (2004) Anatomic variants and pearls-functional endoscopic sinus surgery. Otolaryngol Clin North Am 37(2):221–42.

15. Rice DH, Schaefer SD, Anatomy of the Paranasal Sinuses. In: Rice DH, Schaefer SD (2004) Endoscopic Paranasal Sinus Surgery. Lippincott Williams & Wilkins, 3rd edn.

16. Sethi DS, Stanley RE, Pillay PK (1995) Endoscopic anatomy of the sphenoid sinus and sella turcica. J Laryngol Otol 109(10):951–5.

17. Stammberger H (1989) History of rhinology: anatomy of the paranasal sinuses. Rhinology 27(3):197–210.

18. Stammberger HR, Kennedy DW (1995) Paranasal sinuses: anatomic terminology and nomenclature. The Anatomic Terminology Group. Ann Otol Rhinol Laryngol Suppl Oct;167:7–16.

19. Van Cauwenberge P, Sys L, De Belder T et al (2004) Anatomy and physiology of the nose and the paranasal sinuses. Immunol Allergy Clin North Am 24(1):1–17.

20. Wormald PJ (2003) The agger nasi cell: the key to understanding the anatomy of the frontal recess. Otolaryngol Head Neck Surg 129(5):497–507.

Chapter 3

Frontal Sinus Instrumentation

3

Frederick A. Kuhn, Christopher T. Melroy, Marc G. Dubin,
Shridhar Ventrapragada

Core Messages

- Using endoscopic methods, surgeons treat chronic inflammatory disease in a functional manner rather than in an extirpative or obliterative manner. They seek to preserve the anatomy and enhance the natural drainage pathways of the paranasal sinuses.

- Frontal sinus instrumentation has evolved symbiotically with endoscopic management of the paranasal sinus disorders.

- Specialized instruments allow the surgeon to follow the tenets of functional frontal sinus surgery: complete removal of the frontal recess cells, enlarging the internal frontal ostium, and preserving frontal recess mucous membrane. This maximizes favorable patient outcomes.

- A description of each instrument and its proper use is detailed herein.

Contents

Introduction

In the era of external sinus surgery, access to the frontal sinus was very straightforward. Its position high in the frontal bone allowed relatively safe approaches to the anterior table, which would be removed in a variety of fashions. The osteoplastic flap with obliteration gained acceptance in the 1950s as the standard of management in chronic frontal sinus inflammatory conditions [11]. Its purpose was to make the sinus nonfunctional and no longer an issue. From an instrumentation standpoint, no specialized equipment was needed to approach this relatively superficial structure. The first specialized instrument designed specifically for use in the frontal sinus was the Van Alyea cannula (Fig. 3.1), which was used for transnasal irrigation of the frontal sinus in patients that had not been operated on.

The introduction of endoscopic sinus surgery brought about a paradigm shift in sinus surgery and a renaissance to the study of sinus anatomy and physiology. Using endoscopic methods, surgeons began to treat chronic inflammatory disease in a functional manner rather than in an extirpative or obliterative manner. They sought to preserve the anatomy and enhance the natural drainage pathways of the paranasal sinuses [28]. As all prior transnasal sinus instrumentation was designed to be used with a speculum and headlight, the advent of endoscopic sinus surgery necessitated the development of new instrumentation, which would complement endoscopy.

While the maxillary, ethmoid, and sphenoid sinuses can be approached with straight instrumentation and 0° endoscopes, the frontal sinus drainage pathway lies at an upward angle to the anteroposterior axis of the ethmoid sinuses. It is above and behind the insertion of the middle turbinate attachment to the lateral nasal wall. Standard instrumentation would allow neither access nor safe removal of tissue in this area. In 1989, Kuhn and Bolger developed frontal sinus instruments with Karl Storz (Tuttlingen, Germany) that would allow safe dissection in this area. This set, known as the Kuhn-Bolger Frontal Sinus Instrument Set, consists of two frontal sinus curettes, one

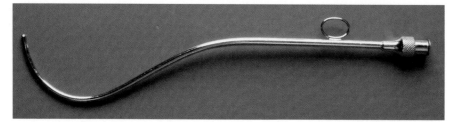

Fig. 3.1. Van Alyea cannula. This was originally designed for transnasal irrigation of the frontal sinus in the 1930s. It is currently used for irrigation of the frontal sinus in patients who had previously been operated on, especially when topical antibiotic or steroid instillation is desired

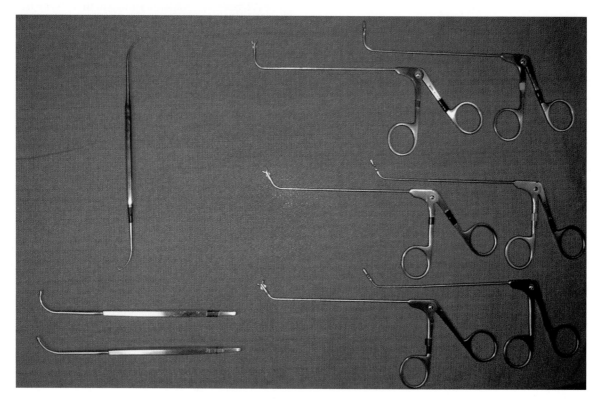

Fig. 3.2. Kuhn–Bolger frontal sinus instrument set

frontal ostium seeker, and six frontal recess giraffe forceps (Fig. 3.2). These advances in instrumentation and the operative techniques associated with them [2, 3, 7, 12, 14, 16, 18, 19, 21, 27] allowed better success in the frontal recess, and endoscopic frontal sinusotomy became the standard for the primary operative management of chronic frontal sinusitis.

The anatomy of the frontal recess is discussed elsewhere in this publication;, it is an inverted funnel-shaped area, which extends from the internal frontal ostium down along the skull base ending at the anterior ethmoid artery (Fig 3.3). It is extensively and variably pneumatized by a variety of frontal recess cells – the agger nasi cell, four types of frontal cells, supraorbital ethmoid cells, suprabullar and frontal bullar cells. These cells, originally described by Van Alyea, have been revisited and defined over the last 15 years [1, 17, 24, 25]. Anatomically speaking, this is a narrow and confined area that is bordered medially by the anterior aspect of the middle turbinate, laterally by the lamina paprycea, anteriorly by the agger nasi region, and posteriorly by the skull base. The ease of endoscopic access to this small and intensely pneumatized area is in stark contrast to the facile external approach to the frontal sinus.

Several tenets of functional frontal sinus surgery are particularly germane to dealing with dissection of the frontal recess. One is to remove the frontal recess cells completely, taking full advantage of the medial frontal sinus floor to enlarge the ostium and there-

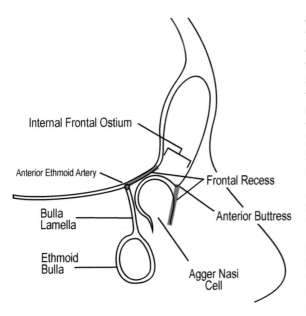

Internal Frontal Ostium

Anterior Ethmoid Artery

Frontal Recess

Bulla
Lamella

Anterior Buttress

Ethmoid
Bulla

Agger Nasi
Cell

Fig. 3.3. Frontal recess anatomy

by relieve potential sources for frontal recess obstruction. Enlarging the frontal sinus outflow tract below the ostium allows more efficient mucociliary clearance from the frontal sinus and reduces the likelihood of frontal recess narrowing secondary to edema and scarring. Most importantly, however, is preservation of all frontal recess mucosa; this allows restoration of function without scarring. Fibrin clot does not adhere to intact mucosa. There is less likelihood of granulation tissue, fibrous scarring, and frontal sinus contracture. Any frontal recess mucosa inadvertently removed increases the likelihood of these problems. Anything which improves enlarging the drainage pathway while preserving the mucosa and mucociliary clearance is advantageous to patient outcomes.

The operative technique for endoscopic frontal sinus and frontal recess surgery is detailed elsewhere in this book at great length. The purpose of this chapter is to detail the instrumentation that has advanced frontal sinus surgery and review the proper use of this instrumentation in light of these tenets of frontal sinus surgery.

Endoscopes

Historically, the anatomy of the nasal cavity and paranasal sinuses has intrigued mankind, and this rudimentary anatomical knowledge of the anatomy dates back to tomb inscriptions from 1500 BC [28]. The ancient Egyptians created fistulae between the cranial and sinonasal cavities in order to remove intracranial

contents from the recently deceased. Improved access to the nasal cavity and other orifices of the body was obtained by the Roman development of the speculum, which dates to the first century AD From this time of speculae and mirror illumination, no meaningful advances occurred in the visualization of the body's cavities until the time of Philipp Bozzini (1773–1809), who developed the first rigid endoscope [5]. Although Bozzini was a urologist, he developed a system for rigid endoscopy, suitable for use in many body areas, including the nasal cavity [26].

Subsequently, the candle illumination provided by Bozzini's system was enhanced by another urologist, Maximillian Nitze, who developed an endoscope in 1877 with engineer Joseph Leiter that used a glowing platinum wire for illumination [26]. Nitze also integrated an optical system in the body of his endoscope that involved a series of glass lenses separated by airspaces. Thus, the first conventional optical rod was engineered. Hirschmann [20] is credited as the first to modify one of Nitze's cystocopes and utilize it for nasal endoscopy; however, this was short-lived because of low illumination and access to the sinonasal cavities [20].

The next major advance was the development of the Hopkins rod lens system, developed by Harold Hopkins in 1960 [13], which modified Baird's design [13] for sending light and images down a flexible glass cable. His rod incorporated glass fibers for the transmission of light as well as a series of airspaces separated by glass lenses; these improvements increased optical efficiency ninefold. This novel technology was fostered and manufactured by Karl Storz, who coupled Hopkins's endoscope with cold-light illumination. Today, Hopkins rod lens telescopes are the standard for rigid nasal endoscopy, and their coupling with a remote xenon light source provides excellent illumination without the morbidity of "hot light" from the scope's tip.

An array of endoscopes are needed for proper operative and postoperative care:

- Most manufacturers offer scopes with 4- and 2.7-mm ("pediatric") diameters.
- The largest possible scope should be used as each 10% increase in diameter results in a 46% increase in illumination [5].

A variety of telescopes are available that allow field-of-view illumination and visualization at a fixed angle from the telescope axis. Although the endoscope itself is straight, an angle-of-view prism is incorporated into the distal tip of the scope that allows visualization and illumination of the field of view at a defined angle from the working axis of the endoscope.

The 0° endoscope is the telescope of choice for ethmoid and sphenoid sinus surgery. Since the working axis of the scope is straight ahead and in line with the instruments, disorientation is not as much of an issue; however, when working from a monitor, the image must be kept vertical to avoid disorientation. Although the 0° telescope is easier to maneuver than the angled telescopes, it is limited by its inability to visualize areas that are not directly in line with the telescope's axis. Consequently, angled telescopes are very important when working at an angle to the anteroposterior axis of the nose such as in the maxillary and frontal sinuses. In general, the technique for frontal recess dissection begins posteriorly. The skull base is identified at the most posterior aspect of the ethmoid dissection at its junction with the sphenoid face and is then continued from posterior to anterior along the skull base towards the frontal recess. At the frontal recess (as well as at the maxillary sinus ostium) the telescope is changed to one of the angled telescopes to afford better visibility and illumination.

The anterosuperior location of the frontal recess necessitates the use of angled telescopes to look above the "horizontal." Although some surgeons use a 45° endoscope in this area, the 70° telescope is preferred owing to its enhanced visualization of the frontal recess. In addition, the 90° instruments designed for use here are best used in conjunction with this telescope. As mentioned earlier, the conceptual anatomy of the frontal recess resembles an inverted funnel that begins superiorly at the frontal ostium and descends posteroinferiorly (Fig. 3.3). It is bounded by the skull base posteriorly, ending at about the anterior ethmoid artery, and by the agger nasi region anteriorly, ending at the anterior attachment of the middle turbinate to the lateral nasal wall. This vertical component of the recess is complex and is best visualized with the more angled 70° telescope. The availability and use of angled telescopes in the office for postoperative debridements is at least as important as their operative use.

Finally, the use of reverse light post endoscopes is advantageous during frontal sinus surgery. A reverse endoscope is one that has the light cord attachment, "the post," pointed up when in use, 180° from its usual location. This allows the light cable to attach on the superior aspect of the endoscope, thereby freeing up more space underneath the telescope for the surgeon to manipulate other instruments. This is ideal as the instruments for frontal recess dissection are designed to be passed underneath the telescope. However, the superior port location may complicate the use of "line-of-sight" image guidance systems, in which case either an electromagnetic image guidance system or 90° light post offset scopes may be used.

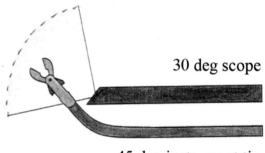

30 deg scope

45 deg instrument tip

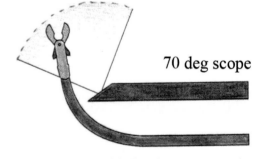

70 deg scope

90 deg instrument tip

Fig. 3.4. Forty-five-degree instruments are designed for the 30° endoscope and the 90° instruments are designed for the 70° endoscope

Fig. 3.5. Angled frontal recess curettes

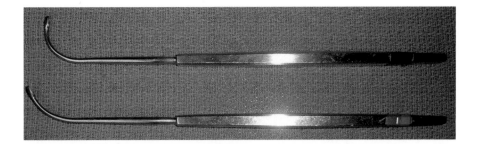

Frontal Curettes

Frontal recess curettes (Fig. 3.5) have been designed with an angled tip that fits the frontal recess. As the skull base is being dissected from posterior to anterior, it begins to slope sharply upward near the anterior ethmoid artery (neurovascular bundle). This is the posterior entrance to the frontal recess. Standard straight sinus instruments, such as the J-curette or the 45° Blaksley forceps, cannot access this area of the skull base owing to the frontal sinus being 90° above the "line of sight." Consequently, the angled frontal recess curettes are used to continue the skull base dissection by sliding them up the posterior frontal recess wall behind the frontal recess cells. The curette and cell walls are then pulled inferiorly and anteriorly with little side-to-side movement. Misdirection of the frontal curette off a parasagittal plane may result in inadvertent injury to the skull base medially or the orbit laterally. Special care should be taken in patients with a Keros type III anatomic variation of the anterior skull base [15] to prevent injury to the lateral cribriform plate lamella (Fig. 3.6). In such a configuration the olfactory groove is deep and creates a tall lateral lamella of the cribriform plate, which is more prone to injury with resultant cerebrospinal fluid leak [16].

Suction Kuhn frontal sinus curettes (Fig. 3.7) available in 45° and 90° angles are useful if blood obscures the field of view in the frontal recess. A suction is incorporated into the distal tip of the curette without adding bulk to the tip and allows the instrument to remove blood from the operative field during the dissection. The proximal end of the curette has a toggle connector which attaches to the suction tubing. This allows better maneuverability by using lightweight intravenous connecting tubing interposed between the instrument and the main suction tubing. The handle has a low profile and is hollow to permit suction at the tip; however it can be bent if much force is applied to it.

The primary goal of the frontal recess curette is to fracture the bony cellular elements of the frontal recess. Overaggressive use of the curette in the frontal recess may damage the mucosa and compromise the frontal sinus outflow tract. Therefore, after disrupt-

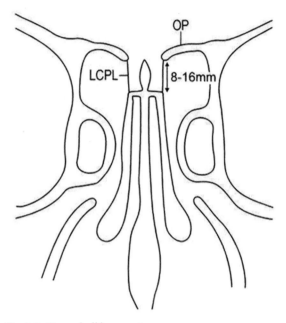

Fig. 3.6. Keros skull base anatomy

ing the cell walls with the curette, bony partitions can be manipulated with the frontal sinus seekers and removed with a tissue debrider using an angled blade or frontal sinus giraffes (see later). These delicate giraffes were engineered to remove fragments of bone and mucosa that have already been disrupted by more aggressive means.

Frontal Sinus Seekers

Dissection of frontal recess cells entails the manipulation of small fragments of bone and mucosa in a difficult anatomic area.

Tips and Pearls
■ Fractured frontal recess cell walls must be manipulated and removed in a careful and meticulous fashion in order to maximize the functional result and minimize scarring and mucosal injury to surrounding structures.

3

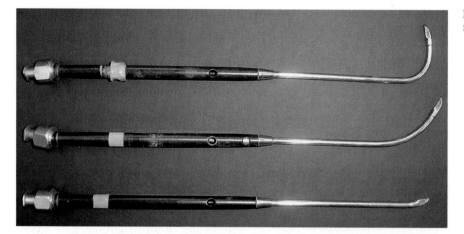

Fig. 3.7. Kuhn suction frontal sinus curettes

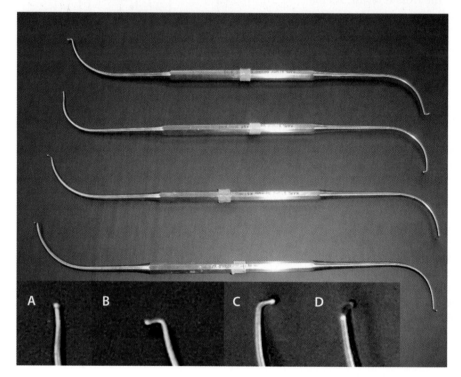

Fig. 3.8. Frontal sinus seekers

Frontal sinus seekers were designed to fit the anatomy "around the corner" and manipulate bone and mucosa with their fine ball-ended tips. These seekers were created in two angles, 77° and 90°, in order to work on different anatomical variants of the frontal recess. The 90° frontal sinus seeker is more commonly used in the frontal recess as its angle works well with the slope of the skull base in the frontal recess and complements the 70° endoscope well.

Each set of frontal sinus seekers (Fig. 3.8) has five discrete tips, one straight and four bent at 90° to the shaft, which allow the surgeon to work in all four quadrants of the frontal recess or sinus. The set is composed of five separate handles with two tips each,

two straight at 77° and 90° and four with the tips bent to the four quadrants. They have been named the "inny," "outty," "lefty," and "righty" seekers, the names of which reference (the umbilicus and baseball pitchers, as well as) the direction of the tip in relation to the handle. These were engineered to seek and probe the frontal recess as well as to remove frontal sinus bone fragments and redrape mucosa around the ostium. They are also valuable in the gentle manipulation of frontal recess mucosa after underlying bone has been removed. This allows mucosa to be "teased" from bone and maneuvered into its desired position; this is done to cover any areas of exposed bone with viable mucosa. Frontal sinus seekers are indispens-

Fig. 3.9. Kuhn-Bolger frontal sinus giraffes

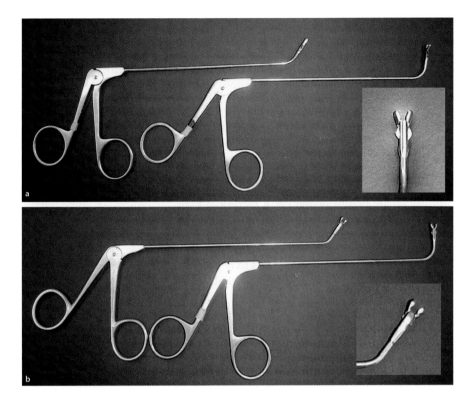

able when performing the frontal sinus rescue procedure [19] as they are used to elevate mucosa off the lateral aspect of a middle turbinate remnant. After the bony vertical middle turbinate remnant is resected from the skull base with its medial nasal mucosa, the elevated lateral flap of frontal recess mucosa is rotated medially to the nasal vault with the seeker to break up the circular geometry of the scar and to cover exposed bone where the middle turbinate remnant was resected.

Kuhn–Bolger Frontal Sinus Giraffes

After a frontal recess cell has been disrupted and its bony partitions teased from their mucosa with frontal sinus seekers, frontal sinus giraffes (Fig. 3.9) are helpful in removing the loose pieces of bone. The distal tip of these instruments is a "double spoon," or cup forceps configuration used as a grasping instrument, which is angled to fit up into the frontal recess. The handle and shaft design is similar to that of the Kuhn frontal sinus punches described in the next section. There are three pairs of frontal giraffe forceps; each pair consists of front-to-back and side-to-side biting forceps. They come in 45° 2- and 3-mm cups and 90° 2-mm cups. Their design allows careful manipulation and removal of bone fragments left in the frontal recess after dissection.

Tips and Pearls

■ Understanding the proper use of frontal recess giraffes will avoid inadvertent injury to the anterior skull base.

These instruments were not designed to remove bony cell walls still attached to the skull base because their tips are not through-cutting. Twisting a frontal recess cell remnant still attached to the anterior skull base with a frontal recess giraffe would run the risk of a skull base CSF leak. The partition could only be fractured if the giraffe were incorrectly used to twist or rock the partition from the skull base. This could lead to skull base fracture and CSF leak, since the bone may be only 0.1–0.2-mm thick. The weakest point of the entire anterior skull base in fact is the point where the ethmoid roof is penetrated by the anterior ethmoid artery [27].

Kuhn Frontal Sinus Punches

The frontal sinus punches were designed in conjunction with Karl Storz to allow more removal of frontal recess/sinus cell walls while preserving the mucous membranes. Although upon cursory inspection these punches appear similar to the frontal sinus giraffes, their use is very different. Their tips are through-cut-

3

tion of the dental drill) reach the anterior frontal sinus ostium, which the straight drill cannot, but visualization around the right-angle tip is very difficult. Angled drills are now commercially available for the microdebrider hand piece and are easier to manipulate in the frontal recess. Gyrus (Bartlett, TN, USA) manufactures an angled drill with a shaft that is rotatable, but has a fixed tip. The angled drill made by Xomed (Jacksonville, FL, USA) has an independently rotatable tip, but has a less ergonomic hand piece. The surgeon must be careful with the use of drills in order to avoid circumferential injury, as this leads to osteoneogenesis, scarring, and frontal recess stenosis [16].

Stereotactic Computer Assisted Navigation Instruments

A full discussion of stereotactic computer assisted navigation or image guided surgery systems is beyond the scope of this chapter [8]. These systems were initially designed with the ability to correlate a patient's anatomy with the computed tomography (CT) images on a computer screen. The early systems tracked a simple probe that the surgeon intermittently inserted into the sinonasal cavity for reference. As the systems evolved, certain instruments and suctions were developed that could be detected and tracked by the system in addition to the probes. This allowed the surgeon to correlate his or her anatomical location with the sinus CT images, while actively using an instrument or suction without having to interrupt dissection, remove the instrument, aspirate blood to clear the field, and then insert the probe.

Different systems have a different armamentarium of instruments that can be tracked. Systems that rely on line of sight for tracking, such as BrainLab (Munich, Germany), Xomed (Jacksonville, FL, USA), and Stryker (Kalamazoo, MI, USA), allow a clamp-on reference array to be placed on almost any instrument. This allows the active tracking of multiple instruments simultaneously. Actively tracking a frontal sinus curette can be very valuable while dissecting the frontal recess. Electromagnetic tracking systems, such as General Electric's Instatrak (Boston, MA, USA), utilize a variety of proprietary straight and angled suctions and curettes attached to the system. The 45° Fried and 90° Kuhn Instatrak suctions (Fig. 3.11) are key for tracking in the frontal recess with this system. These suctions all have a ball-tip at the end of the suction tube, which is used to register the suction to the headset. This tip also allows it to be used as a dissector to maneuver bone and mucosa within the sinuses, particularly the frontal recess. Cranial pins allow the electromagnetic transmitter (Fig. 3.12) or reference array to be attached to the head and eliminate the headset or headband.

Other Instrumentation

There are several other instruments commonly used during frontal recess dissections that were not detailed in the previous sections. The frontal mushroom developed by Stammberger (Fig. 3.13) has a handle, shaft, and overall appearance similar to the frontal sinus giraffes; however, the distal tip is a mushroom punch. This is a through-cutting instrument that has the advantage of being able to work circumferentially,

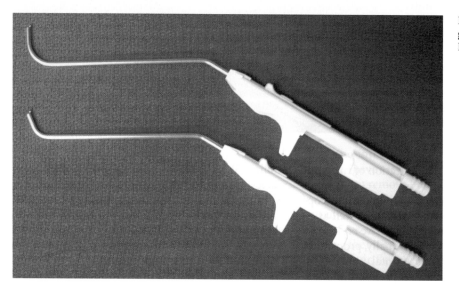

Fig. 3.11. Forty-five-degree Fried and 90° Kuhn Instatrak suctions

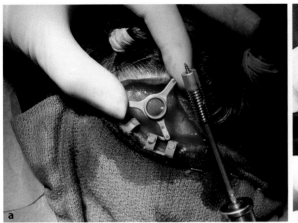

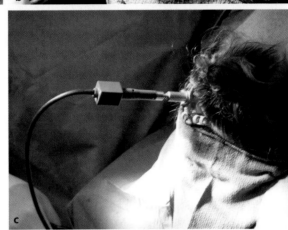

Fig. 3.12. Electromagnetic transmitter affixed to the skull with pins

Fig. 3.13. Frontal mush-
room

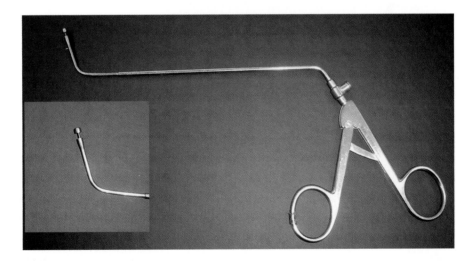

which is especially important around the frontal sinus ostium. Although it removes loose pieces of bone
well, it is used on mucosa sparingly as it has the tendency to strip rather than cut. This could lead to circumferential mucosal injury.

The Rosa frontal Kerrison (Fig. 3.14) and Hosemann frontal mushroom punches (Fig. 3.15) are more
substantial instruments and can be used in the frontal recess to remove heavier bone than the more delicate Kuhn frontal sinus punches and the frontal
mushroom punch. These are commonly used to remove osteitic bone from the frontal recess and may
be used instead of drills during Draf type IIb and III
procedures [7].

Balloon catheters are the newest of the frontal sinus instruments and are addressed in Chap. 25.

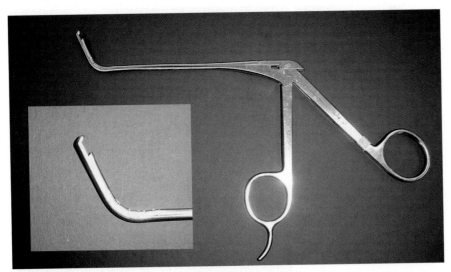

Fig. 3.14. Frontal Kerrison (Rosa)

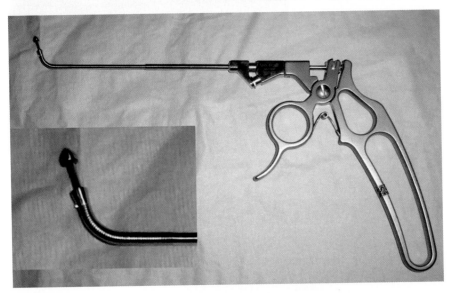

Fig. 3.15. Hosemann frontal mushroom punch

Conclusion

The development of new frontal sinus instruments, techniques, and procedures has allowed a renaissance of intranasal frontal sinus surgery to the extent that it has virtually replaced all other frontal sinus surgical procedures over the last 15 years. The focus has shifted from the frontal sinus itself to the real source of frontal sinus disease, namely, the frontal recess – the frontal sinus drainage pathway. The rare instances where it is not sufficient are limited to those few patients who must be obliterated, reexplored after obliteration, have a frontal sinus tumor, or have some other lesion which cannot be reached from below.

Endoscopic management of the frontal sinus has enabled therapies that preserve the function of the sinus rather than obliterate it. Keeping the tenets of functional frontal sinus surgery in mind, instruments have been engineered to enable careful dissection of this area and to restore physiologic function while preserving the normal anatomic structures. The application of these instruments and principles has expanded the realm of frontal sinus surgery to treat conditions other than chronic inflammatory disease and to decrease the need for external and open operations.

References

1. Bent JP, Cuilty-Siller C, Kuhn FA (1994) The frontal cell in frontal sinus obstruction. Am J Rhinol 8:185–91.
2. Bumm K, Wurm H, Bohr C, et al. (2005) New endoscopic instruments for paranasal sinus surgery. Otolaryngol Head Neck Surg 133(3):444–9.
3. Chandra RK, Kennedy DW, Palmer JN (2004) Endoscopic management of failed frontal sinus obliteration. Am J Rhinol 18(5):279–84.
4. Christmas DA, Krouse JH (1996) Powered instrumentation in dissection of the frontal recess. Ear Nose Throat J 75(6):359–64.
5. DeDivitiis E, Cappabianca P (eds). Endoscopic endonasal transsphenoidal surgery. Springer-Verlag, New York, 2003. Leonhard M, Cappabianca P, DeDivitiis E. The endoscope, endoscopic equipment and instrumentation. pp. 9–19.
6. Draf W (1991) Endonasal microendoscopic frontal sinus surgery: the Fulda concept. Otolaryngol Head Neck Surg 2:234–40.
7. Dubin MG, Kuhn FA (2005) Endoscopic modified Lothrop (Draf III) with frontal sinus punches. Laryngoscope 115(9):1702–3.
8. Dubin MG, Kuhn FA (2005) Stereotactic computer assisted navigation: state of the art for sinus surgery, not standard of care. Otolaryngol Clin North Am 38(3):535–49.
9. Graham SM, Nerad JA (2003) Orbital complications in endoscopic sinus surgery using powered instrumentation. Laryngoscope 113:874–878.
10. Gross CW, Zachmann GC, Becjer DG, et al. (1997) Follow-up University of Virginia experience with the modified Lothrop procedure. Am J Rhinol 11:49–54.
11. Hardy JM, Montgomery WV (1976) Osteoplastic frontal sinusotomy: an analysis of 250 operations. Ann Otol Rhinol Laryngol 85(4 Pt 1):523–32.
12. Hoseman W, Herzog D, Beule AG, Kaftan H (2004) Experimental evaluation of drills for extended frontal sinusotomy. Otolaryngol Head Neck Surg 131(3):187–191.
13. Jennings CR. Harold Hopkins (1998) Archives of Otolaryngology Head and Neck Surgery 124:1042.
14. Kang SK, White PS, Lee M, et al. (2002) A randomized control trial of surgical task performance in frontal recess surgery: zero degree versus angled telescopes. Am J Rhinol 16:33–6.
15. Keros P (1962) On the practical value of differences in the level of the lamina cribrosa of the ethmoid. Z Laryngol Rhinol Otol 41:809–13.
16. Kuhn FA (1996) Chronic frontal sinusitis: the endoscopic frontal recess approach. Operative Tech Otolaryngol Head Neck Surg 7:222.
17. Kuhn FA, Bolger WE, Tisdal RG (1991) The agger nasi cell in frontal recess obstruction: an anatomic, radiologic, and clinical correlation. Oper Tech Otolaryngol Head and Neck Surg 2:226–31.
18. Kuhn FA, Javer AR (2001) Primary endoscopic management of the frontal sinus. Otolaryngol Clin North Am 34(1):59–75.
19. Kuhn FA, Javer AR, Nagpal K, Citardi MJ (2000) The frontal sinus rescue procedure: early experience and three-year follow-up. Am J Rhinol 14(4): 211–6.
20. Lesserson JA, Schaefer SD (1994) Instrumentation for endoscopic sinus surgery. Ear Nose Throat J 73(8):522–31.
21. Loury MC (1993) Endoscopic frontal recess and frontal sinus ostium dissection. Laryngoscope 103:455–8.
22. May M (1991) Frontal sinus surgery: endonasal endoscopic osteoplasty rather that expternal osteoplasty. Oper Tech Otolaryngol Head and Neck Surg 2:226–31.
23. McLaughlin RB, Hwang PH, Lanza DC (1999) Endoscopic trans-septal frontal sinusotomy: the rationale and results of an alternative technique. Am J Rhinol 13(4):279–87.
24. Merritt R, Bent JP, Kuhn FA (1996) The intersinus septal cell. Am J Rhinol 10: 299–302.
25. Owen RG, Kuhn FA (1997) The supraorbital ethmoid cell. Otolaryngol Head Neck Surg 116:254–61.
26. Sircus W, Flisk E (2003) Milestones in the evolution of endoscopy: a short history. J R Coll Physicians Edinb 33:124–34.
27. Stammberger H (1991) Functional endoscopic sinus surgery. Philadelphia, BC Decker.
28. Stammberger H (1989) History of rhinology: anatomy of the paranasal sinues. Rhinology 27:197–210.

Chapter 4

Injection and Anesthetic Techniques

4

Subinoy Das, Brent A. Senior

Core Messages

- Proper injection and anesthetic techniques are essential for enhancing visualization, minimizing complications, and maximizing patient outcomes.

- General anesthesia is preferred for most endoscopic procedures. Good communication with the anesthesiologist is important for optimizing the surgical field.

- Volatile anesthetics cause vasodilatation, which can increase bleeding and should be minimized. Total intravenous anesthesia may improve the surgical field and minimize postoperative nausea and vomiting.

- Heart rate is an independent variable which affects the surgical field. Preoperative and/or intraoperative beta blockade may enhance visualization.

- Reverse Trendelenburg position reduces the intracranial mean arterial blood pressure without reducing cerebral perfusion pressure and may decrease bleeding.

- The intraoral greater palatine block, intranasal sphenopalatine block, and uncinate injection is routinely used to minimize bleeding and postoperative pain. Topical anesthetics and/or decongestants should be used liberally.

- The surgeon holds the primary responsibility to minimize anesthetic complications for the patient. This includes the awareness of patient allergies, maximal doses, contraindications, and side effects of all materials administered to the patient.

Contents

Introduction

Proper anesthesia and injection techniques are critical to safely and effectively perform endoscopic sinus surgery. These techniques when used properly minimize pain and provide for maximal vasoconstriction. Mastery of and attention to these topics can significantly enhance the safety and quality of endoscopic sinus surgery.

Anesthesia

Endoscopic sinus surgery can be performed under local anesthesia with/without sedation or general anesthesia. Local anesthesia with sedation avoids some of the risks inherent with general anesthesia, allows for monitoring of vision and pain, and may provide for an additional level of safety. Previous studies have reported that patients undergoing endoscopic sinus sur-

4

gery under local anesthesia with sedation have a satisfaction level comparable to that of patients receiving general anesthesia [15]. Also, many surgeons report decreased bleeding and decreased operative times under local anesthesia compared with general anesthesia [5]. However, modern general anesthetic techniques have improved considerably and remain the authors' preference. Furthermore, general anesthesia is helpful when using computer-assisted navigation, as head movement may disrupt the reference headbands for the guidance system.

General anesthesia results in a state of total unconsciousness with resultant loss of airway reflexes, amnesia, and analgesia. Volatile agents are used for the maintenance phase of anesthesia; however, these agents cause vasodilatation, which is deleterious to the surgical field, particularly during endoscopic sinus surgery. Techniques such as controlled hypotension have been developed to assist in the surgical field; however, these are typically accomplished with higher concentrations of these volatile agents, with resultant increased vasodilatation, rebound tachycardia, and equivocal effects on the quality of the surgical field. In addition, controlled hypotension poses a risk to end-organ function [9].

In 1989, AstraZeneca Corporation introduced propofol [16], the first of a new class of intravenous anesthetics known as alkyl phenols. Propofol is an intravenous sedative-hypnotic agent that can be used for the induction of general anesthesia as well as the maintenance of general anesthesia via a continuous infusion.

Tips and Pearls

- Propofol induces arterial hypotension without significant reflex tachycardia but does not appear to have the peripheral vasodilatory effects comparable with those of the volatile agents.

In addition, propofol appears to cause less postoperative nausea and vomiting. However, propofol does cause pain on injection and it is delivered as a lipid emulsion; thus, strict aseptic technique must always be maintained to prevent a bloodstream infection. It also has a distribution half-life of 2–4 min, but it readily distributes to peripheral fat and has an elimination half-life of 2–4 h and therefore may build up in a patient if used during a long operation.

The advent of propofol and remifentanil, a very short-acting narcotic, and target-controlled infusion pumps, which greatly simplify maintenance of a steady blood level, allowed for the development of total intravenous anesthesia (TIVA). TIVA is a form of general anesthesia and has many advantages over traditional general anesthesia using volatile anesthetics [4].

Tips and Pearls

- Wormald et al. [17] performed a prospective, randomized, controlled trial comparing TIVA with traditional anesthesia with sevoflurane and found a significant improvement in a validated grading system of the surgical field that was independent of heart rate or mean arterial blood pressure. As a result, the authors recommend the use of TIVA whenever deemed reasonable by the anesthesia team for each particular patient.

In addition, multiple studies [1, 11] have confirmed the effect of heart rate on the surgical field, and have shown that beta-blocker premedication improves the surgical field. Placing the patient in the reverse Trendelenburg position [14] also has been shown to reduce intracranial mean arterial blood pressure without reducing cerebral perfusion pressure. Therefore, the reverse Trendelenburg position is used in all of the authors' procedures.

As the field of anesthesiology continues to evolve, various strategies and protocols will emerge that provide the optimal anesthesia for patients undergoing sinus surgery. Because of the profound effect that anesthesia can have on the surgical field, it behooves the rhinologist to develop a close working relationship with their anesthesiology colleagues and remain informed of developments that affect sinus surgery.

Local Anesthetics, Vasoconstrictors, and Injection Locations

Local anesthetics [3] and vasoconstrictors [12] also play an important role in minimizing postoperative pain and improving the surgical field during endoscopic sinus surgery. There are a myriad of mixtures and protocols used for local anesthesia and vasoconstriction. Two basic classes for local anesthetics exist: the amino esters and the amino amides. Cocaine, a naturally occurring amino ester, was the first anesthetic to be discovered and was introduced into Europe in the 1800s. Lidocaine, an amino amide, is the most widely used cocaine derivative and was developed during World War II.

Amino esters and amino amides differ in several important aspects:

- Esters are metabolized in plasma via pseudocholinesterases, whereas amides are metabolized in the liver.
- Esters are unstable in solution, whereas amides are very stable.

■ Esters are more likely to cause true allergic reactions.

All esters and amides are vasodilators with the exception of cocaine, which is a vasoconstrictor; thus, the combination of anesthesia and vasoconstriction makes cocaine an ideal anesthetic for intranasal surgery [6]. However, the euphoria and highly addictive nature of cocaine have made it one of the most widely abused recreational drugs and thus made it illegal in most countries. As a result, cocaine is more difficult to use for legitimate medical purposes. Cocaine is also known to cause cardiac arrhythmias and many have recommended its abandonment [10] and the use of safer mixtures.

Epinephrine, a human adrenergic catecholamine, is commonly added to the local anesthetics at a variety of concentrations. Epinephrine induces peripheral vascular resistance via alpha-receptor stimulated vasoconstriction. The authors commonly use 1% lidocaine with 1:100,000 epinephrine for their local injections.

Tips and Pearls
■ Oxymetazoline is a potent alpha-agonist that causes rapid vasoconstriction of nasal arterioles, resulting in profound vasoconstriction with minimal systemic absorption. However, it causes rebound vasodilatation and therefore is physiologically addictive; repeated use can cause chemical dependence with diminishing effect.

The greater palatine foramen injection [2] is an effective method for controlling bleeding and providing anesthesia during paranasal sinus surgery; however, concerns for intraorbital and intracranial complications have limited its widespread acceptance among sinus surgeons. The greater palatine foramen is located posteromedially to the third maxillary molar and anteromedially to the maxillary tuberosity and pterygoid hamulus. It is the opening to the greater palatine canal, which courses in a posterosuperior direction and leads superiorly into the pterygopalatine fossa. Here in the pterygopalatine fossa lies the internal maxillary artery and its multiple branches which supply blood to the nose and paranasal sinuses. The closed space and bony walls of the pterygopalatine fossa make it readily amenable to local anesthesia.

Multiple mechanisms of hemostasis are obtained with a greater palatine canal injection. These include:

■ Epinephrine-induced vasoconstriction
■ Mechanical tamponade of the vessels
■ Parasympathetic block allowing unopposed sympathetic activity

The optimal injection is delivered at the level of the sphenopalatine foramen, which corresponds to the level of the internal maxillary and sphenopalatine arteries. Superiorly, the pterygopalatine fossa is limited by the anterior basal portion of the greater wing of the sphenoid bone. The inferior orbital fissure is located anterosuperiorly in the pterygopalatine fossa and contains orbital fat and fascia. The optic foramen lies approximately 2 cm above the inferior orbital fissure. The foramen rotundum is located posteriorly, superiorly, and laterally to the sphenopalatine foramen. The mean distance of the greater palatine foramen to the sphenopalatine foramen is 28 mm in men and 27 mm in women. The mean distance of the greater palatine foramen to the inferior orbital fissure is 40 mm in men and 37 mm in women.

Tips and Pearls
■ The authors inject the greater palatine foramen at a conservative depth of 25 mm in all adults to minimize the risk of intraorbital penetration.

The sphenopalatine foramen can also be injected transnasally [8]. Here, the sphenopalatine artery and nerve pass interiorly into the nose. A combination of the sphenopalatine block with the greater palatine block leads to profound vasoconstriction in the posterior portion of the nasal cavity and significantly reduces bleeding.

Technique

General Anesthesia

Prior to the start of each operation, the overall anesthetic plan is discussed with the anesthesiologist. In many cases, the anesthesiologist may be new or unfamiliar with the specific issues involved in maintaining the surgical field during endoscopic sinus surgery. Developing a collegial relationship with the anesthesiologist is essential and is facilitated by sharing literature reviewing the anesthetic issues involved with sinus surgery. The vasodilatory effects of volatile anesthetics and the merits of TIVA and beta blockade are discussed. The anesthesiologist then develops a plan customized for each individual patient. Monitors are provided for the anesthetist to view the surgical field so that the effects of intraoperative adjustments on the surgical field may be witnessed. This is important for enfranchising the anesthetist to the team approach for

4

optimizing the surgical field and so that they may learn from their intraoperative decisions. The patient is then placed in reverse Trendelenburg position, which elevates the head approximately 10–20°.

Intraoral Greater Palatine Block

The authors utilize bilateral greater palatine blocks (Fig. 4.1, Video 4.1) in nearly all cases as previously described [2]. A 3-ml aliquot of 1% lidocaine with 1:100,000 epinephrine is drawn into a 3-ml Luer-lock syringe. Before obtaining this fluid, the expiration date and the proper concentration of the lidocaine and epinephrine on the stock container are confirmed by the surgeon. A 1.5-in. 25 gauge needle is measured with a ruler and bent at a 60° angle at a length of 25 mm for all adults. This needle is placed on the syringe. After the patient has been intubated and the bed turned, two tongue blades are placed in the mouth and used to palpate the hard palate–soft palate junction. The greater palatine foramen will be located just anterior to the border of this junction. It can often be seen as a subtle depression in the hard palate mucosa and/or can be palpated with a gloved finger.

Tips and Pearls

■ Although historically described as next to the second maxillary molar, the greater palatine foramen is next to the third molar approximately 50% of the time.

The needle is placed into the greater palatine foramen and advanced to the bend of the needle. Occasionally, the needle is marched anteriorly from the hard palate border when the greater palatine foramen is difficult to find. The needle is then aspirated for blood to prevent an intravascular injection. If no blood is obtained, then 1.5 ml of the anesthetic is delivered slowly to the canal. If the needle is properly placed, there is moderate resistance to the fluid being delivered into the canal. If there is very minimal resistance, it is likely that the needle went through the soft palate into the nasopharynx, and is not correctly placed in the canal. The same procedure is repeated for the contralateral canal.

Topical Decongestion with Oxymetazoline

The patient's nose is sprayed 1 h preoperatively with topical oxymetazoline. After the patient has been draped, a 0° rigid endoscope is immediately obtained,

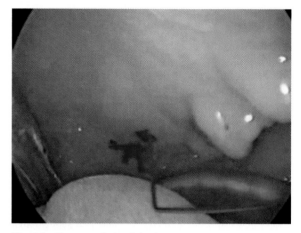

Fig. 4.1. Greater palatine injection

and under endoscopic visualization, oxymetazoline-soaked cotton pledgets are placed anteriorly into each nasal cavity to decongest the nasal septum and turbinate mucosa. This is a critical step that is performed carefully under endoscopic visualization to prevent trauma to the septal mucosa or middle turbinate that can occur with blind placement of the pledgets. This prevents nuisance bleeding from an anterior mucosal laceration that can seriously hamper an entire operation. After these pledgets have been placed, attention is given to completing the preparation for the operation, including installing a camera and setting up a microdebrider. The authors routinely use an endoscope irrigation system to wash away minor bleeding at the scope tip and always sit during the operation with an armrest for the left arm to help stabilize the scope. This also minimizes anterior nasal bleeding by reducing arm fatigue throughout the operation. Pledgets are repositioned deeper into the nose as necessary. This is particularly valuable when it is initially necessary to medialize a turbinate.

Sphenopalatine Injection

The sphenopalatine foramen is then injected transnasally posterior and superior to the horizontal portion of the basal lamella at the posterior aspect of the middle turbinate (Fig. 4.2, Video 4.2). A solution of 1% lidocaine with 1:100,000 epinephrine is used. This is a technically difficult injection that is performed by placing a 30° bend in the first centimeter of a spinal needle or by using an angled tonsil needle. The tip of the needle is used to palpate the foramen. The needle is placed in an upward and lateral direction and used to bleb up the mucosa adjacent to the sphenopalatine foramen. Typically, blanching of the epithelium is already seen by a properly injected greater pala-

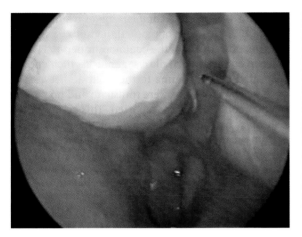

Fig. 4.2. Sphenopalatine foramen injection

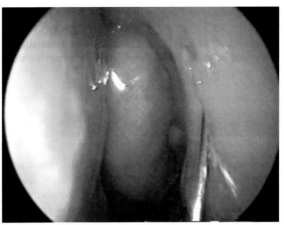

Fig. 4.3. Uncinate process injection

tine foramen block, and the sphenopalatine injection augments this blanching. If the foramen is unable to be reached, then a well-placed bleb near the foramen will diffuse to the foramen and cause vasospasm of the sphenopalatine branches. Alternatively, the injection can be placed medially at the rostrum of the septum between the middle turbinate and the inferior turbinate to minimize bleeding from the posterior nasal artery.

Tips and Pearls

- As always, care should be taken to aspirate before injecting to prevent an intravascular injection.

Lateral Nasal Wall Injections

Next, the lateral nasal wall is injected with 1% lidocaine with 1:100,000 typically with a 25-gauge needle with a slight bend at the tip. The optimal injection is superior and anterior to the anterior attachment of the middle turbinate. The inferior border of the middle turbinate, the septum, the superior turbinate, and other supplemental injections are utilized depending on the disease process and type of operation. The uncinate process is injected after topical oxymetazoline decongestion with 1% lidocaine with 1:100,000 epinephrine. Multiple spots along the uncinate process are typically injected (Fig. 4.3, Video 4.3).

Tips and Pearls

- Using TIVA (with propofol and remifentanil) instead of volatile agents may enhance the surgical field.
- Control heart rate with beta blockade whenever possible.

- Use reverse Trendelenburg position.
- Communicate and work together with the anesthesia team. Allow the anesthesiologist to watch the operation.
- For a greater palatine block, bend the needle at 25 mm by 60°.
- The greater palatine foramen is commonly visible and palpable. It is more commonly next to the third molar.
- Use a bent spinal needle or angled tonsil needle to perform the sphenopalatine block.
- Gently place topical pledgets initially under endoscopic visualization to prevent anterior nasal trauma.
- The maximal concentration of lidocaine is 4 mg/kg without epinephrine and 7 mg/kg with epinephrine.
- The first signs of lidocaine toxicity mimic alcoholic inebriation.

Complications

General Anesthesia

General anesthesia has significantly become safer every decade since Crawford W. Long first used ether in 1842. Currently, the risk of death attributable to general anesthesia is quoted at 1:10,000, though this combines elective surgeries and emergency surgeries. Minor side effects of anesthesia are common, with sore throat in 25% of patients intubated, dizziness and headaches in 15%, fever in 5–15%, and postoperative nausea and vomiting in 5–15%. TIVA appears to cause less nausea and vomiting, but propofol carries the risk of pain with injection and a real sepsis risk due to the lipid emulsion used to deliver propofol. Other risks of anesthesia include malignant

Chapter 5

Septal and Turbinate Surgery

Parul Goyal, Peter H. Hwang

5

Core Messages

■ Accurate diagnosis of the site(s) of obstruction in the preoperative evaluation is the key to formulating the appropriate surgical plan.

■ Nasal endoscopy allows evaluation of the nasal valve area with minimal distortion.

■ Endoscopic surgical techniques allow improved illumination and visualization compared with traditional headlight methods

■ Rhinomanometry and acoustic rhinometry often do not correlate with subjective complaints and are less clinically useful than physical examination and endoscopy

Indications

■ Symptoms of nasal obstruction with corresponding findings of septal deviation and/or turbinate hypertrophy

■ Nasal septal deviation leading to impaired access to middle meatus for endoscopic sinus surgery

■ Contact point headaches due to septal spurs

Tips and Pearls

■ Taking extra time to identify the subperichondrial plane at the start of a septoplasty will minimize the bleeding during surgery.

■ Early identification of a flap tear during septoplasty can allow the surgeon to work beyond the tear without enlarging it further.

■ Mucosa-preserving techniques for inferior turbinate reduction allow the physiologic properties of the turbinate to be maintained.

Contents

Preoperative Evaluation

Nasal septal and turbinate procedures are commonly performed for a variety of indications, including nasal obstruction, need for surgical access during endoscopic sinus surgery, and contact point headaches.

In patients with complaints of nasal obstruction, accurate determination of the cause of the nasal obstruction is critical in formulating a surgical plan. This is best accomplished by a combination of a thorough physical examination and nasal endoscopy. The evaluation begins with an external nasal examination in order to assess the structure and strength of the cartilaginous framework of the nose. A twisted external nasal deformity or weakness of the external or in-

5

ternal nasal valves may signify the need for adjunctive external nasal procedures in addition to planned endonasal approaches. Specifically, the internal nasal valve, which represents the narrowest region of the nasal airway, requires careful examination. Observation during both gentle and forced respiration, in addition to palpation of the upper and lower lateral cartilages, may reveal nasal valve weakness.

Anterior rhinoscopy and nasal endoscopy are integral to the evaluation of patients with nasal obstruction.

Tips and Pearls

- Anterior rhinoscopy should be performed before decongestants are applied in order to assess the inferior turbinates in their native state, which is necessary to evaluate the contribution of the turbinates to the patient's nasal obstruction.

Caudal and anterior septal deviations can be readily seen on anterior rhinoscopy; however, in patients with significant turbinate hypertrophy or septal deviation, nasal endoscopy may be required to visualize the full extent of septal and turbinate anatomy.

Rigid nasal endoscopy is an important part of the routine evaluation of patients with nasal obstruction. In addition to facilitating the diagnosis of more posterior septal and turbinate abnormalities, nasal endoscopy allows detection of other obstructive causes such as polyposis or neoplasms. Rigid endoscopy also offers an excellent means for evaluating the nasal valve in its native state, without the distortion of the valve region that can occur when a nasal speculum is placed during anterior rhinoscopy.

Patients undergoing endoscopic sinus surgery may require concurrent surgical treatment of the septum if middle meatal access is impaired owing to septal deviation. While it may be possible to work around a septal deviation after aggressive intraoperative decongestion of the mucosa intraoperatively, one should consider that an uncorrected septal deviation may limit access for postoperative debridement and surveillance.

Rhinomanometry and acoustic rhinometry are two tests of nasal function that can offer numerical measurements of nasal resistance and cross-sectional area, respectively. While these methods are reproducible and scientifically valid, the clinical utility of these measures has been debated. Improvement in these objective parameters after septal and turbinate surgery has been demonstrated, but there has been poor correlation with patients' subjective assessment of nasal patency [13, 23, 28]. Owing to this lack of correlation, these measures are not routinely carried out in patients undergoing septal or turbinate surgery.

Turbinate Reduction

A variety of techniques have been used for inferior turbinate reduction. These include:

- Partial or complete turbinectomy
- Electrocautery
- Laser cautery and reduction
- Radiofrequency tissue reduction
- Submucosal reduction
- Turbinate lateralization via outfracture

Varying degrees of success have been reported with these techniques. The authors' preferred techniques for management of hypertrophic inferior turbinates is the combination of submucosal resection and turbinate outfracture. Many turbinate procedures can be performed in an office setting under local anesthesia [7].

Turbinate procedures may be subdivided into those procedures addressing soft-tissue aspects of turbinate hypertrophy, and those addressing bony aspects of turbinate hypertrophy.

Soft-Tissue Reduction

Submucosal Soft-Tissue Resection

The technique of submucosal inferior turbinate resection has been shown to lead to long-lasting improvement of nasal patency with a low risk of complications [19]. Elevation of a mucosal flap requires precise technique to prevent flap perforations. The technique has been greatly facilitated by the introduction of special microdebrider blades designed specifically for submucosal turbinate resection.

Prior to initiating the procedure, the nose is decongested and the inferior turbinate is infiltrated with 1% lidocaine with epinephrine. Although the technique can be performed without an endoscope, use of an endoscope greatly improves visualization. Microdebrider blades of 2 and 2.9 mm are available with a dissecting tip on the leading edge of the blade. The tip allows a stab incision to be made along the anterior aspect of the inferior turbinate. With the cutting face of the microdebrider blade facing laterally towards the turbinate bone, the tip of the blade can be used to dissect a submucosal flap. Dissection is performed along the lateral nasal wall and the medial and inferior aspects of the inferior turbinate. If special turbinate blades are not available, the procedure may be performed with a standard pediatric microdebrider blade. A stab incision is made with a no. 15 blade scalpel, and the mucosal flap is developed with a Cottle elevator. The microdebrider blade can then be introduced for submucosal resection.

After flap elevation, the cutting face of the blade is turned towards the mucosal surface. The submucosal soft tissue is resected (Fig. 5.1b).

Tips and Pearls

■ In submucosal tissue resection, emphasis is placed on the anterior aspect of the turbinate and along the lateral nasal wall because these areas contribute the most to clinical nasal obstruction.

Resection of the turbinate bone can also be accomplished using this technique. When resection of a portion of the turbinate bone is planned, a subperiosteal dissection is performed to facilitate resection of a portion of the bone [14]. Placement of packing is not necessary.

The microdebrider submucosal resection technique has the advantage of allowing the surgeon to sculpt the turbinate, allowing accurate intraoperative assessment of the degree of reduction obtained [14]. Preservation of the mucosa allows the functional properties of the turbinate to be maintained [19]. Submucosal resection may also be performed without the use of a microdebrider.

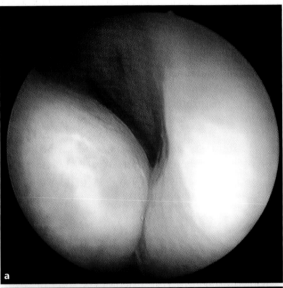
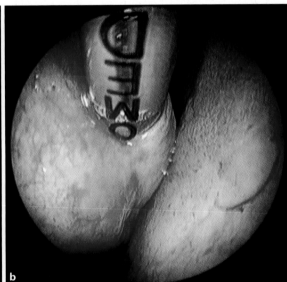
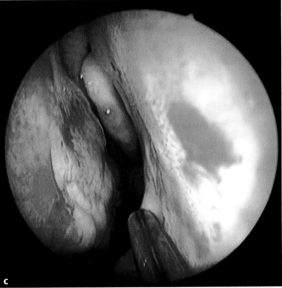

Fig. 5.1. **a** Preoperative view of a hypertrophic inferior turbinate shows contact between the turbinate and nasal septum. **b** Intraoperative view shows microdebrider being used to perform submucosal resection of soft tissue along the medial and inferior aspects of the inferior turbinate. **c** Intraoperative view showing significant improvement in the nasal airway after microdebrider submucosal resection and turbinate lateralization

5

Thermal/Radiofrequency Soft-Tissue Reduction

Another strategy to achieve tissue reduction of the inferior turbinates is through the delivery of exogenous electrical or radiofrequency energy to coagulate the submucosal soft tissue. Options include monopolar electrocautery, bipolar electrocautery, and radiofrequency tissue reduction (Somnoplasty® and Coblation®).

The goal of these techniques is to induce controlled submucosal coagulative necrosis that ultimately leads to fibrosis of the lesion, contracture, and tissue volume reduction.

Monopolar electrocautery is typically applied to a spinal needle inserted longitudinally into the submucosal tissue of the inferior turbinate. Cautery is applied as the needle is slowly withdrawn [5]. Special hand pieces are available for bipolar electrocautery and radiofrequency reduction of the inferior turbinates. In each of these techniques, the probe is inserted in a submucosal plane in order to achieve reduction of targeted portions of the inferior turbinate. Because the maximal temperatures produced using radiofrequency are much lower than those produced using electrocautery, the risk of thermal injury to the overlying mucosa is decreased [2]. Some radiofrequency devices (Somnus Medical Technologies, Bartlett, TN, USA) allow for quantification of the energy delivered in joules. Advantages of thermal and radiofrequency soft-tissue reduction include a mucosal-sparing technique, and good patient tolerance under local anesthesia. Short-term results demonstrate clinical efficacy. Disadvantages include the possibility of mucosal injury if excessive energy is applied, and the relative lack of efficacy data in long-term results.

Laser techniques using CO_2, Nd:YAG, KTP, and argon lasers have also been used for inferior turbinate reduction [4]. These techniques involve the surface coagulation of soft tissue using a variety of laser hand pieces adapted for intranasal use. Although laser techniques can be performed with little patient discomfort, they involve significant mucosal injury and thus may be potentially disruptive of turbinate function [21].

Bone Reduction

Inferior Turbinate Lateralization

While typically insufficient as a standalone procedure, turbinate lateralization by outfracture can be an excellent complement to soft-tissue reduction in improving nasal airway patency. A Boies elevator is used to direct force laterally and inferiorly along the attachment of the inferior turbinate to the lateral nasal wall. Successful displacement is typically noted by audible fracturing of the turbinate bone. To avoid a greenstick fracture, it can occasionally be helpful to first infracture the turbinate by placing the elevator in the inferior meatus, then medializing the turbinate. Subsequent outfracture will typically be more thorough and secure. Adding inferior turbinate lateralization to submucosal resection has been shown to lead to improved long-term results [19]. Figure 5.1a and c shows the preoperative and immediate postoperative views in a patient treated with the combination of microdebrider submucosal resection and turbinate lateralization.

Submucosal Bone Resection

In patients with hypertrophic or osteitic inferior turbinate bone, submucosal resection of the bone may be indicated. A longitudinal incision along the ventral aspect of the turbinate allows elevation of the medial turbinate mucosa and exposure of the turbinate bone. Since elevation of mucosa lateral to the turbinate bone may be difficult, some authors have described resection of the turbinate bone and lateral turbinate mucosa. The preserved medial mucosa is then used to cover the turbinate remnant [1].

Turbinectomy

Various forms of partial or complete inferior turbinate resection have been described [26]. Most involve resection of the full thickness of the turbinate using heavy scissors. One may expect prolonged crusting during the postoperative period, owing to the exposed bone resulting from full-thickness resection.

Tips and Pearls

■ While conservative resection of the anterior-most aspect of the inferior turbinate is unlikely to result in adverse sequelae, complete turbinate resection may be associated with untoward outcomes, including atrophic rhinitis and paradoxical nasal obstruction.

It may be beneficial to reserve full-thickness resection techniques for patients who have failed more conservative methods of reduction.

Results

High success rates have been reported using the entire gamut of turbinate reduction methods [4, 5, 8, 17, 20, 26]; however, few studies have directly compared results using the different methods of reduction. Passali et al. [19] performed a prospective randomized clinical trial comparing different methods of inferior turbinate reduction. The authors enrolled 382 patients who underwent inferior turbinate reduction by one of the following procedures: turbinectomy, laser cautery, electrocautery, cryotherapy, submucosal resection, and submucosal resection with lateral displacement.

On the basis of this work, the authors found that submucosal resection combined with lateral displacement of the turbinates led to the greatest symptomatic improvement.

Furthermore, patients with submucosal reduction achieved values closest to normal with regard to measures of nasal physiology.

In general, preservation of turbinate mucosa is desirable. The surgical techniques of turbinectomy, laser cautery, surface electrocautery, and cryotherapy can lead to significant mucosal injury and damage. Use of these types of techniques has been shown to lead to greater disruption of nasal physiology in comparison with mucosa-preserving techniques [19, 21].

Cavaliere et al. [2] presented data on short-term follow-up of two different surgical techniques used for turbinate reduction. One group of patients underwent submucosal resection of a portion of the turbinate bone under microscopic visualization. The other group underwent radiofrequency volumetric tissue reduction of the inferior turbinates. The authors found significant improvement in nasal obstruction in both groups. The submucosal resection group had a temporary increase in mucociliary transport time, but both groups had normalization of the transport time at 1 month follow-up.

Complications

Aggressive resection of the inferior turbinates using techniques that sacrifice turbinate mucosa has been associated with atrophic rhinitis. This is characterized by excessive nasal crusting, malodorous rhinorrhea, and paradoxical complaints of nasal obstruction.

Tips and Pearls
- Of 190 cases of secondary atrophic rhinitis, Moore and Kern [16] found that 80% were associated with a prior history of partial or complete inferior turbinectomy.

The safety of aggressive turbinate resections has been debated in the literature, with reports on the incidence of crusting and atrophic rhinitis varying from 3 to 89% of patients undergoing total inferior turbinectomy [16, 26]. Despite this controversy, most authors agree that there is greater disruption of nasal physiology with more extensive resections. Impairment of the functional properties of the turbinates has been demonstrated by increased mucociliary transport times and lower secretory Immunoglobulin A concentrations with aggressive mucosal resection techniques [19, 21]. Modern surgical techniques that emphasize mucosal preservation allow less disruption of physiologic function, and allow the risk of atrophic rhinitis to be minimized.

The risk of bleeding in patients undergoing turbinate reduction varies depending on the technique used. The risk has been reported to be highest with laser reduction, with rates as high as 16% [6]. The rates of bleeding for turbinectomy and submucosal resection have been reported to be 1–2% [6, 26]. Submucosal thermal reduction methods have even lower risk of bleeding because of their minimally invasive nature.

Septoplasty

Nasal septal deviation is a frequent cause of nasal obstruction. Surgical correction by means of a septoplasty allows for definitive treatment. An adequate knowledge of nasal and septal anatomy is very important in understanding the surgical techniques used for correction.

The nasal septum consists of cartilaginous and bony components. The anterior aspect of the nasal septum is composed of the quadrangular cartilage. The bony components of the septum include the perpendicular plate of the ethmoid bone superiorly, the maxillary crest anteroinferiorly, and the vomer and perpendicular portion of the palatine bone posteroinferiorly.

The cartilaginous and bony structural components of the septum are lined by perichondrium or periosteum, and a layer of respiratory mucosa. Dissection during septoplasty is performed in the subperichondrial and subperiosteal planes to allow an avascular plane of dissection. In addition, subperichondrial and subperiosteal dissection allows maximal preservation of flap strength and blood supply [10].

The quadrangular cartilage articulates with the maxillary crest and the vomer inferiorly. At the ar-

5

ticulation of the cartilage to these bony components of the septum, the mucoperichondrial layer and the mucoperiosteal layer are not contiguous owing to the presence of dense decussating fibers. The perichondrium and periosteum each pass around the edge of the cartilage or bone, remaining continuous with the corresponding layer from the opposite side. For that reason, it is often difficult to extend the dissection inferiorly over the region of the maxillary crest and the vomer. Because spurs and deviations often occur at the junction of the cartilage and these bony components, it is frequently necessary to carry the dissection beyond these regions. This requires sharp dissection through the decussating fibers.

The quadrangular cartilage is an important contributor to nasal dorsum and tip support. In performing nasal septal surgery, it is important to preserve adequate amounts of the cartilage to prevent loss of nasal dorsum and tip support. It is traditional to preserve at least a 1-cm dorsal and caudal strut of cartilage to prevent tip collapse.

Surgical Technique

Septoplasty has traditionally been performed using a headlight. Advances in endoscopic techniques have allowed the use of the endoscope in performing septoplasty, leading to improved illumination and magnification.

Both the endoscopic and the nonendoscopic techniques start in a similar fashion. A hemitransfixion incision (along the caudal margin of the septal cartilage) or a Killian incision (10–15 mm posterior and parallel to the caudal margin) is used. The incision is carried through the mucosa, underlying soft tissue, and perichondrium to identify the subperichondrial plane. After the mucoperichondrial flap has been elevated 1–2 cm, the endoscope may be introduced under the flap to continue elevation further posteriorly. The use of a scope irrigator and suction Freer elevator can facilitate dissection by helping to clear blood in the field. The endoscope can sometimes give the surgeon a narrow field of vision, so it is important to elevate broadly enough to obtain adequate superior and inferior exposure. When an endoscopic approach is used, the initial hemitransfixion incision and flap elevation are performed on the side of the greater septal deviation.

If the septal deviation involves a portion of the cartilaginous septum, selective resection of the quadrangular cartilage is performed. Care must be taken to retain an adequate dorsal and caudal strut of septal cartilage to prevent alteration of the nasal tip support mechanisms. After the cartilage is incised with a Freer elevator just anterior to the site of the deviation,

flap elevation is continued on the contralateral side in a similar subperichondrial plane (Fig. 5.2). Flap elevation is continued until the deviated portions of the cartilaginous and bony septum are adequately exposed. A sharp Freer elevator is helpful to disarticulate the bony-cartilaginous junctions at the margins of the quadrangular cartilage. Deviations are commonly identified at the junction between quadrangular cartilage and the perpendicular plate of the ethmoid, but deflections can also occur at the junctional zones with the vomer and the maxillary crest.

The deviated portions of the septum can then be removed using a variety of instruments. Endoscopic scissors and Jansen Middleton forceps allow cuts to be made superiorly and inferiorly along the exposed portion of the septal cartilage and bone. The piece can then be removed using Takahashi forceps.

Tips and Pearls

- It is important to use cutting instruments superiorly in the region of the perpendicular plate of the ethmoid bone because excessive manipulation in this area can potentially disrupt the integrity of the skull base and result in CSF leak.

Since the bony septum does not provide significant structural support to the nasal dorsum and tip, large portions of the bony septum can be resected without adverse sequelae.

Alternatives to cartilage resection include cartilage scoring and shaving. In some patients, release of the cartilaginous septum from its bony articulations and perichondrial attachments allows for release of the forces contributing to the deviation of the cartilage. In these instances, the cartilage deviation may resolve after the cartilage is disarticulated from its bony attachments. In other instances, scoring may be necessary even after releasing these attachments. Scoring of the cartilage can be performed along the concave side of the cartilage. This may allow straightening of a curved portion of the cartilage.

It is important to remember that the periosteum over the maxillary crest is divided from the perichondrium of the quadrangular cartilage by thick decussating fibers. Thus, in order to address deformities involving the maxillary crest, flap dissection must be carried through the decussating fibers to the floor of the nasal cavity. Alternatively, the classic "two tunnel" technique may be used to approach prominent spurs along the maxillary crest. In this technique, a superior "tunnel" is elevated over the cartilaginous septum above the spur, and a second tunnel is elevated below the spur, along the nasal floor and the inferior aspect of the maxillary crest. The dissection is then joined at the apex of the spur, with great care being

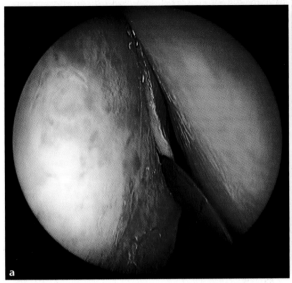
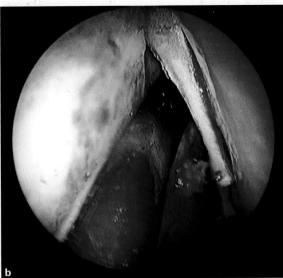

Fig. 5.2. **a** Endoscopic view of incision of the septal cartilage just anterior to the bony-cartilaginous junction. **b** After incising the cartilage, mucoperichondrial flap elevation is performed on the contralateral side in order to isolate the deviated portions of the septal cartilage and bone

taken to avoid tearing the thin mucosa overlying the apex of the spur (Fig. 5.3). The maxillary crest bone is often very thick, and may be difficult to remove. After elevation of bilateral mucoperiosteal flaps, it can be helpful to use a small osteotome or rongeurs to remove the deviated portions of the crest.

After the deviated portions of the bony and cartilaginous septum have been addressed, the hemitransfixion (or Killian) incision is closed using a plain gut suture. A variety of packs and splints have been described for use after septoplasty, but in the authors' experience these can be avoided by using a quilting suture to reapproximate the flaps. A plain gut suture on a straight Keith needle is used as the quilting suture. This suture decreases the likelihood of blood collection between the septal flaps, and allows the patient to recover without the burden of nasal packing.

Isolated Septal Deflections

Endoscopic techniques are particularly helpful in addressing isolated septal deformities. Occasionally, septoplasty may be required to address a solitary septal deflection at the bony-cartilaginous junction at the perpendicular plate of the ethmoid. In such cases, a limited endoscopic septoplasty may be performed to minimize soft-tissue dissection and operative morbidity. A vertical septal incision may be placed along the mucosa immediately anterior to the septal deflection. A limited perichondrial flap can then be raised to isolate and resect the bony-cartilaginous deviation,

subsequently laying the flap back to its native position. A single plain gut mattress suture, or no suture, is typically sufficient for closure.

The endoscopic technique is also useful if an isolated septal spur is to be addressed. An incision can be made longitudinally along the apex of the spur, without the need for a caudal septal incision. Flaps are then elevated superiorly and inferiorly to expose the spur. Resection can be performed using through-cutting sinus instruments, an osteotome along the base of the spur, or powered instruments. Typically, there is enough redundancy of the overlying mucosal flaps after spur removal that the flaps cover the surgical defect well when laid back down. Suturing is not required if the flaps are well approximated [9].

Caudal Septal Deviation

Deviation of the caudal septum can contribute significantly to nasal obstruction.

Tips and Pearls

■ Deviations in this area can be difficult to manage, and generally cannot be addressed adequately via endoscopic techniques [3].

Caudal septal deviations are best treated using traditional septoplasty techniques, sometimes in conjunction with endonasal or open rhinoplasty approaches.

5

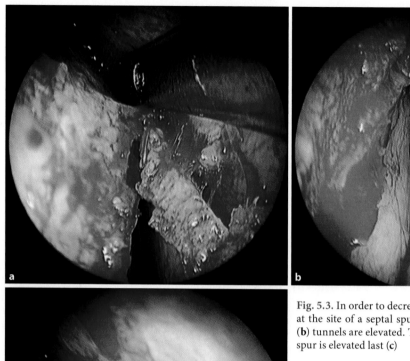

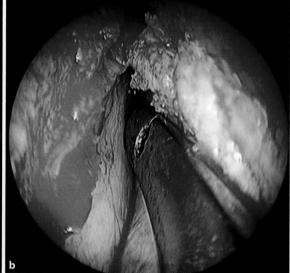

Fig. 5.3. In order to decrease the likelihood of flap perforation at the site of a septal spur, separate superior (**a**) and inferior (**b**) tunnels are elevated. The mucosa overlying the apex of the spur is elevated last (**c**)

Resection of cartilage in this area must be performed with caution given the contribution of this area to nasal tip support.

A variety of techniques have been described to deal with caudal deformities. It may be useful to expose the entire caudal aspect of the septum via a transfixion incision. Elevation of bilateral mucoperichondrial flaps allows the entire caudal portion of the septum to be exposed. After the cartilage is exposed, several options are available to treat the deviation.

In some cases, the caudal aspect of the septum is scrolled, where the scrolled portion does may not contribute significantly to tip support. In such cases, conservative resection of the scrolled portion may be adequate in relieving the caudal deviation. Deviation of the caudal strut due to excess length may be managed by shortening the caudal septal strut, allowing it

to rest at the midline along the nasal spine [22]. The cartilaginous strut can then be secured to the spine with suture to stabilize it in its new position. Some authors have advocated the creation of a "groove" between the medial crura into which the caudal septum can be anchored [12]. Surgical manipulation of the caudal septum may lead to changes in nasal appearance, and thus it is important to counsel patients with caudal deviations prospectively about possible aesthetic outcomes.

Nasal Valve

The internal nasal valve, comprising the angle between the septum and the caudal border of the upper lateral cartilage, is the narrowest aspect of the nasal airway and is a primary site of nasal airway resistance. Preoperative evaluation of the integrity of the nasal valve is important to determine whether concurrent surgical correction of the nasal valve will be needed. A thorough discussion of nasal valve procedures is beyond the scope of this chapter; techniques available for the management of the nasal valve include the placement of spreader grafts, batten grafts, onlay butterfly grafts, or flaring sutures. Management of high septal deviations in the region of the nasal valve can be difficult because resection of cartilage in this region may compromise dorsal and caudal support. Cartilage shaving and scoring techniques may allow correction without significant cartilage resection.

elevation and disruption. Dolan [3] compared the techniques of endoscopic septoplasty and traditional septoplasty. The efficacy and complication rates were found to be equivalent between the two types of techniques.

Surgical intervention for contact point headaches has also been shown to be successful. A study assessing long-term outcomes in patients who underwent surgical management of contact point headaches revealed significant improvement in 85% of patients at 2 years and 65% of patients at 10 years after surgery [27]. Because contact points may be due to factors other than septal deviations and spurs, accurate preoperative examination and patient selection are important factors when considering surgical intervention for these patients.

Results

Many studies have found septoplasty to be effective in the treatment of nasal obstruction [20]. There has been poor correlation between subjective perception of nasal airflow and objective measures of nasal resistance and cross-sectional areas [24]; therefore, patient-reported outcomes of symptom improvement may be the best indicators of success in septal and turbinate surgery. For a variety of outcome measures, success rates for septoplasty have been reported to range from 63 to 85% [20, 24].

Siegel et al. [24] compared preoperative and postoperative quality-of-life scores in patients who underwent septoplasty. In their study of 93 patients, these authors found statistically significant improvements in nasal specific health as measured by the Nasal Health Survey. No significant changes were found in preoperative and postoperative general health status scores. A multi-institutional study using a validated outcomes instrument [nasal obstruction septoplasty effectiveness (NOSE) scale] showed significant improvement in symptoms of nasal obstruction in patients who had undergone septal surgery. Patients underwent either septoplasty alone or septoplasty in conjunction with turbinate reduction. Statistically significant improvements were found in symptom scores for patients in both groups [25]. The authors reported that 94% of their patients were pleased with the results of the surgery.

Hwang et al. [9] reviewed 111 cases of endoscopic septoplasty, and found complications to be rare. The authors felt the endoscopic approach allowed improved visualization and was a valuable teaching tool when compared with traditional headlight septoplasty. In addition, the ability to place incisions adjacent to sites of focal deviation and spurs allows the surgeon to reduce the amount of mucosal

Complications

Tears of the mucosal flaps occur most frequently at the sites of septal spurs. An important factor in management of mucosal tears is early intraoperative identification. In our experience, the magnification provided by endoscopic techniques allows identification of any tears when they are very small. This can allow the surgeon to elevate beyond the tear without enlarging it further. Early identification will also allow the surgeon to take additional care in avoiding an adjacent tear on the contralateral side.

Septal perforations most commonly occur when there are corresponding tears in both flaps at sites where the intervening cartilage or bone has been removed. When opposing flap tears are noted during surgery, repair using absorbable suture can be performed to decrease the risk of long-term perforation. Placement of cartilage between the torn portions of the flaps also helps to decrease the likelihood of a perforation [11]. Perforation rates have been reported to be as high as 9% for submucous resection techniques. With modern cartilage-preserving techniques, the rate has been reported as being much lower, at approximately 1% [15].

Aggressive resection of septal cartilage can lead to impaired support to the nasal dorsum and tip. Current surgical techniques emphasize conservative resection of cartilage, decreasing this risk. The risk of postoperative bleeding significant enough to require intervention is low in patients undergoing septoplasty alone, and has been reported as less than 1% [15]. Less common risks of septoplasty include septal hematoma and CSF leak [18]. Use of quilting sutures or splints may help decrease the likelihood of hematoma formation. Hematomas may progress to septal abscess and may lead to cartilage necrosis, so early recognition and drainage is very important.

The complications of septoplasty can be summarized as follows:

- Septal perforation
- Bleeding
- Septal hematoma
- Septal abscess
- Loss of nasal dorsum and tip support
- CSF leak

5

Postoperative Management

Septoplasty and turbinate reduction procedures are performed on an outpatient basis, with patients being discharged after a short recovery period. Since we do not use packing or splints routinely, we advise patients to expect small amounts of bloody drainage over the first few days. Saline nasal irrigations begun on the first postoperative day can help to clear clots and to minimize formation of crusts. The first office visit occurs 1 week postoperatively. At this visit, nasal endoscopy is performed. There is often persistent septal and turbinate edema, but early improvement in the patency of the nasal airway is usually evident. Patients who have undergone septal or turbinate procedures alone generally do not need significant debridement in the postoperative period. In rare instances, there may be synechia formation between the septum and inferior turbinates. These can be easily divided using through-cutting forceps or suction tips. Patients who have undergone concurrent sinus surgery may undergo more extensive debridement of their sinus cavities. By 4 weeks postoperatively, patients may expect to notice symptomatic improvement, and endoscopic examination will typically reveal an improved nasal airway with macroscopic resolution of mucosal edema.

References

1. Bielamowicz S, Hawrych A, Gupta A (1999) Endoscopic inferior turbinate reduction: a new technique. Laryngoscope 109:1007–1009
2. Cavaliere M, Mottola G, Iemma M (2005) Comparison of the effectiveness and safety of radiofrequency turbinoplasty and traditional surgical technique in treatment of inferior turbinate hypertrophy. Otolaryngol Head Neck Surg 133:972–978
3. Dolan RW (2004) Endoscopic septoplasty. Facial Plast Surg 20:217–221
4. Ferri E, Armato E, Cavaleri S, Capuzzo P, Ianniello F (2003) Argon plasma surgery for treatment of inferior turbinate hypertrophy: a long-term follow-up in 157 patients. ORL J Otorhinolaryngol Relat Spec 65:206–210
5. Fradis M, Malatskey S, Magamsa I, Golz A (2002) Effect of submucosal diathermy in chronic nasal obstruction due to turbinate enlargement. Am J Otolaryngol 23:332–336
6. Friedman M, Tanyeri H, Lim J, Landsberg R, Caldarelli D (1999) A safe, alternative technique for inferior turbinate reduction. Laryngoscope 109:1834–1837
7. Goyal P, Hwang PH (2006) In-office surgical treatment of sinus disease: Office-based surgical procedures in rhinology. Op Tech Otolaryngol Head Neck Surg 17:58–65
8. Gupta A, Mercurio E, Bielamowicz S (2001) Endoscopic inferior turbinate reduction: an outcomes analysis. Laryngoscope 111:1957–1959
9. Hwang PH, McLaughlin RB, Lanza DC, Kennedy DW (1999) Endoscopic septoplasty: indications, technique, and results. Otolaryngol Head Neck Surg 120:678–682
10. Kim DW, Egan KK, O'Grady K, Toriumi DM (2005) Biomechanical strength of human nasal septal lining: comparison of the constituent layers. Laryngoscope 115:1451–1453
11. Kridel RW (2004) Considerations in the etiology, treatment, and repair of septal perforations. Facial Plast Surg Clin North Am 12:435–450, vi
12. Kridel RW, Scott BA, Foda HM (1999) The tongue-in-groove technique in septorhinoplasty. A 10-year experience. Arch Facial Plast Surg 1:246–256; discussion 257–248
13. Larsson C, Millqvist E, Bende M (2001) Relationship between subjective nasal stuffiness and nasal patency measured by acoustic rhinometry. Am J Rhinol 15:403–405
14. Lee KC, Hwang PH, Kingdom TT (2001) Surgical management of inferior turbinate hypertrophy in the office: three mucosal sparing techniques. Oper Tech Otolaryngol Head Neck Surg 12:107–111
15. Marks S, Nasoseptal Surgery. In: Marks S (2000) Nasal and Sinus Surgery. W.B. Saunders Philadelphia, PA
16. Moore EJ, Kern EB (2001) Atrophic rhinitis: a review of 242 cases. Am J Rhinol 15:355–361
17. Nease CJ, Krempl GA (2004) Radiofrequency treatment of turbinate hypertrophy: a randomized, blinded, placebo-controlled clinical trial. Otolaryngol Head Neck Surg 130:291–299
18. Onerci TM, Ayhan K, Ogretmenoglu O (2004) Two consecutive cases of cerebrospinal fluid rhinorrhea after septoplasty operation. Am J Otolaryngol 25:354–356
19. Passali D, Passali FM, Damiani V, Passali GC, Bellussi L (2003) Treatment of inferior turbinate hypertrophy: a randomized clinical trial. Ann Otol Rhinol Laryngol 112:683–688
20. Rowe-Jones J (2004) Nasal surgery: evidence of efficacy. Septal and turbinate surgery. Rhinology 42:248–250
21. Sapci T, Sahin B, Karavus A, Akbulut UG (2003) Comparison of the effects of radiofrequency tissue ablation, CO2 laser ablation, and partial turbinectomy applications on nasal mucociliary functions. Laryngoscope 113:514–519
22. Sedwick JD, Lopez AB, Gajewski BJ, Simons RL (2005) Caudal septoplasty for treatment of septal deviation: aesthetic and functional correction of the nasal base. Arch Facial Plast Surg 7:158–162
23. Shemen L, Hamburg R (1997) Preoperative and postoperative nasal septal surgery assessment with acoustic rhinometry. Otolaryngol Head Neck Surg 117:338–342
24. Siegel NS, Gliklich RE, Taghizadeh F, Chang Y (2000) Outcomes of septoplasty. Otolaryngol Head Neck Surg 122:228–232

25. Stewart MG, Smith TL, Weaver EM, Witsell DL, Yueh B, Hannley MT, Johnson JT (2004) Outcomes after nasal septoplasty: results from the Nasal Obstruction Septoplasty Effectiveness (NOSE) study. Otolaryngol Head Neck Surg 130:283–290

26. Talmon Y, Samet A, Gilbey P (2000) Total inferior turbinectomy: operative results and technique. Ann Otol Rhinol Laryngol 109:1117–1119

27. Welge-Luessen A, Hauser R, Schmid N, Kappos L, Probst R (2003) Endonasal surgery for contact point headaches: a 10-year longitudinal study. Laryngoscope 113:2151–2156

28. Yaniv E, Hadar T, Shvero J, Raveh E (1997) Objective and subjective nasal airflow. Am J Otolaryngol 18:29–32

Chapter 6

Endoscopic Middle Meatal Antrostomy and Ethmoidectomy

6

Seth J. Kanowitz, Joseph B. Jacobs, Richard A. Lebowitz

Core Messages

- The concept of ostiomeatal complex (OMC) obstruction as the underlying etiologic factor in the development of rhinosinusitis has been well established in the literature [5, 17].

- As the OMC is the final common drainage pathway for the maxillary, anterior ethmoid, and frontal sinuses, adequate ventilation and continued patency of this area is paramount in maintaining physiologic drainage of these sinuses.

- Preoperative review of the paranasal sinus (PNS) computed tomography (CT) scans for the relevant anatomy is paramount in surgical planning.

- Adequate decongestion, vasoconstriction, and relative hypotension during surgery are critical for maintaining a dry operative field for proper visualization.

- Intraoperatively the surgeon should define the lateral (lamina papyracea), medial (middle turbinate), and superior (skull base) limits of dissection.

- The angle and plane of dissection should be at the level of the orbital floor when proceeding posteriorly toward the face of the sphenoid sinus.

- Palpate behind vertically oriented ethmoid bony partitions prior to removal in order to distinguish them from the skull base.

- The skull base is identified by its relatively increased thickness, solid feel, smooth contour, and whiter bone color.

Contents

Preoperative Preparation

Preoperative preparation includes:

- Antibiotics
- Steroids
- CT PNS
- Management of allergic rhinitis and comorbid nasal conditions
- Stopping aspirin, nonsteroidal anti-inflammatory agents (NSAIDS), and anticoagulant vitamin supplements

Before being considered a candidate for endoscopic sinus surgery, a patient should have failed "maximal medical therapy," the definition of which may vary among practitioners, and is beyond the scope of this chapter. Once a decision to proceed with surgery has been made, preoperative management generally consists of the following:

- *Antibiotics*: Preoperative antibiotics are administered in cases where mucopurulent drainage is present, or if antibiotic prophylaxis is medically indicated. Amoxicillin/clavulanate (Augmentin) for 5–7 days, or a cephalosporin or quinolone is generally prescribed.
- *Steroids*: In an attempt to reduce mucosal inflammation, preoperative oral steroids (30–50 mg Prednisone daily for 3–5 days) are used in cases of nasal polyposis, or significant polypoid/hyperplastic mucosal disease. In patients with reactive lower airway disease (asthma), preoperative steroids are prescribed as per the recommendations of the patient's primary care physician or pulmonologist.
- *CT PNS*: Indications for the use of intraoperative image guidance are discussed elsewhere in this textbook. If a decision is made to perform computer-assisted sinus surgery, a CT scan is obtained using the protocol appropriate for the image guidance system. In all cases, 3 mm coronal images through the PNS are obtained, and must be present in the operating room. Sagittal reformatted images of the frontal sinus outflow tract are obtained when endoscopic frontal sinusotomy is planned.
- *Management of allergic rhinitis and comorbid nasal conditions*: When present, allergic rhinitis and other comorbid nasal conditions must be properly treated as part of appropriate "maximal medical therapy."
- *Stopping aspirin, NSAIDS, and anticoagulant vitamin supplements*: Any nonessential medications which might contribute to bleeding and impair visualization are stopped 10 days prior to surgery. Patients requiring anticoagulation therapy are managed in accordance the recommendations of the treating physician.

Endoscopic Middle Meatal Antrostomy

Indications

- Isolated chronic maxillary sinusitis or complicated acute maxillary sinusitis
- In conjunction with an anterior ethmoidectomy for disease of the OMC
- Endoscopic visualization of maxillary sinus for biopsy or surgical management of a maxillary sinus or OMC tumor
- Approach to pterygomaxillary space or orbital floor

Relative Contraindications

- Aplastic or markedly hypoplastic maxillary sinus
- Vascular lesions
- Abnormalities within the anteroinferior or lateral quadrants of the maxillary sinus unable to be accessed by angled telescopes or instruments
- Dehiscent orbital floor or lamina papyracea with evidence of fat or rectus muscle protrusion
- Advanced noninflammatory disease
- Medical contraindications to elective anesthesia/surgery

Technique

The technique is demonstrated in Video 6.1.

Tips and Pearls

1. Review the preoperative PNS CT scans.
   (a) Identify the superior attachment of the uncinate process (skull base, lamina papyracea, or middle turbinate).
   (b) Identify the position of orbital floor relative to the maxillary ostium, and the attachment of the inferior turbinate (i.e., the "height" of the infundibulum).

(c) If there is previous trauma, be mindful of a dehiscent or displaced infraorbital nerve.

(d) Identify the anterior ethmoid artery traversing the skull base from the orbit.

(e) Identify septal deviations or spurs narrowing the OMC.

(f) Inspect the lamina, and the skull base for any area of dehiscence, particularly if there is a history of prior surgery or trauma, and in cases of sinus neoplasm, mulocele, allergic fungal sinusitis, or long standing sinonasal polyposis.

(g) Evaluate for the presence of an infraorbital ethmoid cell (haller cell).

2. Decongest the turbinates and anesthetize the lateral nasal wall (see Chap. 4).

3. Gently medialize the middle turbinate using a Freer elevator.

4. Retract the uncinate anteriorly using the angled end of a Woodsen elevator and incise the mucosa of the uncinate process along its anterior attachment to the lateral nasal wall in a posteroinferior to anterosuperior direction.

5. Detach the uncinate from its posteroinferior attachment using straight through-cutting forceps or endoscopic scissors. Remove the uncinate process using 45° up-biting forceps and a gentle rocking motion from anterosuperior to posteroinferior.

6. Visualize the maxillary sinus ostium, bulla ethmoidalis, and orbital floor using a 30° rigid fiberoptic endoscope.

7. Widen the maxillary sinus ostium using a combination of appropriately angled through-cutting forceps and powered instrumentation.

After the patient is brought into the operating room, general anesthesia is administered in a standard fashion. We prefer to perform our procedures under general anesthesia with a laryngeal masked airway, though intubation for patients with more tenuous upper or lower airways is always considered preoperatively and should be at the discretion of the anesthesiologist [3]. The nasal cavity is then decongested and anesthetized in a standard fashion and is addressed separately in this book (see Chap. 4). In general 0.5-in. Codman neuropledgets (cottonoids) (Johnson & Johnson, Raynham, MA, USA) soaked with 4% oxymetazoline are placed into the patient's nose using a headlight and a small nasal speculum prior to prepping the patient. After approximately 10 min of decongestion, the lateral nasal wall is injected for hemostasis with 1% lidocaine with 1:100,000 epinephrine using a 22G 1.5-in. needle [14]. The 4-mm 0° rigid fiberoptic endoscope (Karl Storz, Culver City, CA, USA) is used for visualization during the injections and subsequent procedure. The patient's head should be elevated approximately 30° to decrease venous engorgement of the nasal and sinus cavities. Finally, the eyes should be taped closed laterally, using a Steri-Strip or clear tape, and never hidden under towels or drapes. This allows the operating surgeon to visualize and palpate the orbits at all points during the procedure.

If necessary, we perform submucosal resection of the nasal septum prior to addressing the maxillary or ethmoid sinuses to allow for better endoscopic visualization of these areas (see Chap. 5). If access is not limited by the septum, all endoscopic procedures are performed before addressing the nasal septum. If the inferior turbinate is large enough to impede instrumentation in the nasal cavity despite adequate decongestion, then we also perform a gentle outfracture and/or turbinoplasty at the outset. It is important to remember that if the inferior turbinate bone is outfractured the uncinate process may inadvertently be displaced laterally into the maxillary sinus, thus making the subsequent uncinectomy more difficult. Any obstructing middle meatal or nasal polyps are resected with the use of the microdebrider and the tissue is sent as a specimen for histology examination. Finally, in the rare instance when the middle turbinate is significantly obstructing the middle meatus, then a partial middle turbinectomy is performed [6]. In the case of a concha bullosa, the lateral portion of the pneumatized turbinate is resected by first incising the anterior tip of the turbinate in a vertical fashion using the straight end of a Woodson elevator. Endoscopic scissors or straight Blakesley through-cutting forceps (Karl Storz, Culver City, CA, USA) are then used to resect the lateral lamella of the middle turbinate, with preservation of the superior attachment and medial portion of the turbinate. The scissors/forceps should be directed inferiorly and posteriorly to avoid avulsing the turbinate from its attachment at the skull base, as significant bleeding or creation of an iatrogenic CSF leak may occur. If necessary, the middle turbinate remnant can then be gently medialized with the Freer elevator to create additional space and access to the middle meatus. If a paradoxically curved or otherwise significantly obstructing middle turbinate is present, a curved hemostat clamp is used to crush the middle turbinate along its lower third, and then the turbinate is partially resected along this line using the endoscopic scissors, with preservation of the superior attachment.

The angled tip of a Woodsen elevator (Fig. 6.1) (Karl Storz, Culver City, CA, USA) is then placed within the hiatus semilunaris and used to palpate the free posterior edge of the uncinate process (Fig. 6.2a) [10]. Gentle anterior traction is then applied and the anterior insertion of the uncinate process into the lateral nasal wall is identified. The angled tip of the Woodsen elevator (or angled tip of the incisor) (Fig. 6.1) is then used to in-

6

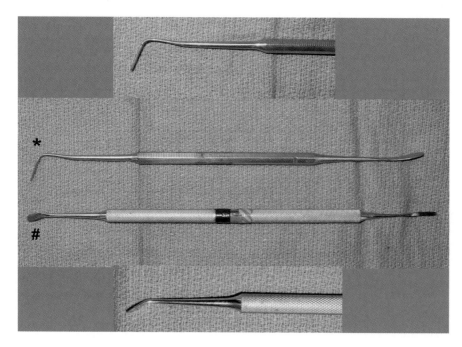

Fig. 6.1. Incisor (asterisk) and Woodsen elevator (pound sign) (Karl Storz, Culver City, CA, USA). Magnified views of the angled ends of the incisor (top) and the Woodsen elevator (bottom)

cise the lateral nasal wall along the anterior aspect of the uncinate process from posteroinferior to anterosuperior (Fig. 6.2b). The inferior attachment of the uncinate process is then cut using the endoscopic scissor. The uncinate is then grasped at its remaining superior insertion using Blakesley forceps and displaced medially and inferiorly using a gentle rocking motion (Fig. 6.2c). If the procedure is performed properly, the uncinate should be able to be removed in its entirety. Remnants of the uncinate process, superiorly and inferiorly, are removed with Blakesley through-cutting forceps or the microdebrider [1,9]. Alternatively, side-biting punch forceps (opening to the right for the patient's left side, and opening to the left for the patient's right side) (Karl Storz, Culver City, CA, USA) can be placed within the infundibulum and the uncinate remnants can be removed in a piecemeal fashion. The dissection of the thin bony remnants should proceed anteriorly until the thick lacrimal bone is approached. This bone is usually identified when the side-biting instrument meets added resistance. At this point the dissection should be stopped to avoid damage to the nasolacrimal system.

Once the uncinate process has been removed, the maxillary sinus ostium can be visualized best with a 30° rigid fiberoptic endoscope (Karl Storz, Culver City, CA, USA) just above the insertion of the inferior turbinate and halfway between the anterior and posterior ends of the turbinate (Fig. 6.2d) [13]. Furthermore, the bulla ethmoidalis and orbital floor can be identified as well. If the natural ostium is too small to visualize owing to obstruction by mucosal disease, it can be palpated as a soft depression using an angled olive-tipped suction or a curved maxillary sinus seeker (Karl Storz, Culver

City, CA, USA). Often a trail of mucous or an air bubble can be visualized emanating from the ostium. The maxillary sinus ostium is then further enlarged using a 0° and 30° rigid fiberoptic endoscope and a combination of backbiting and through-cutting instruments to remove diseased bone and free mucosal remnants. The Stammberger down-biting punch (Karl Storz, Culver City, CA, USA) can also be utilized to open the ostium along its inferior edge. The 60° angled microdebrider can also be used to widen the ostium. The natural ostium should be widened to include the posterior fontanelle to prevent a postoperative mucous recirculation phenomenon. If at any time during the procedure visualization is obscured by bleeding, the middle meatus can be repacked with oxymetazoline-soaked 0.5-in. Codman neuropledgets or additional injections with 1% lidocaine with 1:100,000 epinephrine can be performed.

After the antrostomy is complete, the maxillary sinus should be easily visualized with the 30° rigid fiberoptic endoscope. The 70° rigid fiberoptic endoscope (Karl Storz, Culver City, CA, USA) can be employed if abnormalities are located in the inferior or far lateral recesses of the sinus. If a retention cyst is present it can be marsupialized using the giraffe forceps or angled microdebrider blade. Any mass or suspicious lesion can be biopsied at this point using appropriately angled forceps.

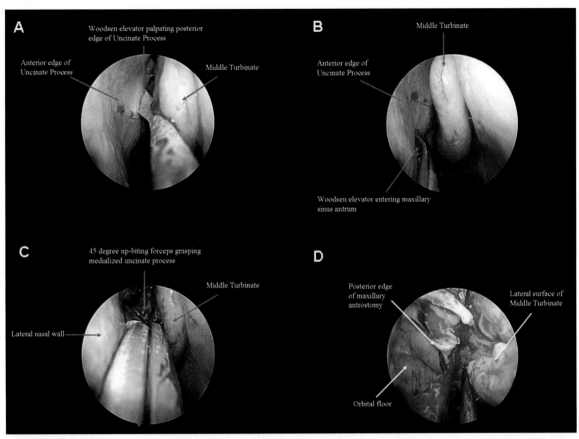

Fig. 6.2. Maxillary antrostomy. **a** Palpation of the posterior edge of the uncinate process with the angled end of the Woodsen elevator. **b** Entering the maxillary sinus ostium with the an-gled end of the Woodsen elevator. **c** Forty-five-degree up-biting forceps grasping the medialized uncinate process. **d** Completed maxillary antrostomy with visualization of the maxillary sinus

Endoscopic Anterior Ethmoidectomy

Indications

- In conjunction with a middle meatal antrosto-my for disease of the OMC
- Chronic anterior ethmoid rhinosinusitis
- In conjunction with frontal sinusotomy for disease of the frontal recess and frontal sinuses
- Approach to the anterior skull base
- Approach to the medial orbital wall for endo-scopic orbital abscess drainage
- Biopsy or surgical management of an anterior ethmoid tumor

Relative Contraindications

- Potential skull base involvement by inflamma-tory or noninflammatory disease

- Large encephaloceles with or without cerebral vasculature herniation
- Dehiscent lamina papyracea with fat or rectus muscle herniation
- Vascular lesions
- Orbital involvement by inflammatory or non-inflammatory disease

Technique

The technique is demonstrated in Video 6.2.

Tips and Pearls

1. Review the preoperative PNS CT scans
   (a) Identify the height and slope of the skull base from anterior to posterior.
   (b) Identify the location of the anterior ethmoid artery (a small nipplelike dehiscence in the lamina papyracea in the area where the

artery exits the orbit and traverses the skull base). The anterior ethmoid artery marks the posterior aspect of the frontal recess.

(c) Examine the skull base and lamina papyracea for any evidence of dehiscence, particularly in patients with a history of trauma or prior surgery and in cases of sinus neoplasm mucocele, allergic fungal sinusitis, or long standing sinonasal polyposis

2. Enter the inferomedial aspect of the anterior face of the ethmoid bulla

3. Identify the lamina papyracea as the lateral limit of dissection, the middle turbinate as the medial limit of dissection, and the skull base superiorly

4. Visualization of the maxillary antrum allows for identification of the height of the orbital floor and the sagittal plane of the lamina papyracea.

5. Remove ethmoid partitions in a systematic fashion

6. Maintain excellent hemostasis and visualization

With the advent of modern-day rigid fiberoptic endoscopes and large digitally enhanced monitors, it is easy to forget that the ethmoid labyrinth is a relatively small space situated between many vital structures of the anterior skull base and orbits. Each ethmoid labyrinth is approximately 4–5 cm in length, 2.5–3 cm in height, and 0.5 cm in width anteriorly to 1.5 cm in width posteriorly [12]. With these dimensions in mind it is imperative to proceed through the dissection in a controlled and systematic manner while keeping all known landmarks in view [2, 4, 7, 15, 16, 18, 19].

After the completion of the uncinectomy and middle meatal antrostomy as outlined above, the bulla ethmoidalis can be easily visualized in the middle meatus with a 0° rigid fiberoptic endoscope. The bulla is initially entered along its medial and inferior aspect with a curette, straight Blakesley forceps, a straight suction, or the tip of the microdebrider (Fig. 6.3a). The lateral partitions can then be removed with up-biting or straight through-cutting instruments to identify the lamina papyracea. The remaining partitions of the anterior ethmoid sinus, usually one to four cells, can then be sequentially removed in an anterior to posterior direction using similar instruments to

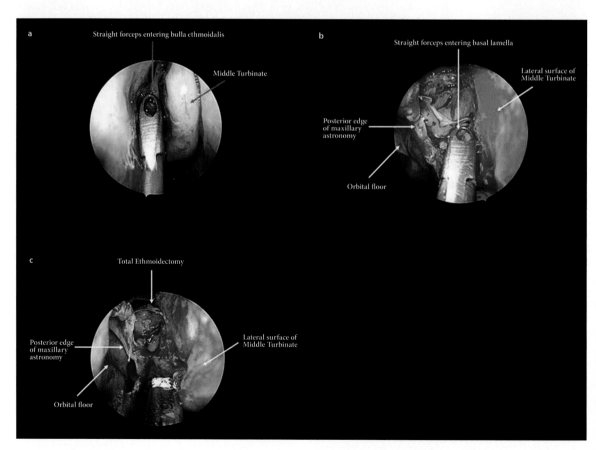

Fig. 6.3. Anterior and posterior ethmoidectomy. **a** Straight forceps entering the bulla ethmoidalis. **b** Straight forceps entering the basal lamella after completion of the anterior ethmoidectomy. **c** Completed maxillary antrostomy and total ethmoidectomy

avoid excessive shearing forces and mucosal stripping [12]. The microdebrider can be used as well, making sure to angle the blade medially away from the orbit. When the bulla is removed, the suprabullar and retrobullar recesses can be visualized as well as the basal lamella [8]. Polyps within the anterior ethmoid chamber can be removed with either appropriately angled forceps or the microdebrider after retrieving a specimen for pathology study.

As the bony partitions are removed, the lamina papyracea, middle turbinate, and skull base should be identified and the 0° rigid fiberoptic endoscope should be positioned such that a wide field of view is maintained. The plane and angle of dissection should proceed along the level of the orbital floor, which can be visualized through the maxillary antrostomy. This will prevent a steep angle of dissection and accidental violation of the anterior skull base. It is also important to remember that the lateral skull base adjacent to the orbit is 10 times thicker than the medial skull base as it slopes downward and attaches to the vertical strut of the middle turbinate [8]. Although concentrating the dissection medially avoids orbital penetration, the risk of skull base injury is significantly increased. The skull base is identified by its relatively increased thickness, solid feel, smooth contour, and whiter bone color. As the dissection proceeds posteriorly, the anterior ethmoid artery is usually identified traversing immediately below the anterior skull base posterior to the supraorbital ethmoid cells [8]. Its position usually demarcates the posterior aspect of the frontal recess. It may be enclosed in a bony conduit or may be dehiscent along its entire course; thus, dissection is this area must proceed with caution

Endoscopic Posterior/Total Ethmoidectomy

Indications

- In conjunction with a middle meatal antrostomy and anterior ethmoidectomy for inflammatory mucosal disease of the PNS
- Chronic posterior ethmoid rhinosinusitis
- Disease of the sphenoethmoid recess
- Approach to the sphenoid sinus for sphenoidotomy
- Approach to the sphenoid sinus for endoscopic transsphenoidal surgery
- Approach to the medial orbital wall and orbital nerve for endoscopic orbital decompression
- Biopsy or surgical management of a posterior ethmoid or sphenoid sinus mass

Relative Contraindications

- See the relative contraindications in the section "Endoscopic Anterior Ethmoidectomy"
- Significant extension of disease into the sphenoid sinus with possible involvement of carotid arteries, optic nerves, or the anterior skull base

Technique

The technique is demonstrated in Video 6.3.

Tips and Pearls
- Review the preoperative PNS CT scans as done for an anterior ethmoidectomy and evaluate for potentially complex posterior ethmoid pneumatization patterns lateral and superior to the sphenoid sinus (onodi cell)
- Enter the inferomedial aspect of the basal lamella.
- Preservation of the inferior aspect of the basal lamella serves as a "strut" to help support the middle turbinate in a medial position.
- Remove the inferior aspect of the posterior ethmoid partitions in a systematic fashion.
- Palpate behind each vertical ethmoid bony partition to verify that it is not the skull base and proceed from posterior to anterior.
- The anterior face of the sphenoid marks the posterior limit of dissection.
- The posterior ethmoid artery lies 2–3 mm anterior to the anterior sphenoid sinus wall.
- The skull base is thicker, feels more solid, has a smooth contour, and a whiter color.

The basal (ground) lamella represents the division between the anterior and posterior ethmoid air cells. In general the posterior ethmoid cells are relatively larger and fewer in number (between two and six cells) [12]. After removal of the anterior ethmoid cells, the basal lamella can be easily visualized oriented in a horizontal position. It is entered medially and inferiorly in the same manner as the anterior face of the ethmoid bulla, although the bone of the basal lamella is thicker (Fig. 6.3b). Blakesley 45° up-biting through-cutting forceps are then used to remove the inferior aspects of the bony partitions in a systematic fashion while maintaining the same anatomic landmarks used during the anterior ethmoidectomy [2, 4, 7, 15, 16, 18, 19]. The vertically oriented bony partitions can be distinguished from the horizontally oriented skull base. The forceps or an

6

angled bone curette is placed behind each partition to verify that it lies below the skull base. The dissection along the skull base should proceed from posterior to anterior with palpation of the skull base posterior to the bony partition about to be removed. Once again, the skull base can be distinguished by its relatively increased thickness, solid feel, smooth contour, and whiter bone color. The posterior limit of dissection is the anterior face of the sphenoid sinus. It also usually marks the anterior edge of the most posterior ethmoid cell [11]. However, if identification of the skull base remains difficult at this point, a sphenoidotomy should be performed and the skull base should be identified within the sphenoid sinus [8]. The goal of surgery is to remove as many bony partitions and diseased mucosa until the ethmoid cavity has a smooth contour along the skull base and lamina papyracea (Fig. 6.3c). However, it is imperative not to strip mucosa from the skull base or medial orbital wall during dissection.

Complications and Management

Surgical complications include:

- Orbital injury (fat herniation, rectus muscle damage, optic nerve damage, orbital hema-toma, anterior and posterior ethmoid artery bleed)
- Sphenopalatine artery bleed
- Nasolacrimal system injury
- Iatrogenic frontal or ethmoid sinusitis
- Postoperative maxillary sinus mucous recirculation phenomenon
- Violation of the skull base with CSF leak and/or brain parenchymal injury

Orbital Injury (Fat Herniation, Rectus Muscle Damage, Optic Nerve Damage, Orbital Hematoma, Anterior and Posterior Ethmoid Artery Bleed)

The proximity of the orbit to the operating field places it at risk during endoscopic sinus surgery. Damage to the orbital contents is more likely when surgical landmarks are obscured by abnormalities or bleeding. In all cases of orbital penetration, prompt recognition and appropriate management will help to minimize the potential morbidity. Violation of the lamina papyracea in and of itself is not an absolute indication to prematurely end the procedure. Palpation of the globe while visualizing the medial orbital wall with an endoscope should allow for visualization of herniated orbital contents. If orbital fat is encountered it should be identified, protected with a cottonoid, and all dissection should remain medial to it. Attempts to remove exposed orbital fat should be avoided as this will likely cause bleeding. Furthermore, attempts to push it back into the orbit are often unsuccessful. Use of the microdebrider after violation of the lamina papyracea and/or periorbita should proceed with utmost caution, especially in the hands of a novice, as the simultaneous suction and cutting mechanism can remove the fat or muscle and rapidly make matters worse. If the microdebrider is used, the cutting side of the tip should always be angled medially away from the orbital contents. Postoperatively patients should be advised to avoid nose-blowing and strenuous activities for 2 weeks to help minimize periorbital emphysema, and a prophylactic course of antibiotics should be prescribed to minimize the risk of orbital cellulitis. If the medial rectus muscle is identified or damaged, surgery should be stopped and an ophthalmology consult obtained immediately, as these injuries are very difficult to repair after muscle retraction, scarring, and denervation.

Orbital hematomas can often be managed without adverse sequelae; however, increased intraocular pressure can prove devastating if not recognized early. Violation of the lamina papyracea with slow venous oozing may only cause periorbital ecchymosis and can be managed conservatively. However, rapid arterial bleeding with retrobulbar hematoma may cause proptosis with vascular compromise of the optic nerve. Suctioning at the bleeding site (i.e., anterior or posterior ethmoid artery) should be immediately performed and the nose should *not* be packed to allow for egress of blood into the nose as opposed to the orbit. If the bleeding site can be easily identified, it should be appropriately controlled with bipolar or suction cautery. Epinephrine-soaked pledgets can also be employed to help slow the bleeding and allow for identification of the offending vessel. Orbital pressures should be checked with a tonometer and an ophthalmology consult should be obtained immediately. Decompression of the orbit should proceed immediately, as irreversible visual loss can occur within 1 h. A lateral canthotomy and cantholysis should be performed using fine straight scissors or a no. 15 surgical blade. In order to fully decompress the orbit, it is important to retract the lower lid inferiorly to identify and cut the lateral canthal ligament. Mannitol (1 g/kg intravenously over 30 min) dehydrates the orbital fat and vitreous body and should be administered in conjunction with acetazolamide (500 mg intravenously; may be repeated in 4 h), which reduces aqueous humor production. Visual acuity and light perception (afferent papillary defect) should also be serially documented. If lateral decompression fails to adequately decompress the orbit, then endoscopic medial orbital wall decompression with periorbitia release shoud be prformed.

filtration is begun as posterior as possible, preferably into the anterior sphenoid wall and superior turbinate, moving anteriorly on both the nasal septum and the medial aspect of the middle turbinate.

Under endoscopic guidance with a 0° telescope, the middle turbinate may be gently displaced laterally. Only the inferior part of the turbinate is displaced. There is no need to push on the superior aspect of the turbinate as this may cause skull base injury and it does not add to the exposure. Rarely, the middle turbinate is so large that it may interfere with adequate exposure and, therefore, limited removal of its anteroinferior tip is required. It is the author's experience that this applies only to the relatively inexperienced surgeon. As we gain experience and confidence, partial middle turbinectomy is almost never required. Again, if it is performed, only the inferior aspect of the turbinate is removed without actual entry into the infundibulum (Fig. 7.1). Depending on the exposure provided so far and the comfort of the surgeon, a self-retaining speculum such as a long nasal speculum or the Hardy pituitary speculum may be inserted now. However, if only limited intrasphenoidal work is needed, the entire procedure can be performed without a speculum.

Long bipolar forceps are now inserted into the superior meatus. We currently use endoscopic coaxial forceps. If they are not available, long Bayonette forceps may be used, but they is more difficult to maneuver within a narrow space. The bipolar jaws are introduced on both sides of the superior turbinate, thus "hugging" the superior turbinate, as superior as possible and as posterior as possible. The superior aspect of the superior turbinate is now cauterized (Fig. 7.2). Next, endoscopic scissors are used to transect the superior turbinate superiorly, relatively close to its skull base attachment through the cauterized area (Fig. 7.3) The tip of the turbinate is gently pulled down and, with a combination of bipolar cautery and endoscopic scissors, the posterior attachment of the superior turbinate is separated from the anterior sphenoid wall without significant bleeding (Fig. 7.4). Alternatively, a microdebrider may be used to remove the superior turbinate.

If the sphenoid sinus ostium has not been identified before, it is usually apparent now. It is used as the starting point for wide sphenoidotomy (Fig. 7.5). However, if the ostium is difficult to identify, the sphenoid sinus may be entered medially, about halfway between the skull base and the choana. Different instruments may be used for anterior sphenoid wall removal. They include sphenoid punch, drill or microdebrider. The author prefers the Kerrison rongeurs. They are safe, predictable, reliable, and come in different sizes and angulations (Fig. 7.6). Again, as mentioned in the "Transnasal–Transethmoid Approach" section, proceeding laterally and superiorly

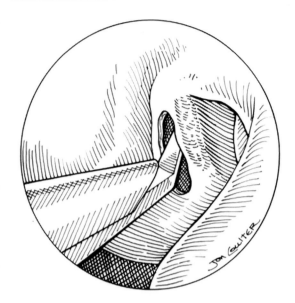

Fig. 7.5. Wide sphenoidotomy is begun through the natural ostium. (Reprinted with permission from Har-El [6])

should be done with caution. Palpation with up-biting forceps or a neurosurgical nerve hook before bone removal is recommended (Fig. 7.7). Insertion of a 70° telescope into the sphenoid cavity will allow the surgeon to evaluate the lateral wall and the roof before bone removal.

The surgeon must remember that the posterior division of the sphenopalatine artery, the nasoseptal division, runs across the anterior wall of the sphenoid sinus from lateral to medial [5, 17]. Depending on the extent of sphenoidotomy required, it is safer to cauterize the inferior aspect of the anterior sphenoid wall before bone removal. The extent of anterior sphenoid wall removal depends on the exact disease process and the planned procedure. By approaching the sphenoid sinus after removing the superior turbinate, we usually have room for an 8 mm × 12 mm sphenoid sinus opening. This is certainly adequate for decompression or for exposure required for centrally located lesions such as pituitary tumors. However, if additional exposure is required, the surgeon may extend the sphenoidotomy laterally and/or medially. Lateral exposure may be obtained by performing limited posterior ethmoidectomy through the superior meatus. This is followed by additional bone removal of anterior sphenoid wall in a medial-to-lateral direction. Again, positive identification of the carotid artery and the optic nerve should be achieved before this maneuver.

For medial and contralateral extension of the sphenoidotomy, one of two maneuvers may be used. The surgeon may elect to insert a backbiting bone punch into the sphenoid sinus and then remove the posterior aspect of the nasal septum in a posterior-to-anterior

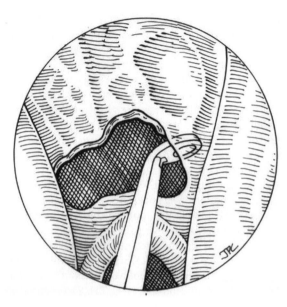

Fig. 7.7. Up-biting forceps (or any other curved instrument) are used to palpate laterally and superiorly before bone removal. (Reprinted with permission from Har-El [6]).

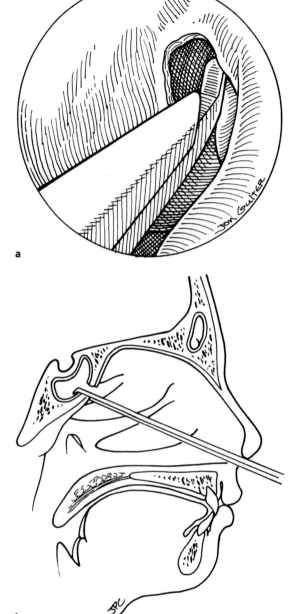

Fig. 7.6. Kerrison rongeurs are used to perform wide sphenoidotomy. **a** Surgeon's view, left sphenoid sinus. **b** Sagittal view, left sphenoid sinus. (Reprinted with permission from Har-El [6])

Takahashi forceps are then used to remove the remaining strut of the nasal septum and then proceed into the sphenoid sinus by removing the sphenoid rostrum and the intrasphenoidal septum (Fig. 7.8b). The end result is a very wide sphenoidotomy which includes the midline and, if required, the contralateral anterior sphenoid wall.

For pituitary surgery, the intrasphenoidal septum is usually removed. The bulging pituitary usually makes the identification of the sella turcica quite easy [10, 11]. Confirmation of the exact location of the sella may be also achieved with the use of an intraoperative computerized navigation system or the C-arm image intensifier.

If it is not destroyed by the pituitary tumor, the leading bony wall of the sella turcica is removed with fine Kerrison rongeurs and the dura is exposed. Pituitary surgery is now performed in cooperation with the neurosurgical team. Depending on the amount of bleeding at the end of the procedure, intranasal packing may or may not be required. As for pituitary surgery, if there is no evidence of CSF leakage, there is no need for extensive intrasphenoidal packing.

The superior turbinectomy approach does not add any specific complications to the list mentioned above for the transethmoid approach. We have not seen any evidence of olfactory deficiency after unilateral turbinectomy. We did, however, see an incidence of posterior septal necrosis and perforation despite the fact that transseptal surgery was not performed. This was attributed to bilateral cauterization of the nasoseptal divisions of the sphenopalatine artery combined with a tight, prolonged, bilateral intranasal packing

direction. Only limited, 2–5-mm, bone removal is required. Alternatively, especially when the intrasphenoidal septum and/or the midline sphenoid rostrum are very thick and do not allow the use of the backbiting forceps, the sharp end of a Freer elevator is used to penetrate through the posterior septum about 3–5 mm anterior to the sphenoid sinus, into the contralateral posterior nasal cavity (Fig. 7.8a). Heavy straight

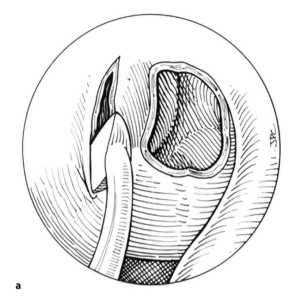

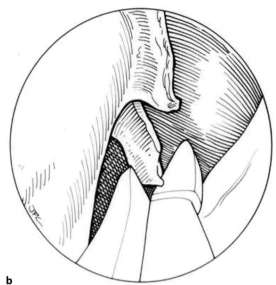

a   b

Fig. 7.8. Medial/contralateral extension of the sphenoidotomy. **a** Transseptal penetration into the contralateral posterior nasal cavity. **b** Straight forceps are used to remove the posterior nasal septal strut and proceed posteriorly to remove the intrasphenoidal septum. (Reprinted with permission from Har-El [6])

because of CSF leakage. Shah and Har-El [19] studied patient outcome after pituitary surgery. They compared the endoscopic direct transnasal approach with the conventional sublabial transseptal approach. They found a significantly shorter operative time, shorter hospital stay and lower incidence of immediate diabetes insipidus. There was no difference in the incidence of long-term diabetes insipidus.

References

1. Anon JB, Rontal M, Zinreich SJ (1996) Anatomy of the paranasal sinuses, Thieme, New York.
2. Cakmok O, Shohet MR, Kern EB (2000) Isolated sphenoid sinus lesions. Am J Rhinol 14:13–19.
3. Goldsmith AJ (1999) The traspalatal approach for juvenile angiofibroma. Oper Tech Otolaryngol Head Neck Surg 10:98–100.
4. Hardy J (1969) Transphenoidal microsurgery of the normal and pathological pituitary. Clin Neurosur 16:185–217.
5. Har-El G (1994) The anterior wall of the sphenoid sinus. Ear Nose Throat J 73:446–448.
6. Har-El G (2002) Approaches to the sphenoid sinus. In: Bluestone CD, Rosenfeld RM (eds) Surgical atlas of pediataric otolaryngology, 2nd edn. BC Decker, Hamilton, pp 353–365.
7. Har-El G (2003) Extracraial approaches to the sphenoid sinus. In: Har-El G, Weber PC (eds) Rhinologic and otologic aspects of skull base medicine and surgery. American Academy of Otolaryngology-Head and Neck Surgery, Alexandria, pp 53–64
8. Har-El G (2003) Overall review of extracranial approaches to the sphenoid sinus. Oper Tech Otolaryngol Head Neck Surg 14:174–177.
9. Har-El G (2003) Endoscpic direct transnasal sphenoidotomy. Oper Tech Otolaryngol Head Neck Surg 14:185–187.
10. Har-El G, Todor R (2003) Endoscopic transnasal approach to the pituitary gland. Oper Tech Otolaryngol Head Neck Surg 14:205–206.
11. Har-El G, Todor R (2003) Endoscopic pituitary surgery. In: Har-El G, Weber PC (eds) Rhinologic and otologic aspects of skull base medicine and surgery. American Academy of Otolaryngology-Head and Neck Surgery, Alexandria, pp 114–130.
12. Har-El G (2005) Combined endoscopic transmaxillary – transnasal approach to the pterygoids, lateral sphenoid and retrobulbar orbit. Ann Otol Rhinol Laryngol 114:439–442.
13. Kennedy DW (1985) Functional endoscopic sinus surgery technique. Arch Otolaryngol 111:643–649.
14. Levine HL, May M, Rontal M, Rontal E (1993) Complex anatomy of the lateral nasal wall: simplified for the endoscopic sinus surgeon. In: Levine HL, May M (eds) Endoscopic sinus surgery. Thieme, New York, pp 1–28.
15. Proetz AW (1949) Operation on the sphenoid. Trans Am Acad Ophthalmol Otolaryngol 53:538 –541.
16. Rice DH (1995) Embryology. In: Donald PJ, Gluckman JL, Rice DH (eds) The sinuses. Raven Press, New York, pp 15–23.
17. Schwartz JS, Har-El G (2003) Posterior septal perforation after nontransseptal sphenoid sinus surgery. Oper Tech Otolaryngol Head Neck Surg 14:221–222.
18. Sethi D, Stanley RE, Pillay PK (1995) Endoscopic anatomy of the sphenoid sinus and sella turcica. J Laryangol Otol 109:951–955.
19. Shah S, Har-El G (2001) Diabetes insipidus after pituitary surgery: incidence after traditional versus endoscopic transsphenoidal approaches. Am J Rhinol 15:377–379.
20. Van Alyea OE (1949) Discussion of operation on the sphenoid sinus. Trans Am Acad Ophthalmol Otolaryngol 53:542–545.

Chapter 8

Endonasal Micro-endoscopic Frontal Sinus Surgery

8

Wolfgang Draf, Amir Minovi

Core Messages

■ With the help of endonasal type I–III drainages it is possible to adjust frontal sinus surgery to the underlying abnormality.

■ From types I–III upwards, surgery is increasingly invasive.

■ Type III median drainage [5] is identical with the endoscopic modified Lothrop procedure [7].

■ The concept of endonasal drainages of the frontal sinus implicates preservation of bony boundaries of frontal sinus outlet in contrast to the classic external frontoorbital procedure [12, 13, 17, 23]. This means less danger of shrinking and reclosure with development of mucocele. It is a surgical strategy, not just a technique. The frontoorbital external operation should not be used anymore for treatment of inflammatory diseases.

■ If type III drainage is technically not possible (anteroposterior diameter of the frontal sinus of less than 0.8 cm) or failed, the osteoplastic frontal sinus obliteration must be considered.

Contents

Introduction

Modern external and endonasal surgery of the paranasal sinuses began roughly at the turn of the twentieth century [8, 25]. At the beginning of this new period only a few surgeons were able to perform a successful endonasal ethmoidectomy and simple drainage of the frontal sinus. In the preantibiotic and preendoscopic period, endonasal surgery of the paranasal sinuses was a life-threatening treatment with a high incidence of catastrophic complications like meningitis, brain abscess and encephalitis. This was the reason why for many decades most of rhinologists preferred the external approach for paranasal sinus surgery. With the development of new optical aids, mainly endoscopes and the operating microscope, a new revolutionary era started between the 1950s and the 1970s. Further improved understanding of the pathophysiology of paranasal sinus mucosa played an important role in the rebirth of endonasal sinus surgery [3, 9, 20].

In the beginning of the 1980s a new concept for endonasal micro-endoscopic frontal sinus surgery was established. The results concerning different types of frontal sinus drainage were published in several studies where comprehensive experience with this surgical concept had been achieved [5, 28]. Meanwhile, by doing a high number of frontal type III drainages, wide-ranging knowledge with this technique could be gained [6].

Indications

The following are indications for endonasal frontal sinus drainage types I–III:

1. Indications for type I drainage
   - (a) Acute sinusitis
     - Failure of conservative surgery
     - Endocranial and orbital complications
   - (b) Chronic sinusitis
     - Primary surgery
     - No risk factors (aspirin hypersensitivity, asthma, and nasal polyposis)
     - Revision after incomplete ethmoidectomy
2. Indications for type II drainage
   - (a) Type IIa drainage
     - Serious complications of acute sinusitis
     - Medial mucopyocele
     - Tumor surgery (benign tumors)
     - Good-quality mucosa
   - (b) Type IIb drainage – all indications of type IIa, if the resulting type IIa is smaller than 5×7mm. For type IIb a drill is necessary.
3. Indications for type III drainage
   - (a) Difficult revision surgery
   - (b) Primarily in patients with prognostic risk factors and severe polyposis, particularly patients with
     - Samter's triad
     - Mucoviscidosis
     - Kartagener´s syndrome
     - Ciliary immotility syndrome
     - Benign and malignant tumors

Preoperative Workup

The most important aim of any surgical procedure is to relieve the patients' symptoms. Not all symptoms of chronic sinusitis can be eliminated with surgical treatment. It is, therefore, of utmost importance to take the time to listen to patients and to establish their main problems. A discussion is then required to make clear to the patient what can be achieved with surgery and which symptoms are likely to be improved.

Tips and Pearls

- It is also necessary to remember that sinus surgery is not about treating what is found on a CT scan, but is part of the management of a well-informed patient.

In general, the history taken should include the following aspects:

1. *Symptoms of the present illness.* Patients frequently present to the surgeon with their diagnosis, instead of describing their signs and symptoms. Detailed questioning about the symptoms is required, concentrating on the duration, time of onset and any symptom-free intervals. The patient should also be asked for the most common symptoms of chronic sinusitis.

Common symptoms of chronic sinusitis include:

- Nasal obstruction
- Postnasal drip
- Headache and location
- Facial pressure
- Hyposmia

2. *Past medical and surgical history.* Most patients who are referred for sinus surgery have been treated medically in the past. Many of them have had several courses of antibiotics in conjunction with systemic and/or topical corticosteroids. It is mandatory to ask all patients about any previous sinus surgery.

The following questions during the taking of the medical history require particular attention:

- Episodes of antibiotic therapy?
- Duration of local/systemic corticosteroid treatment?
- Previous surgery?
- Success of previous surgery and symptom-free intervals after surgery?
- Any other medication, particularly agents which can cause mucosal swelling as a side effect, such as antihypertensive drugs?
- Presence of Samter's triad (polyps, asthma, aspirin intolerance)?

3. *Physical examination and endoscopy.* Routine physical examination includes anterior rhinoscopy and rigid/flexible nasal endoscopy. Anterior rhinoscopy gives the surgeon a first impression of the sinonasal condition.

The following features should be noted from the physical examination:

- Septal deviation
- Color, texture and turgor of the mucosa
- Size and shape of the turbinates

Endoscopic examination of the nasal cavity with rigid and flexible endoscopes is now the gold standard in the preoperative evaluation of chronic sinusitis. In our hospital we prefer the flexible endoscope as it is well tolerated, even in children, and most patients do not even require local anesthesia. A 0° or 30° rigid endoscope can also be used to examine the nasal cavity. Before using a rigid endoscope, a mixture of topical anesthetic and a vasoconstrictor should be applied to the nasal mucosa. By displaying the endoscopic image on a TV monitor, we can demonstrate any abnormality to the patient.

During nasal endoscopic examination, the following anatomical structures should be evaluated routinely:

- Relationship between the middle turbinate and the nasal septum
- Paradoxical middle turbinate (a medially rather than a laterally concave middle turbinate)
- The extent of resection of a previously trimmed middle turbinate
- The presence of a concha bullosa (an air-filled, pneumatized middle turbinate)
- The extent and size of any polyps

Operative Technique

The procedure is performed with the patient under combined general and local anesthesia. Nasal vibrissae are cut to get a better view of the nasal cavity when using the microscope. To minimize bleeding, topical decongestant is applied by packing the inferior and middle portions of the nasal meatus with gauze strips soaked in naphazoline hydrochloride and 2 ml of 10% cocaine solution. Injection with 1% Xylocaine with 1:120,000 units of epinephrine is performed in the region of the agger nasi and uncinate process. At least 10 min should be allowed for local vasoconstriction. Packing of the throat is also performed. Bleeding is a major concern during endonasal sinus surgery. In many cases, bleeding can be minimized with the support of anesthetic techniques. The anesthesiologist should be informed continuously about the actual bleeding condition, and should follow surgery on a monitor. Intraoperative communication between the surgeon and the anesthesiologist is essential.

If the comorbidities of the patient provide no contraindication, the anesthesiologist should intraoperatively aim at a mean arterial pressure of 60 mmHg and a heart rate of 50–60 beats per minute. Arterial hypotension will minimize hemodynamic causes for bleeding.

The influence of various anesthetics on bleeding is continuously under discussion. A total intravenous technique may have advantages with regard to bleeding on the microcirculatory level. In the case of diffuse bleeding, adrenaline-soaked pledgets (1:1,000 adrenaline) may be applied intraoperatively [1]. We recommend starting the surgery on the right side, with the surgeon staying on the same side. Because of the positioning of the surgeon, the surgical approach is more difficult on the right side than on the left. The combined endonasal micro-endoscopic surgery is performed by using a Zeiss operating microscope with a 250- or 275-mm objective lens and a 45° rigid telescope with a suction/irrigation handle (Fig. 8.1). The shaver is very useful for gentle tissue removal and also for drilling in the frontal sinus. Surgery on the frontal recess is usually preceded at least by an an-

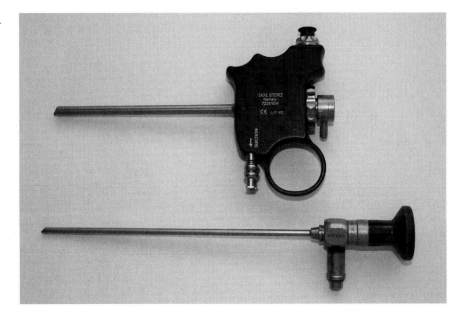

Fig. 8.1. Combined irrigation/suction handle with 45° rigid telescope

8

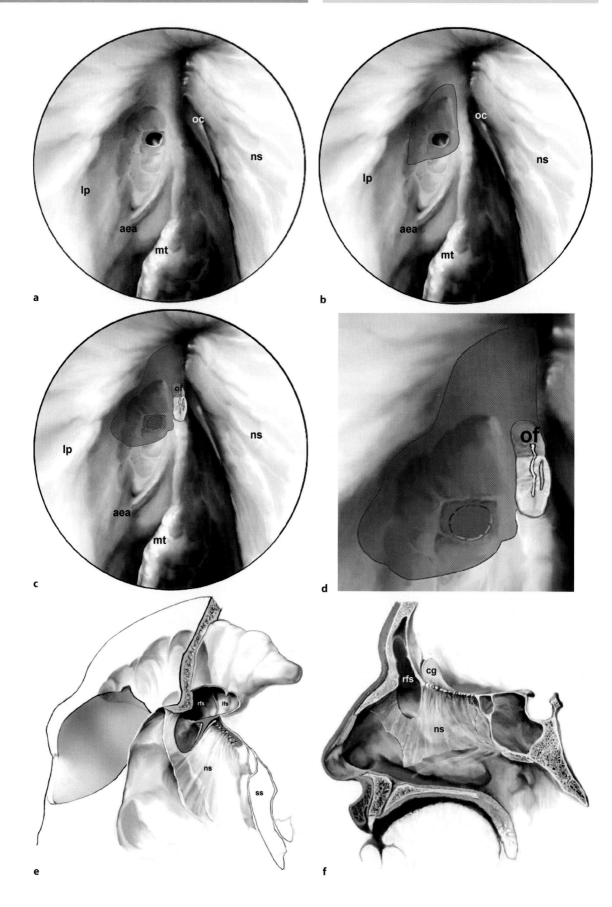

terior ethmoidectomy, but more often than not by a complete ethmoidectomy. Exceptions are those cases where a complete ethmoidectomy has already been performed. It is important to remove agger nasi cells and to visualize the attachment of the middle turbinate medially, the lamina papyracea laterally, and the anterior skull base with the anterior ethmoid artery superiorly.

Type I: Simple Drainage

The type I drainage (Fig. 8.2a) is established by ethmoidectomy including the cell septa in the region of the frontal recess [14]. The inferior part of Killian's infundibulum and its mucosa remain untouched. This approach is indicated when there is only minor abnormality in the frontal sinus and the patient does not suffer from "prognostic risk factors" like aspirin hypersensitivity and asthma, which are associated with poor quality of mucosa and possible problems in outcome. In the majority of cases the frontal sinus heals because of the improved drainage via the ethmoid cavity.

Type IIa/IIb: Extended Drainage

Extended drainage is achieved after ethmoidectomy by resecting the floor of the frontal sinus between the lamina papyracea and the middle turbinate (type IIa; Fig. 8.2b) or the nasal septum (type IIb; (Fig. 8.2c, d)) anterior the ventral margin of the olfactory fossa.

Hosemann et al. [10, 11] showed in a detailed anatomical study that the maximum diameter of a neo-ostium of the frontal sinus (type IIa), which could be gained using a spoon or a curette, was 11 mm, with an average of 5.6 mm. They also presented an excellent critical evaluation and results [11].

If one needs to achieve a larger drainage opening like type IIb, one has to use a drill because of the increasing thickness of the bone going more medially towards the nasal septum. During drilling with the diamond burr in a classic drill hand piece, bone dust

may fog the endoscope, demanding repeated cleaning. At this point the microscope is useful as it allows one to work with two hands, while an assistant holds a simple self-retracting speculum. The endoscopic fourhand technique as an alternative was developed by May (1990) and was popularized recently by several authors [18]. Sinus surgery is carried out by the surgeon and an assistant. The rigid telescope is held by the assistant, thereby enabling the surgeon to work with both hands. The surgeon is able to control the suction with one hand and perform dissection with the other hand; hence he/she will be able to achieve good visualization when there is more bleeding. A detailed description of this technique is given by Simmen and Jones [24].

A great help for drilling in the frontal sinus is achieved with new straight and differently curved drills used with the shaver providing simultaneous suction and irrigation, thus reducing fogging of the telescopes (Fig. 8.3).

As soon the frontal recess is identified using the middle turbinate and, where identifiable, the anterior ethmoid artery as landmarks, the frontal infundibulum is exposed and the anterior ethmoid cells are resected. During surgery, repeated considerations of the CT scan will establish the presence of so-called frontal cells [14], which can develop far into the frontal sinus giving the surgeon the erroneous impression that the frontal sinus has been properly opened. Sagittal CT slices and navigation may be helpful in difficult situations. In the case of frontal cells, a procedure called by Stammberger [26] "uncapping the egg" using a 45° telescope may be necessary, resulting in a type IIa drainage.

If after a type IIa drainage has been performed, further widening to produce a type IIb drainage is required, the diamond burr is introduced into the clearly visible gap in the infundibulum and drawn across the bone in a medial direction. Care is taken to ensure that the frontal sinus opening is bordered by bone on all sides and that mucosa is preserved at least on one part of the circumference. In case one feels the type IIa drainage is too small with regard to the underlying abnormality, it is better to perform the type IIb drainage. At the end, a rubber finger stall can be introduced into the frontal sinus for about 5 days.

Fig. 8.2. Different kinds of endonasal frontal sinus drainage. **a** Type I drainage after anterior ethmoidectomy. **b** Type IIa drainage. Removal of the frontal sinus floor from the lamina papyracea and middle turbinate. **c** Type IIb drainage with extension of the drainage from the lamina papyracea to the nasal septum. **d** Type IIb drainage detail with identification of the first olfactory fiber. (Reprinted from [5] with kind permission from Springer Science+ and Business Media). **e** View from left inferior. Type III drainage with "frontal T" and first olfactory fiber on both sides. **f** Sagittal view of the type III drainage with resection of the frontal sinus floor anterior to the olfactory cleft. *aea* anterior ethmoid artery, *cg* crista galli, *lfs* left frontal sinus, *lp* lamina papyracea, *mt* middle turbinate, *ns* nasal septum, *oc* olfactory cleft, *of* olfactory fiber, *rfs* right frontal sinus, *ss* sphenoid sinus. (Reprinted from [5] with kind permission from Springer Science+Business Media)

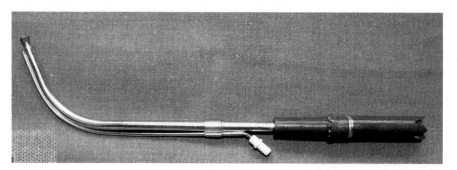

Fig. 8.3. A 70° diamond burr for performing resection work on the floor and septum of the frontal sinuses

Type III: Endonasal Median Drainage

The extended type IIb opening is enlarged by removing portions of the superior nasal septum in the neighborhood of the frontal sinus floor (Fig. 8.2e, f, Video 8.1). The diameter of this opening should be about 1.5 cm. This is followed by resection of the frontal sinus septum or septa, if there is more than one. Starting on one side of the patient, one crosses the midline until the contralateral lamina papyracea is reached.

To achieve the maximum possible opening of the frontal sinus, it is very helpful to identify the first olfactory fibers on both sides: the middle turbinate is exposed and millimeter by millimeter cut from anterior to posterior along its origin at the skull base. After about 1.5 mm and just medial to the origin of the middle turbinate, one will see the first olfactory fiber coming out of a little bony hole. The same is done on the contralateral side. After completing the resection of the perpendicular plate back to the first olfactory fibers, one can identify the "frontal T" [5], which is a result of surgical dissection, like the "bridge" in ear surgery. Its long crus is represented by the posterior border of the perpendicular ethmoid lamina resection; the shorter wings on both sides are provided by the posterior margins of the frontal sinus floor resection (Fig. 8.2e, f). After that, the ethmoidectomy on the left side is completed in the same way as on the right.

To perform the type III drainage in the technically most efficient way, it is helpful to change between the use of an endoscope and a microscope. Alternatively, this procedure can be done with the endoscope alone, though it is more time-consuming. Curved drills of different angles used with the shaver motor are helpful. They allow one to go more superiorly with the resection of the interfrontal sinus septum and to perform a more complete removal a possible frontal cell. These measures help to create excellent landmarks for the anterior border of the olfactory fossa on both sides, which makes the completion of frontal sinus floor resection to its maximum until the first olfactory fiber easier and safer (Fig. 8.2e, f).

In difficult revision cases, one can begin the type III drainage primarily from two starting points, either from the lateral side, as already described, or medially. The primary lateral approach is recommended if the previous ethmoid work was incomplete and the middle turbinate is still present as a landmark. One should adopt the primary medial approach, if the ethmoid has been cleared and/or if the middle turbinate is absent.

The medial approach begins with the partial resection of the perpendicular plate of the nasal septum, followed by identification of the first olfactory fiber on each side, as already described.

After surgery the patient is put on antibiotics until the packing is removed on the seventh postoperative day. The long lasting packing allows reepithelialization of most parts of the surgical cavity, which makes the postoperative treatment more comfortable. Recently we started to fill the frontal sinus and upper anterior ethmoid with a new gel (Stammberger Sinus Dressing, Rapidrhino Company) and put only two rubber finger stalls underneath into the nose. This seems to reduce the time of packing to 5 days without compromising the high long-term opening rate.

The endonasal median drainage is identical to the nasofrontal approach IV [19] and the "modified Lothrop procedure" [7]. Lothrop [15, 16] himself warned against using the endonasal route, judging it as too dangerous during his time and he performed the median drainage via an external approach. In 1906, Halle [8] created a large drainage from the frontal sinus directly to the nose using the endonasal approach with no more aids than a headlight and the naked eye.

The principal difference between the endonasal median frontal sinus drainage and the classic frontoorbital external Jansen [13], Lothrop [16], Ritter [23], Lynch [17] and Howarth [12] operation is that the bony borders around the frontal sinus drainage are preserved. This makes it more stable in the long term and reduces the likelihood of reclosure by scarring [2], which may lead to recurrent frontal sinusitis or a mucocele, not to mention the avoidance of external scar.

The endonasal median drainage (type III) is indicated after one or several previous sinus operations have not resolved the frontal sinus problem, including an external frontoethmoidectomy. It is also justified as a primary procedure in patients with severe polyposis and other prognostic "risk factors" affecting outcome, such as aspirin intolerance, asthma, Samter's triad (aspirin hypersensitivity, asthma and allergy), Kartagener's syndrome, mucoviscidosis and ciliary dyskinesia syndrome. Its use in patients with severe polyposis without these risk factors is undetermined and needs to be evaluated. It seems that patients with generalized polyposis but who still show in the periphery of the sinuses along the skull base air on a coronal CT scan ("halo sign") have a comparatively better prognosis than those without, and can be managed by a more conservative technique. It is useful also for removal of benign tumors in the frontal sinus

(Fig. 8.4) and the ethmoid as long as the main part of the tumor in the frontal sinus is medial to a postoperative vertical line through the lamina papyracea. In addition the use of the type III drainage makes the removal of malignant tumors which are just reaching the frontal sinus safer.

Tips and Pearls

- Early identification of lamina papyracea and middle turbinate as the most important anatomic landmarks.
- Control of the eye bulb during the whole surgery by the surgeon and the operating nurse.
- A bulb pressing test after Draf [4] and Stankiewicz [27] can be helpful when there is suspicion of injury to the lamina papyracea.

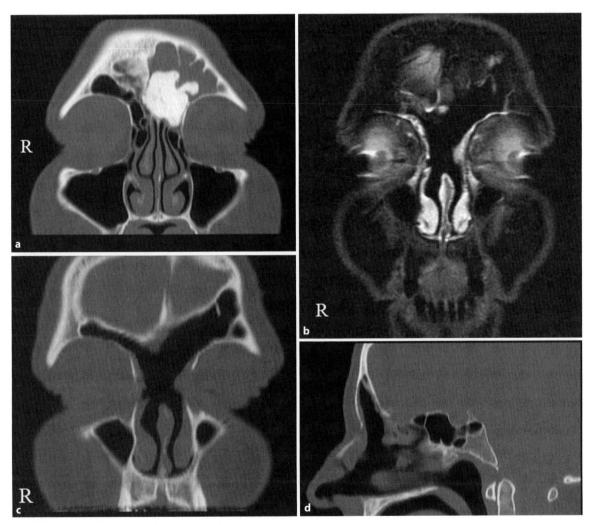

Fig. 8.4. Patient with an osteoma of the left frontal sinus complaining of unilateral frontal headaches. **a** Preoperative coronal CT scan with total opacification of the left frontal sinus. Magnetic resonance tomography (**b**) and CT (**c, d**) 6 months after tumor removal in combination with a type III frontal sinus drainage showing a wide-open left frontal sinus without any evidence of tumor recurrence

- Always dissect laterally to the middle turbinate, never medially and superiorly.
- The middle meatal antrostomy should be performed just above the inferior turbinate and should not go further anteriorly than the lacrimal sac and the nasolacrimal duct.
- If middle turbinate surgery is needed, the superior part should be preserved as an anatomic landmark.

Postoperative Care

No uniform recommendations concerning postoperative care exist in the literature. We would like to offer some general recommendations for postoperative treatment. We have learned by experience that local aftercare should concentrate on removal of mobile obstructive material only, not on crusts protecting mucosal wounds.

Local aftercare of the surgical area by the ENT surgeon:
1. In the postoperative days after removal of packing and with continuously expanding interval based on each individual patient for about 3 months
2. Local aftercare should consist of:
   (a) Removal of mobile fibrin clots and crusts only
   (b) Separation of synechiae and adhesions
   (c) Suction of secretion from the nasal cavity

Daily local care of the operative area by the patient:
1. Minimum of 3 months
2. Application of topical steroids
3. Inhalation and irrigation of the nose
4. Application of ointments

Systemic aftercare:
1. *Antibiotics:* They are indicated in the postoperative period for 1–2 weeks in cases of acute sinusitis or chronic purulent sinusitis. In type III drainage, we recommend prophylactic antibiotic use, as long as the packing is in place.
2. *Antiallergic medical therapy*: This is recommended for 6 weeks postoperatively if allergy has been diagnosed by history or specific tests. In less severe cases, we prescribe day antihistamines. In patients with severe allergy (e.g., Samter's triad), the combination of antihistamines with low-dose corticosteroid medication for 6 weeks helps to prevent early recurrence of polyps.

Results of Endonasal Frontal Sinus Surgery

Judging the results of endonasal frontal sinus surgery requires a postoperative follow-up of 10 years or more [21, 22]. The failure rate of Neel et al. [21] with a modified Lynch procedure increased from 7% at a mean follow-up of 3.7 years to 30% at 7 years. Weber et al. [30] carried out in 1995 and 1996 two studies. In the first retrospective study, patients who underwent endonasal frontal sinus drainage (471 type I drainages, 125 type II drainages and 52 type III drainages) between 1979 and 1992 were evaluated. From these groups, random patients were examined: 42 patients with type I drainage, 43 with type II drainage and 47 with type III drainage were included into the study. In each patient the indication was chronic polypoid rhinosinusitis, except in five cases with type III drainage in which an orbital complication existed associated with acute sinusitis. The follow-up period was between 1 and 12 years, with a median of 5 years. Application of subjective and objective criteria to evaluate the success of endonasal frontal sinus drainage (grade 1, endoscopically normal mucosa, independent of the subjective complaints; grade 2, subjectively free of symptoms, but with endoscopically visible inflammatory mucosal changes; grade 3, no subjective improvement and pathologic mucosa, i.e., failure) allowed success rates of 85.7% with type I drainage, 83.8% with type II drainage and 91.5% with type III drainage to be achieved. This means that, despite the choice of prognostically unfavorable cases, type III drainages appeared to show the best results, though this was not statistically significant among the three groups.

In a second study [28–30], endoscopic and CT examinations were systematically carried out. After 12–98 months follow-up of patients with type II drainage, 58% of 83 frontal sinuses were ventilated and normal. A ventilated frontal sinus with hyperplastic mucosa was seen in 12% of cases. Scar tissue occlusion with total opacification on the CT scan was evident in 14% of cases. In 16% of cases, total opacification was due to recurrent polyposis. Patients were free of symptoms or had only minor problems in 79% of cases.

After a period of 12–89 months following type III drainage, 59% of 81 frontal sinuses were ventilated and normal. A ventilated frontal sinus with hyperplastic mucosa was seen in 17% of cases. Scar tissue occlusion with total opacification on the CT scan was obvious in 7% of cases and, in 16% of cases there was total opacification due to recurrent polyposis. The patients were free of symptoms or had only minor problems in 95% of cases. Already this first series of reevaluation of long-term results demonstrates the value of the endonasal frontal sinus surgery.

Acknowledgments

The authors thank Prof. Dr. med. Erich Hofmann, Director of the Department of Interventional Neuro-radiology, Klinikum Fulda, Germany, for the radiologic images.

References

1. Anderhuber W, Walch C, Nemeth E, Semmelrock HJ, Berghold A, Ranftl G, Stammberger H (1999) Plasma adrenaline concentrations during functional endoscopic sinus surgery. Laryngoscope 109:204–207
2. Bockmühl U, Kratzsch B, Benda K, Draf W (2006) Surgery for paranasal sinus mucocoeles: Efficacy of endonasal micro-endoscopic management and long-term results of 185 patients. Rhinology 44:62–67
3. Draf W (1983) Endoscopy of the Paranasal Sinuses. Springer, Berlin Heidelberg New York (German edition 1978: Die Endoskopie der Nasennebenhöhlen)
4. Draf W (1986) Kurs endonasale mikro-endoskopische Chirurgie der Nasennebenhöhlen. Academic Teaching Hospital Fulda
5. Draf W (1991) Endonasal micro-endoscopic frontal sinus surgery. The Fulda concept. Oper Tech Otolaryngol Head Neck Surg 2:234–240
6. Draf W, Endonasal frontal sinus drainage Type I-III according to Draf. In: Kountakis S, Senior B, Draf W (2005) The frontal sinus. Springer, Berlin Heidelberg New York
7. Gross WE, Gross CW, Becker D, Moore D, Phillips D (1995) Modified transnasal endoscopic Lothrop procedure as an alternative to frontal sinus obliteration. Otolaryngol Head Neck Surg 113:427–434
8. Halle M (1906) Externe und interne Operation der Nasennebenhoehleneiterungen. Berl Klein Wschr 43:1369–1372
9. Heermann H (1958) Ueber endonasale Chirurgie unter Verwendung des binokularen Mikroskops. Arch Ohr-Nas-Kehlk-Heilk 171:295–297
10. Hosemann W, Gross R, Goede U, Kuehnel T (2001) Clinical anatomy of the nasal process of the frontal bone (spina nasalis interna). Otolaryngol Head Neck Surg 125:60–65
11. Hosemann W, Kuehnel T, Held P, Wagner W, Felderhoff A (1997) Endonasal frontal sinusotomy in surgical management of chronic sinusitis: A critical evaluation. Am J Rhin 11:1–9
12. Howarth WG (1921) Operations on the frontal sinus. J Laryngol Otol 36:417–421
13. Jansen A (1894) Eroeffnung der Nebenhoehlen der Nase bei chronischer Eiterung. Arch Laryng Rhinol (Berl) 135–157
14. Lang J (1989) Clinical anatomy of the nose nasal cavity and paranasal sinuses. Thieme, Stuttgart
15. Lothrop HA (1899) The anatomy and surgery of the frontal sinus and anterior ethmoidal cells. Ann Surg 29:175–215
16. Lothrop HA (1914) Frontal sinus suppuration. Ann Surg 59:937–957
17. Lynch RC (1921) The technique of a radical frontal sinus operation which has given me the best results. Laryngoscope 31:1–5
18. May M, Hoffmann DF, Sobol SM (1990) Video endoscopic sinus surgery: a two-handed technique. Laryngoscope 100:430–432
19. May M, Schaitkin B (1995) Frontal sinus surgery: endonasal drainage instead of an external osteoplastic approach. Oper Tech Otolaryngol Head Neck Surg 6:184–192
20. Messerklinger J (1970) Die Endoskopie der Nase. Monatsschr Ohrenheilk 104:451–56
21. Neel HB, McDonald TJ, Facer GW (1987) Modified Lynch procedure for chronic frontal sinus diseases: Rationale, technique, and long term results. Laryngoscope 97:1274
22. Orlandi RR, Kennedy DW (2001) Revision endoscopic frontal sinus surgery. Otolaryngol Clin North Am 34:77–90
23. Ritter G (1906) Eine neue Methode zur Erhaltung der vorderen Stirnhoehlenwand bei Radikaloperationen chronischer Stirnhoehleneiterungen. Dtsch Med Wochenschr 32:1294–1296
24. Simmen D, Jones N (2005) Surgery of the paranasal sinuses and the frontal skull base. Thieme, New York
25. Spiess G (1899) Die endonasale Chirurgie des Sinus frontalis. Arch Laryngo 9:285–91
26. Stammberger H (2000) F.E.S.S. "uncapping the egg". The endoscopic approach to frontal recess and sinuses. Storz Company Prints
27. Stankiewicz JA (1989) Complications of endoscopic sinus surgery. Otolaryngol Clin North Am 22:749–758
28. Weber R, Draf W, Keerl R, Schick B, Saha A (1997) Micro-endoscopic pansinusoperation in chronic sinusitis. Results and complications. Am J Otolaryngol 18:247–253
29. Weber R, Hosemann W, Draf W, Keerl R, Schick B, Schinzel S (1997) Endonasal frontal sinus surgery with long-term stenting of the nasofrontal duct. Laryngorhinootologie 76:728–734
30. Weber R, Keerl R, Huppmann A, Draf W, Saha A. Wound healing after endonasal sinus surgery in time-lapse video: a new way of continuous in vivo observation and documentation in rhinology. In: Stamm A, Draf W (2000) Micro-endoscopic surgery of the paranasal sinuses and skull base. Springer, Berlin Heidelberg

Endoscopic Modified Lothrop Procedure

Francis T.K. Ling, Ioannis G. Skoulas, Stilianos E. Kountakis

Core Messages

- The endoscopic modified Lothrop procedure is an alternative to an osteoplastic flap procedure.

- The procedure involves endoscopic intranasal removal of the frontal intersinus septum, frontal sinus floor, nasal beak and, anterior superior nasal septum.

- The accessible dimension is the distance between two parallel lines that lie in the parasagittal plane through the midportion of the internal frontal ostium with the first line tangential to the skull base and the second line tangential to the posterior margin of the nasal beak. An accessible dimension less than 5 mm would preclude the patient's candidacy for the endoscopic modified Lothrop procedure.

- Drilling on the posterior area of the frontal recess is avoided in order to prevent postoperative circumferential stenosis, injury to the skull base with possible CSF leak, or injury to the anterior ethmoid artery.

- A large septectomy is made to provide surgical access of instruments from both sides of the nose as well as to help prevent postoperative crusting.

Contents

Introduction

The complex and variable anatomy of the frontal sinus and recess makes the surgical treatment of chronic disease in this area both dangerous and challenging. Pneumatization of the frontal bone by numerous anterior ethmoid air cells during development may effectively block the already narrowed outflow tract of the frontal sinus. In addition, the area of the frontal recess is particularly poorly visualized during endoscopic sinus surgery owing to its anterior and cephalad position. These factors together increase the predilection for scarring and stenosis causing complete sinus obstruction that may be refractory to conventional endoscopic techniques [14, 19]. As well, the potential for injury to intimately associated structures such as the lamina papyracea, cribriform plate, and anterior ethmoidal artery is greater and can make surgery in this area a daunting task for the novice endoscopic surgeon.

Because of the anatomic complexity of the region, Lothrop advocated an external approach for frontal sinus drainage and discouraged an intranasal approach. The Lothrop procedure consisted of bilateral external ethmoidectomy, removal of the frontal sinus floor with communication of both frontal sinuses through a large nasal septectomy. This external procedure required the removal of the lacrimal bone and a portion of the lamina papyracea, which caused medial collapse of the orbital contents and subsequent stenosis of the nasofrontal communication [1]. The procedure did not gain much popularity and with the advent of the osteoplastic flap procedure in the 1960s, the Lothrop procedure was largely abandoned amongst surgeons. Despite being the "gold standard," the osteoplastic procedure with or without frontal sinus obliteration has a reported failure rate of approximately 10%, with a range of 6–25% [3, 15, 16]. It is also associated with postoperative morbidities such as frontal bossing, supraorbital neuralgia, donor site complications, and scarring [17].

In the early 1990s, new advances in endoscopic sinus surgery technology allowed surgeons to revisit

9

the management of recalcitrant frontal sinus disease through a completely intranasal approach. In 1995, Gross et al. [9] first introduced the modification of the Lothrop procedure as an alternative to the osteoplastic flap procedure. Their modification involved a complete endoscopic intranasal removal of the frontal intersinus septum, frontal sinus floor, and anterior superior nasal septum, thus allowing a more precise surgical management of frontal sinus outflow obstruction using advanced drilling technology. Since the first description of the procedure, several surgeons have reported success with the endoscopic modified Lothrop procedure comparable to that with the osteoplastic flap procedure in the management of frontal sinus disease [2, 4, 6, 10, 12, 13, 18]. Because of its numerous advantages, such as improved cosmesis, decreased morbidity, and shorter hospitalization, this procedure is slowly becoming the procedure of choice over the osteoplastic flap procedure in the management of persistent frontal disease after failure of maximal medical management and conservative endoscopic sinus surgery. Indications have also expanded to include other conditions as listed below:

1. Indications
   (a) Failure of appropriate medical therapy and primary endoscopic frontal sinusotomy in the treatment of persistent chronic frontal sinusitis
   (b) Mucoceles of the frontal sinus
   (c) Inverted papilloma invading the frontal recess and sinus
   (d) Select osteomas
   (e) Trauma of the frontal sinus
   (f) Alternative to osteoplastic frontal sinus obliteration
   (g) Revision of a previous endoscopic modified Lothrop procedure in a symptomatic patient demonstrating stenosis
2. Contraindications
   (a) Hypoplastic frontal sinus and frontal recess
   (b) Surgeon inexperience
   (c) Proper instrumentation unavailable
   (d) Sinus disease confined to supraorbital ethmoid air cells and not to the frontal sinus

Preoperative Workup

The endoscopic modified Lothrop procedure is recommended as a surgical option when an external osteoplastic flap procedure is contemplated for the surgical treatment of frontal sinus disease [6, 9]. Candidate patients generally have failed more conservative limited endoscopic sinus surgery and, ideally, have progressed through a protocol of increasingly complex surgeries. In order of more to less conservative, these procedures are as follows: ethmoidectomy with medial maxillary antrostomy without surgery in the frontal recess, frontal recess surgery, endoscopic frontal sinusotomy, unilateral extended frontal sinus surgery (Draf II procedure), endoscopic modified Lothrop procedure, and osteoplastic flap procedure with frontal sinus obliteration [11].

> **Tips and Pearls**
> - Prior to surgery, the patient's underlying condition causing frontal sinus disease is optimized medically.

A selective combination of nasal irrigations, antibiotics, leukotriene antagonists, topical, nebulized and/or oral steroids is often required. Such aggressive preoperative care is mandatory postoperatively as well to prevent restenosis of nasofrontal drainage leading to disease recurrence. This is especially important for patients with more aggressive disease, such as hyperplastic rhinosinusitis, sarcoidosis, Wegener's granulomatosis, and Samter's triad.

> **Tips and Pearls**
> - Anatomic evaluation of the frontal sinus region with a computed tomography (CT) scans is key to the feasibility and safety of the endoscopic modified Lothrop procedure.

The number and the location of frontal recess air cells should be determined as they will dictate the number of barriers that will require removal to reach the internal frontal sinus ostium [5, 19]. Sagittally reconstructed views of the frontal recess are required to determine the important anatomic dimensions needed to allow safe introduction of the drill. The original recommended dimensions [6] were an anteroposterior dimension at the cephalad margin of the frontal recess of at least 1.5 cm, and a nasal beak no thicker than 1 cm. With newer, less bulky powered drills, a recent cadaver study demonstrated that these instruments can be safely introduced into a frontal recess anteroposterior dimension that was less than 1.5 cm [5]. It was determined that an accessible dimension of at least 5 mm is required to allow safe removal of the nasal beak and frontal sinus floor. This accessible dimension is the distance between two parallel lines that lie in the parasagittal plane through the midportion of the internal frontal ostium with the first line tangential to the skull base and the second line tangential to the posterior margin of the nasal beak (Fig. 9.1).

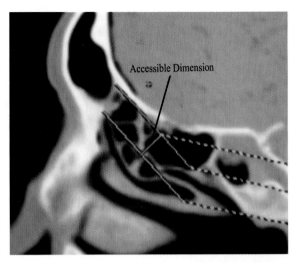

Fig. 9.1. The accessible dimension is the distance between two parallel lines that lie in the parasagittal plane through the midportion of the internal frontal ostium with the first line tangential to the skull base and the second line tangential to the posterior margin of the nasal beak

Tips and Pearls

■ Accessible dimension less than 5 mm would preclude the patient's candidacy for endoscopic modified Lothrop procedure even with the smallest drills that are available today

Surgical Technique

With the patient under general anesthesia, in the supine position, the nasal cavities are first decongested using 4 ml of 4% cocaine solution. The septum and lateral nasal wall at the anterior insertion of the middle turbinate are injected with up to 10 ml of 1% lidocaine and 1:100,000 epinephrine solution. Preoperative antibiotics are given intravenously.

Review of the CT scan and set-up of image-guided navigational equipment is used to help identify the frontal recess, skull base, and floor of the frontal sinus. Rigid endoscopy is then performed to evaluate the nasal cavities and the most approachable frontal recess is chosen to start the procedure. The use of a 30° or 45° endoscope can facilitate visualization of this area.

Identification of the frontal sinus ostium is required next. Medialization of the middle turbinate or its remnant is performed to allow better access to the frontal recess. Various methods can then be used to identify the frontal recess and frontal ostium. One method involves insertion of a wire probe through the frontal isthmus into the frontal sinus to assist in anatomic orientation and to protect posterior structures [1]. Another method to identify the frontal ostium makes use of saline and fluorescein (0.5 ml of 25% fluorescein) irrigations through a minitrephine placed through a stab incision on the medial aspect of the eyebrow into the frontal sinus [17].

Tips and Pearls

■ Anatomically, the frontal ostium is identified posterior and medial to the recessus terminalis, which is the region where the uncinate process most commonly attaches to the lamina papyracea.

Its location can be identified and confirmed with the help of computer-image guidance.

Once the frontal recess has been identified, the superior attachment of the uncinate process remnant is resected using a microdebrider and careful removal of frontal recess air cells is performed to reach the frontal sinus ostium. Once this has been found, mucosa above the insertion of the middle turbinate is removed with the microdebrider and drilling is initiated with a 3.2-mm straight burr in an anterior direction through the anterior insertion of the middle turbinate to enlarge the frontal sinus ostium until the level of the nasal bone is reached. Laterally, drilling is continued until the level of the plane of the lamina papyracea. Drilling is then continued medially until the plane of the nasal septum is reached. This effectively removes the nasal beak (Fig. 9.2).

Drilling must be precise and atraumatic to the surrounding mucosa:

■ Ciliated epithelium over the lateral wall of the frontal recess must be preserved to facilitate mucociliary transport out of the frontal sinus.
■ Mucosa at the posterior margin of the frontal sinus ostium should not be removed in order to prevent postoperative circumferential stenosis.
■ Drilling is directed in an anterior and cephalad direction to avoid injury to the skull base with possible CSF rhinorrhea or hemorrhage from the anterior ethmoid artery.

In order to avoid going through the nasal bones, two fingertips can be placed over the nasal root to feel and sense the closeness of the drill to the nasal bones. This can prevent soft-tissue injury over the nasal root at the glabella and subsequent cosmetic deformity.

After removal of the nasal beak, a septectomy is then performed to allow broad visualization of the operative area and permit greater maneuverability of instruments within the nasal cavity (Fig. 9.3). In

9

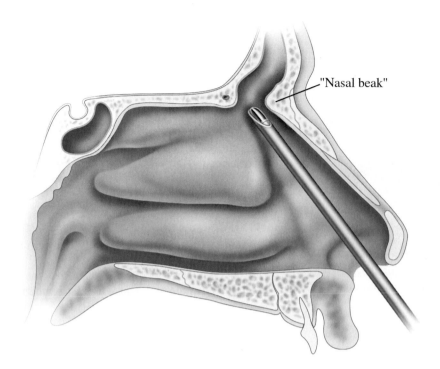

Fig. 9.2. The nasal beak is drilled down. Avoid drilling in the posterior frontal recess to prevent injury to the anterior ethmoid artery and possible CSF leak

"Nasal beak"

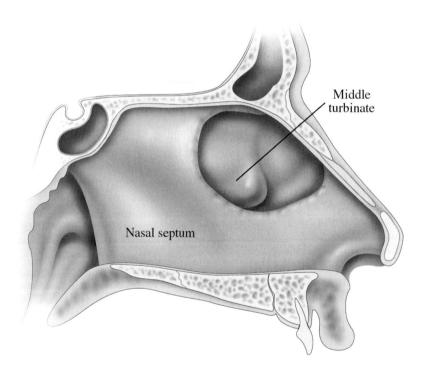

Fig. 9.3. A large septectomy provides access to both nasal cavities and increases maneuverability of endoscopic instruments

Middle turbinate

Nasal septum

addition, its primary purpose is to provide a large common communication for nasofrontal drainage. Using the microdebrider, mucosa is removed over the perpendicular plate of the ethmoid anteri-or to the anterior insertion of the middle turbinate. A 2 cm × 2 cm portion of nasal septum is removed with its posterior aspect level with the anterior end of the middle turbinate. This involves removing the

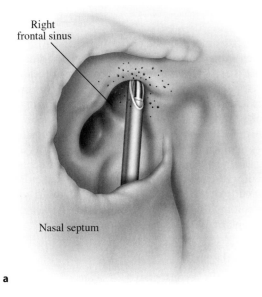
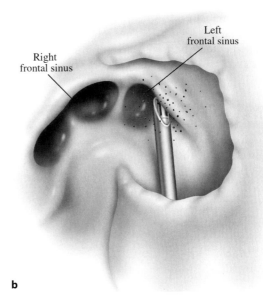

a   b

Fig. 9.4. Drilling is continued through the nasal beak, removing the frontal sinus floor on the opposite side until the opposite lamina papyracea is reached

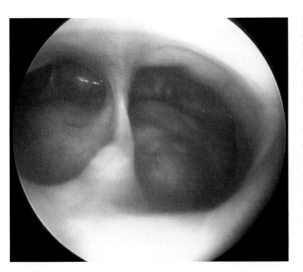

Fig. 9.5. The resultant ostium should provide adequate access for endoscopic surveillance and debridement of the common frontal sinus cavities in the clinic

perpendicular plate of the ethmoid up to the nasal floor of the frontal sinus.

Tips and Pearls

- A larger rather than a smaller septectomy will prevent the accumulation of crusting and de layed healing seen with smaller septal perforations.

Through the septectomy, drilling is then continued through the nasal beak, removing the frontal sinus floor on the opposite side until the opposite lamina papyracea is reached (Fig. 9.4). Again, avoidance of injury to the mucosa laterally and posteriorly is essential. Complete removal of the frontal sinus septum is not necessary and may lead to violation of an anteriorly displaced skull base.

Palpation of the anterior face of the frontal sinus with a curved probe should then be performed to assess the completeness of the procedure. A palpable ledge would indicate incomplete removal of the nasal beak and may compromise nasofrontal outflow. The resultant ostium should be at least 2.0 cm × 1.5 cm at the completion of the operation. This will provide adequate access for endoscopic surveillance and debridement of the common frontal sinus cavities in the clinic (Fig. 9.5).

Postoperative Care

Optimum medical treatment is required to reduce mucosal inflammation and subsequent stenosis or obstruction and hence ensure a successful outcome. A combination of postoperative antibiotics for 10 days, high-dose mucolytics, intranasal steroid sprays and twice daily nasal saline irrigations using syringe or mechanized irrigation devices is recommended. In highly refractory cases such as hyperplastic sinusitis and nasal polyposis, asthma, Samter's triad, or eosinophilia with or without polyposis, patients may benefit from short-term tapering doses of oral steroids. Endoscopic debridement of nasal crusts in the clinic 1 week postoperatively and every 2 weeks thereafter until the wound has been cleaned reduces bacterial and/or fungal load and aids in mucosal healing. Follow-up on a regular basis after mucosal healing is complete should be performed to monitor the disease process and ensure that restenosis does not occur.

Outcomes and Complications

Complications of the endoscopic modified Lothrop procedure are:

- Frontal ostium stenosis
- Orbital injury
- Intracranial injury
- Epistaxis
- Adhesions

Frontal ostium stenosis is the most common complication and it will adversely affect successful outcomes. Although outcomes based on shorter follow-up times have demonstrated frontal ostium patency rates of 90–95% [8, 10, 11], at least 12–18 months is required for stabilization of the operative site. Studies with longer mean follow-up times (20–40 months) have demonstrated reduced patency rates ranging from 57 to 93% [2, 7, 12, 17]. Up to 20% of patients have been reported to require revision surgery secondary to frontal sinus stenosis and failed cases requiring an osteoplastic flap procedure have been reported in up to 18% of patients [12]. If one takes revision surgery and resolution of patient symptoms, the overall success rate of the endoscopic modified Lothrop procedure is on the order of 82–90%. These results are comparable to the success rates of the osteoplastic flap procedure.

Orbital and intracranial injuries are the major complications of this surgery. Owing to the proximity of the surgery to the skull base, the risk of CSF rhinorrhea and pneumocephalus is higher than that associated with standard endoscopic sinus surgery, but is not substantially different from that of the osteoplastic flap procedure [13]. Despite this, none of the studies have reported more than one patient having skull base violations. Minor complications such as epistaxis and adhesions can be seen in up to 25% of cases. This high number reflects the higher degree of complexity and aggressiveness of the endoscopic modified Lothrop procedure.

Future Directions

The endoscopic modified Lothrop procedure is mainly used in patients with recalcitrant frontal sinusitis. Its use is expanded for the treatment of mucoceles, inverted papillomas invading the frontal sinus, osteomas, and frontal sinus trauma. Although short-term results are favorable, longer follow-up is required to determine the efficacy of this procedure especially in cases of mucoceles, where recurrence can occur up to 20 years postoperatively. Although the osteoplastic flap procedure is still considered the "gold standard," the endoscopic modified Lothrop procedure is quickly becoming the procedure of choice for the treatment of complex frontal sinus disease.

Tips and Pearls

1. Sagittally reconstructed CT scans are required to assess a patient's candidacy for the endoscopic modified Lothrop procedure.
   (a) Ideally, an anteroposterior dimension at the cephalad margin of the frontal recess between the nasal bones at the root of the nose and the anterior skull base should be at least 1.5 cm.
   (b) Ideally, the nasofrontal beak should be less than 1 cm.
   (c) If the above dimensions are not ideal, then the accessible dimension should be at least 5 mm.
2. The number and the location of frontal recess cells should be determined in order to know the number of barriers needed to be removed to reach the frontal sinus ostium.
3. When drilling, care is taken not to violate the mucosa on the lateral and posterior wall of the frontal recess in order to prevent complications and postoperative stenosis.
4. A large septectomy is required to provide better instrument access and adequate drainage of frontal sinuses and to prevent postoperative crusting.
5. Aggressive preoperative and postoperative medical management and regular surveillance is required to improve successful surgical outcomes and prevent disease recurrence.

References

1. Becker DG, Moore D, Lindsey WH, Gross WE, Gross CW. (1995) Modified transnasal endoscopic Lothrop procedure: further considerations. *Laryngoscope* 105:1161–1166.

2. Casiano RR, Livingston JA. (1998) Endoscopic Lothrop procedure: the University of Miami experience. *Am J Rhinol* 12:335–339.

3. Catalano PJ, Lawson W, Som P, Biller HF. (1991) Radiographic evaluation and diagnosis of the failed frontal osteoplastic flap with fat obliteration. *Otolaryngol Head Neck Surg* 104:225–234.

4. Chen C, Selva D, Wormald PJ. (2004) Endoscopic modified lothrop procedure: an alternative for frontal osteoma excision. *Rhinology* 42:239–243.

5. Farhat FT, Figueroa RE, Kountakis SE. (2005) Anatomic measurements for the endoscopic modified Lothrop procedure. *Am J Rhinol* 19:293–296.

6. Gross CW, Harrison SE. (2001) The modified Lothrop procedure: indications, results, and complications. *Otolaryngol Clin North Am* 34:133–137.

7. Gross CW, Schlosser RJ. (2001) The modified Lothrop procedure: lessons learned. *Laryngoscope* 111:1302–1305.

8. Gross CW, Zachmann GC, Becker DGet al. (1997) Follow-up of University of Virginia experience with the modified Lothrop procedure. *Am J Rhinol* 11:49–54.

9. Gross WE, Gross CW, Becker D, Moore D, Phillips D. (1995) Modified transnasal endoscopic Lothrop procedure as an alternative to frontal sinus obliteration. *Otolaryngol Head Neck Surg* 113:427–434.

10. Khong JJ, Malhotra R, Selva D, Wormald PJ. (2004) Efficacy of endoscopic sinus surgery for paranasal sinus mucocele including modified endoscopic Lothrop procedure for frontal sinus mucocele. *J Laryngol Otol* 118:352–356.

11. Kountakis SE, Gross CW. (2003) Long-term results of the Lothrop operation. *Curr Opin Otolaryngol Head Neck Surg* 11:37–40.

12. Schlosser RJ, Zachmann G, Harrison S, Gross CW. (2002) The endoscopic modified Lothrop: long-term follow-up on 44 patients. *Am J Rhinol* 16:103–108.

13. Scott NA, Wormald P, Close D, Gallagher R, Anthony A, Maddern GJ. (2003) Endoscopic modified Lothrop procedure for the treatment of chronic frontal sinusitis: a systematic review. *Otolaryngol Head Neck Surg* 129:427–438.

14. Sonnenburg RE, Senior BA. (2004) Revision endoscopic frontal sinus surgery. *Curr Opin Otolaryngol Head Neck Surg* 12:49–52.

15. Ulualp SO, Carlson TK, Toohill RJ. (2000) Osteoplastic flap versus modified endoscopic Lothrop procedure in patients with frontal sinus disease. *Am J Rhinol* 14:21–26.

16. Weber R, Draf W, Kratzsch B, Hosemann W, Schaefer SD. (2001) Modern concepts of frontal sinus surgery. *Laryngoscope* 111:137–146.

17. Wormald PJ. (2003) Salvage frontal sinus surgery: the endoscopic modified Lothrop procedure. *Laryngoscope* 113:276–283.

18. Wormald PJ, Ananda A, Nair S. (2003) The modified endoscopic Lothrop procedure in the treatment of complicated chronic frontal sinusitis. *Clin Otolaryngol Allied Sci* 28:215–220.

19. Wormald PJ, Chan SZ. (2003) Surgical techniques for the removal of frontal recess cells obstructing the frontal ostium. *Am J Rhinol* 17:221–226.

Surgery for Hyperplastic Rhinosinusitis and Nasal Polyposis

Joseph M. Scianna, James A. Stankiewicz

Core Messages

- The typical complaints that a patient with hyperplastic rhinosinusitis presents with polyposis are nasal obstruction and anosmia.

- Important in establishing the history of hyperplastic rhinosinusitis and nasal polyposis is the establishment of previous therapy for the condition.

- Preoperative nasal endoscopy with determination of the extent of disease and visibility of normal anatomic structures such as the uncinate process and middle turbinate is essential.

- Computed tomography evaluation is essential in preoperative planning.

- All risks of surgery should be clear and understood by the patient.

- Successful surgical outcomes require continued postoperative medical therapy.

- The key first step in safe sinus surgery in patients with polyps is establishment of the normal sinus anatomy.

- Constant visualization of instrumentation throughout the surgery will aid in prevention of inadvertent injury to the lamina papyracea or skull base.

- During endoscopic sinus surgery, positioning the microdebrider window at 90° from the lamina papyracea will avoid inadvertent damage to orbital fat and contents in situations with either and iatrogenic or inherent dehiscence of the lamina.

- Identifying the horizontal basal lamella will help avoid damage to the sphenopalatine artery and maintain the structural integrity of the middle turbinate.

- If the frontal recess does not require manipulation, avoid disruption of the mucosa in the area.

- If polyps recur, they first recur in the frontal recess; however, this does not bother most patients.

Contents

Introduction

The term "rhinosinusitis" covers a broad spectrum of disease processes that develop from both environmental and host factors [27]. Rhinosinusitis can be acute, subacute (less than 3 months' duration), or an acute exacerbation of chronic rhinosinusitis [27]. Hyperplastic rhinosinusitis refers to the inflammatory response of normal nasal mucosa and its associated nasal polyp formation [43]. Many theories exist regarding the formation of nasal polyps; however, the exact mechanism of nasal polyp formation is not yet understood [35]. Nasal polyps are present in 5% of nonatopic individuals and only 1.5% of people with allergic rhinitis [16]. No racial or sexual predilection is reported. The prevalence is increased in patients with cystic fibrosis and aspirin-hypersensitivity syndrome (Samter's triad) [19, 22].

10

Preoperative Evaluation

Preoperative evaluation of the sinus patient begins with a complete otolaryngologic history and physical examination [20]. The typical complaints that a patient with hyperplastic rhinosinusitis presents with polyposis are nasal obstruction and anosmia [24]. A significant number of patients will have a history of repeated sinus infections, headache, and may have a medical history significant for asthma and aspirin sensitivity [11]. Environmental allergy may also be prevalent [1]. Since the major complaint associated with hyperplastic rhinosinusitis and nasal polyposis is subjective in nature, many institutions advocate the use a preoperative sinonasal questionnaire. Many different questionnaires exist in the literature and all are focused on defining the baseline symptomatology of the disease as well as the level of exacerbation of the disease process [13].

Important in establishing the history of hyperplastic rhinosinusitis and nasal polyposis is the establishment of previous therapy for the condition [50]. The use of nasal inhaled steroids, oral steroids, prolonged periods of antibiotic use, and history of previous nasal or sinus surgery provide important information and establish the failure of medical therapy for the disease process [9]. In many instances, medical therapy including an oral steroid and 4–8 weeks of antibiotics provided intermittent relief of symptoms, but rapid return to the baseline upon cessation of therapy [14].

A history of nasal trauma, midface trauma, or previous surgery is an important consideration of preoperative planning. Patients with such histories can pose a variety of problems. Dehiscence of the lamina papyracea, or other intranasal anatomic alterations may occur in such traumas [36]. In addition, nasal trauma with severe deviation may necessitate septoplasty in order for surgical resection of nasal polyposis to be performed [23].

As with all patients, a thorough medical history to assess the risk of anesthesia, a propensity for bleeding, and the use of both prescribed anticoagulants as well as herbal supplements which may influence clotting ability is necessary [47]. It is important to establish a social history with emphasis on tobacco use and exposure as well as environmental exposures that may contribute to nasal irritation. A complete review of systems with attention to endocrine disorders such as diabetes, immunologic disorders such as HIV and γ-globulin deficiencies, as well as systemic disorders such as Wegener's granulomatosis provides significant diagnostic information.

A complete head and neck examination is routine in preoperative evaluation [20]. Special attention is taken during the assessment of the nose and nasal structures. Nasal polyposis can rarely lead to visible nasal or facial deformity [28]. Anterior rhinoscopy can demonstrate the extent of polyposis (Fig. 10.1) and the percentage of airway blockage. In addition to visible polyposis, evaluation of the turbinate structures and nasal septum help determine other potential causes for airway obstruction. Evaluation of the

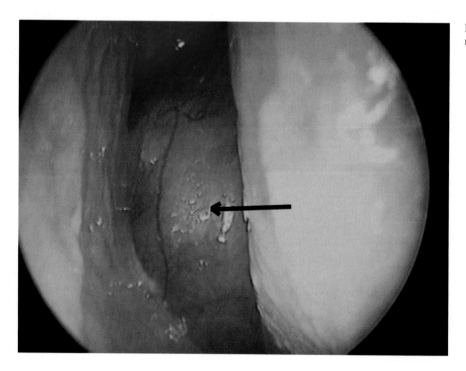

Fig. 10.1. Obstructing nasal polyp (*arrow*)

response of the nasal mucosa of the inferior turbinates to a vasoconstrictive agent such as neosynephrine may also aid in isolating the pathogenesis of nasal obstruction [39].

Nasal endoscopy is very important in the preoperative evaluation of the hyperplastic rhinosinusitis patient [40]. Determination of the extent of disease and visibility of normal anatomic structures such as the uncinate process and middle turbinate are essential. The presence of pus, indicative of active infection, or allergic mucin, thick mucus with a peanut-butter-like appearance and consistency, may be visible [46] (Fig. 10.2).

Laboratory evaluation for hyperplastic rhinosinusitis patients:

- Begins with an allergy screening [17]. Many different allergy-screening tests exist; from the radioallergosorbent test (RAST) to the Multi-Test II skin prick tests. Determining if atopy plays a role in the hyperplastic rhinosinusitis patient is important for postoperative prevention of nasal polyp recurrence [12].
- Evaluation of the total immunoglobulin E level may be indicative of allergic fungal disease, with or without polyposis [38].
- Other laboratory tests that may be beneficial but that are cost-inhibitive include screening for γ-globulin deficiencies [37, 48]. Such tests may be more beneficial in the recalcitrant patient [8].
- The chloride sweat test is a necessary adjunct to the evaluation of the pediatric patient, but is generally not necessary in the adult population [2].

Computed tomography (CT) evaluation is essential in preoperative planning. A screening coronal sinus CT scan (5-mm coronal images) provides essential input into the extent of disease as well as the anatomic structure of the patient [25]. Identification of the level of the skull base and the status of the lamina papyracea is essential prior to operative intervention and prevention of complications [42] (Fig. 10.3). Other important information that can be obtained includes the status of the nasal septum as well as the presence of a concha bullosa that may be contributing to sinonasal obstruction. Heterogenicity of an opacified sinus may be indicative of a fungal ball, whereas bowing of boney structures may be more indicative of mucocele formation [4].

Tips and Pearls

Preoperative CT evaluation:

- Determine the extent of involvement
- Identify the lamina papyracea
- Identify the level of skull base/cribiform plate
- Identify the presence of a concha bullosa

While the screening sinus CT scan provides a cost-efficient evaluation of important bony anatomy, a three-dimensional CT scan such as those used for computerized guidance during surgery may provide additional information in significant detail [44]. While the computer-guided three-dimensional imagery can be an effective adjunct to surgical intervention, it is

Fig. 10.2. Fungal mucin (*arrow*)

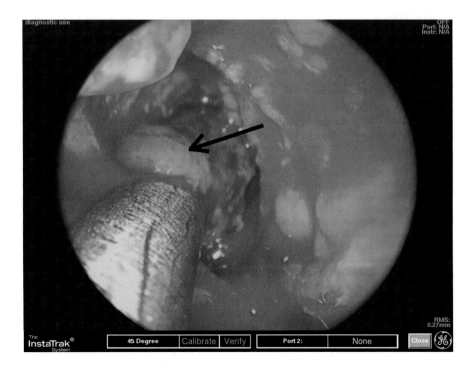

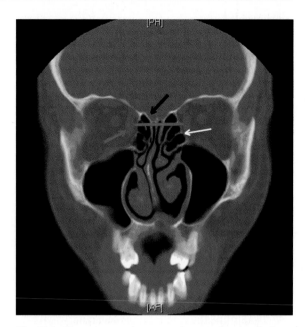

Fig. 10.3. Sinus computed tomography scan showing the lamina papyracea (*white arrow*), medial rectus (*red arrow*), relation of the skull base to the medial rectus (*red line*) and lateral lamella (*black arrow*)

not the standard of care for primary nasal polyp surgery, nor should it be used in lieu of an understanding of the sinonasal anatomy as viewed through an endoscope [33]. Magnetic resonance imaging provides little useful adjunctive information with respect to surgical planning [32].

Indications for sinus surgery for hyperplastic rhinosinusitis/nasal polyposis are as follows:

1. Absolute
   (a) Orbital abscess secondary to acute infection
   (b) Frontal lobe abscess/meningitis secondary to acute infection
   (c) Mucocele
   (d) Fungal mycetoma
2. Relative
   (a) Chronic rhinosinusitis failing medical therapy
   (b) Headaches
   (c) Facial pain
   (d) Recurrent acute sinusitis
   (e) Obstructive nasal polyposis
   (f) Asthma exacerbations in patients with Samter's triad

Operative Procedure

Prior to any operative procedure, a valid and explicit informed consent discussion should occur [29]. Within this discussion, all risks of surgery should be clear and understood by the patient.

Risks of surgery include [45]:

- Recurrent disease requiring repeat or revision surgery
- Entrance into the orbit resulting in blindness
- Double vision
- Violation of the skull base resulting in CSF leak
- Meningitis
- Brain damage
- Death

An understanding that surgical resection of nasal polyps and maintenance of the sinonasal cavity will require continued postoperative medical therapy is also essential.

Tips and Pearls

Surgical goals:

- Define normal anatomy first
- Use maxillary antrostomy to establish the level of the sphenoid ostium and lamina papyracea
- Identify the level of the skull base posteriorly at the sphenoid and proceed from posterior, superior to anterior superior through the ethmoids
- Avoid disruption of the frontal recess if unnecessary
- Preserve normal mucosa

After establishment of informed consent, and prior to preparation in the operating room, an intranasal vasoconstrictive agent such as oxymetazoline begins the operative preparation. The choice of anesthetic used is up to the surgeon and patient. While endoscopic sinus surgery can be performed under local anesthetic or with minimal sedation, general anesthesia is routinely used. General anesthesia is favorable for the comfort of the patient and provides a comfortable teaching environment in educational institutions [10].

After induction of anesthesia, with the patient in a supine position the bed is placed in a slight reverse Trendelenburg position and the bed is rotated to the patient's right. The patient's head is also turned slightly to the right and is placed in a foam headrest to maintain this position. This provides ideal positioning for the right-handed surgeon and helps avoid complications while working in the left nasal cavity.

Nasal preparation then continues with injection of 1% lidocaine with 1:100,000 epinephrine into the nasal cavity. Ideally the medial maxillary wall, anterior and superior to the uncinate process, can be injected. Injections into the middle turbinate as well as any visible polyps are also made. After injection of both nasal cavities, insertion of 4% cocaine pledgets proceeds. Placing of a cocaine-soaked pledget lateral to the middle turbinate in the middle meatus aids in vasoconstriction of this area. This is not always possible depending on the extent of the nasal polyp disease. Several institutions employ pledgets soaked in topical epinephrine at strengths varying from 1:1,000 to 1:100,000 to further aid in hemostasis.

After injection, a throat pack is placed intraorally to dissuade ingestion of blood during the surgery. While the surgeon proceeds to scrub, the patient is prepped and draped by the nursing staff. Care is taken to ensure that both eyes are clearly visible during the surgery. Taping of the lateral canthus will provide eye closure and protection from external abrasion, while providing the surgeon with the opportunity to see orbital transillumination intraoperatively.

Once the surgical field has been established, the 0° endoscope is connected to the operative camera and monitor displays are positioned to the comfort of the surgeon. While monitors are not essential for endoscopic sinus surgery, they allow the surgeon to operate in the upright position and avoid undue strain on the back and neck. If computer-guided imagery is being employed, registration of equipment should take place at this time. Foot pedals operating the microdebrider and endoscope sleeve washers should be positioned appropriately.

While either nasal cavity can be primarily dealt with, a septal deviation to one side may allow for easy access to the contralateral side. The key first step is establishment of the normal sinus anatomy. Specific structures to be identified are the nasal septum, inferior turbinate, middle turbinate, uncinate process, as well as the nasopharynx posterior, inferiorly. If nasal polypoid disease is obstructing these structures,

careful conservative dissection of the polypoid tissues will allow for visualization.

If a concha bullosa is present, it may be contributing to the obstruction of the natural os of the maxillary sinus and hinder surgical progress. The concha bullosa may be resected with every attempt made to maintain the integrity of the middle turbinate [5]. Injection of 1% lidocaine with epinephrine followed by anterior incision of the concha bullosa proceeds with a sickle blade. With an opening into the concha bullosa established, straight punch forceps can be used to remove the lateral wall of the concha bullosa while preserving the mucosa of the lateral aspect of the medial wall of the middle turbinate (Fig. 10.4). Loose fragments of bone can be trimmed with punch forceps or carefully removed with grasping forceps. Care should be taken when using grasping forceps to avoid tearing or shearing of normal sinus mucosa. In general, posterior and inferior directed movements after grasping of bone fragments that may still have a mucosal attachment will help prevent tearing of the mucosa.

Once the middle meatus is visible, attention can be turned to the uncinate process. Often secondary to polyposis, the uncinate process is displaced anteriorly and medially. Care should be taken to identify the uncinate process and ensure that a space exists between the anterior lamina papyracea and the uncinate process. A Lusk probe can be used to palpate this area if necessary. The uncinate process is then cleaved in half with use of the microfranz backbiting forceps. This instrument should only be opened to an acute angle to prevent inadvertent trauma to the lamina papyracea and exposure of orbital contents (Fig. 10.5). The uncinate process should be resected to its anteriormost limit with avoidance of damage to the lacrimal sac. A Lusk probe can then be used to displace the superior and inferior uncinate remnants anteriorly for

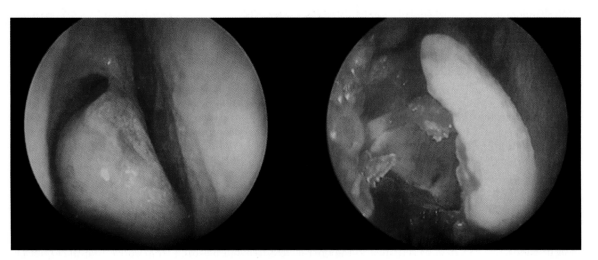

Fig. 10.4. Concha bullosa before resection (*right*) and after entrance (*left*)

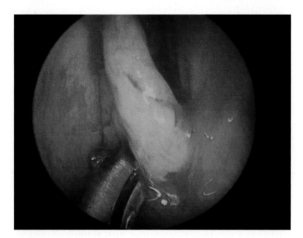

Fig. 10.5. Backbiting forceps at an acute angle

resection with the microdebrider. Care should be taken to avoid damage to the normal mucosa of the maxillary wall behind the uncinate process.

Tips and Pearls

Avoidance of complications:

- Adequate visualization of normal structures
- Careful probing of the uncinate process and natural maxillary os
- Opening of the backbiting instrument at an acute angle
- Avoid the microdebriding window facing laterally
- Maintenance of the relationship of the orbit of the maxillary antrostomy and sphenoid os
- Awareness of the lateral lamella medially along the superior skull base

A 30° telescope can then be used to identify the natural os of the maxillary sinus. Again this may be obstructed by polyps, in which case visible polyps should be removed from the area. Positioning the microdebrider window at 90° from the lamina papyracea will avoid inadvertent damage to orbital fat and contents in situations with either and iatrogenic or inherent dehiscence of the lamina [18]. With careful identification of the natural os of the maxillary sinus, a probe can be introduced and the os can be dilated posteriorly and inferiorly creating a wide maxillary antrostomy (Video 10.1). Remember that the superior limit of the antrostomy is the orbit. Any disease in and around the maxillary sinus can then be removed with either a straight microdebrider or a curved microdebrider (Fig. 10.6). Avoidance of circumferential trauma around the antrostomy will help avoid cicatricial scarring.

A 0° endoscope can then be returned to the operative field. Identification of the ethmoid bulla should

then proceed. Entrance into the bulla with resection of bone and polypoid disease should proceed with preservation of the mucosa overlying the lamina papyracea laterally (Video 10.2). Identifying the horizontal basal lamella will help avoid damage to the sphenopalatine artery and maintain the structural integrity of the middle turbinate.

To enter the posterior ethmoid, the inferior and medial aspect of the vertical basal lamella must be removed with the microdebrider. Preoperative identification on a CT scan of a posterior ethmoid cell lateral and superior to the sphenoid sinus (the Onodi cell) will ensure a complete ethmoidectomy. Once the inferior, posterior ethmoid cells have been adequately removed, the natural os of the sphenoid sinus must be identified. Using a calibrated probe, one can identify the anterior wall of the sphenoid at approximately 7 cm from the nasal sill at a 30° angle. Visualization of the sphenoid os can also be accomplished with resection of the lower third of the superior turbinate. In most cases, the natural os of the sphenoid lies just medial to or directly posterior to the lower third of the superior turbinate [21] (Fig. 10.7).

Again, the calibrate probe can be used and the posterior wall of the sphenoid sinus can be carefully palpated. In an adult the posterior wall of the sphenoid sinus lies 9 cm from the nasal sill at a 30° angle. If available, computer guidance can be used for localization [7]. The natural sphenoid os can be initially widened inferiorly and medially with strict avoidance of disruption of the normal mucosa of the sphenoid sinus (Video 10.3). This initial widening can be accomplished with various punch forceps. Further widening can be accomplished with a microdebrider. Again a wide sphenoidotomy can be created, but avoidance of circumferential damage will prevent postoperative closure secondary to cicatricial scarring.

With the accomplishment of a sphenoidotomy, the posterior aspect of the skull base can be identified (Fig. 10.8). Now with the lamina papyracea and skull base defined, total ethmoidectomy and disease removal can proceed in a posterior to anterior direction. With use of either a curved suction device or other blunt curved instrumentation, the ethmoid cell septations are fractured anteriorly, working tangentially along the skull base. Avoid upward movements of the instrumentation to prevent inadvertent entrance into the skull base and angle the blunt instrument slightly laterally to avoid damage to the lateral lamella of the ethmoid bone. Again, if available, computer localization can be used.

The ethmoidectomy is continued anteriorly and superiorly through the most anterior cells, or suprabullar cells (Video 10.4).

The frontal recess and agger nasi cells are opened last to avoid bleeding from above that may interfere with visualization with the endoscope. To open an

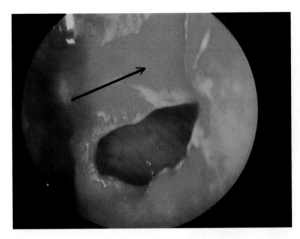

Fig. 10.6. Wide maxillary antrostomy. Note its teardrop shape and the lamina papyracea as the superior limit (*arrow*)

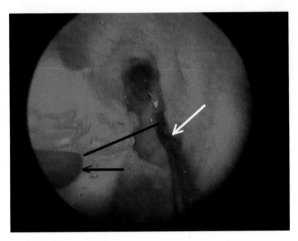

Fig. 10.7. Identification of the sphenoid. The *black arrow* is pointing to the maxillary antrostomy and the *white arrow* is pointing to beaded probe in the sphenoid sinus. The *black line* demonstrates the common level of the maxillary antrostomy and sphenoid os

agger nasi cell which may be contiguous with the lacrimal sac, entrance into the cell in its most inferior medial extent or from a posterior to anterior direction will prevent iatrogenic damage. If the frontal recess does not require manipulation, avoid disruption of this mucosa at all costs. The frontal recess is prone to scarring secondary to the attachment of the middle turbinate [51]. A curved probe or curette can be used to identify the frontal recess. A 30° or 45° endoscope can also be used to aid in its visualization (Video 10.5). Polyps can be removed with up-biting forceps or a curved microdebrider. Simple removal of the back wall of the agger nasi cell will usually suffice. It is important to remember the first place polyps recur is in the frontal recess; however, most patients with nasal polyps are not bothered by their frontal sinus disease. Indications for frontal osteoplastic surgery in patients with polypoid disease are based upon persistent bacterial or fungal disease, complicated chronic sinusitis, and frontal sinus pain refractory to medical therapy. Again, careful avoidance of disruption of normal sinus mucosa will prevent inadvertent scarring.

With all the sinuses open and identified, the microdebrider can be used to remove any residual disease. On occasion, disease may actually be located along the medial aspect of the middle turbinate. This disease should be removed with caution since it is this disease removal which can lead to a CSF leak from the lateral lamella. Careful removal of loose bony fragments will prevent postoperative crusting and bleeding. Conservative use of a suction electrocautery device can minimize postoperative bleeding. If the middle turbinate integrity has been disrupted and concern exists regarding potential for lateralization, a medialization procedure can be performed. With use of a sickle-bladed knife the mucosa of the medial wall of the middle turbinate is damaged. A corresponding mucosal violation occurs along the nasal septum (Video 10.6). The middle turbinate is then held in position with a small pack placed between the anterior aspect of the middle turbinate and the medial wall of the maxillary sinus [15].

In general, extensive packing is not required [34]. Light packing placed in the middle meatus can provide adequate hemostasis for a patient with persistent ooze [30]. Anticoagulant gels are rarely necessary but may be helpful [3, 6]. Lower packs along the floor of the nasal cavity may be temporarily placed if a septoplasty is performed and removed prior to the patient being discharged from the recovery room [49]. The throat pack should then be removed and the stomach suctioned prior to cessation of anesthesia. Once the patient is awake, careful assessment of mental status and vision should occur and be documented appropriately.

Postoperative Care

For patients with extensive hyperplastic rhinosinusitis with nasal polyposis, oral steroids are provided in the immediate postoperative period with a gradual taper over a 1-week period. Patients with obvious fungal disease should be considered for long-term steroid tapers over a 3–4-week period. Postoperative pain medication is provided as well as antibiotic coverage for those patients with nasal packing or for those with evidence of acute infection at the time of surgery. Nasal packing is removed 3–5 days postoperatively with gentle suctioning at the time of packing removal. Nasal saline irrigations can be used to maintain a clear and clean nasal cavity.

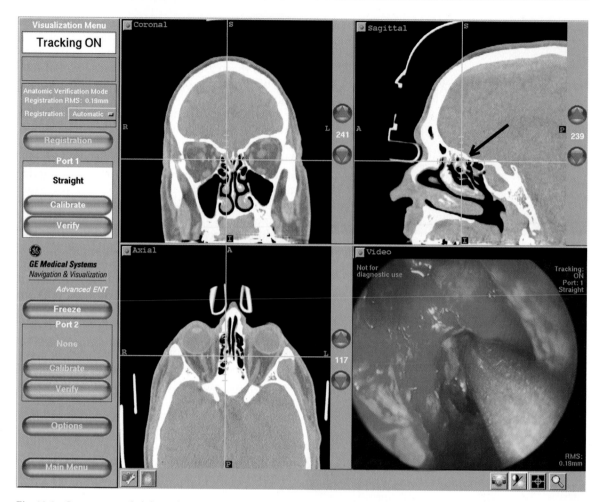

Fig. 10.8. Computer-guided three-dimensional localization of the skull base (*arrow*)

Careful and close follow-up in the postoperative period will help ensure surgical success. Packing may be replaced to help avoid middle turbinate lateralization. Repeat courses of either an oral steroid or antibiotics can be key adjuncts to maintenance of a patent and a healthy nasal cavity. Attenuation of allergic responses with oral or inhaled allergy medication can also prevent recurrence of the hyperplastic response. In most patients with hyperplastic rhinosinusitis with nasal polyps, continued use of a nasal inhaled steroid is required for prevention of recurrent disease [31].

Complications of Surgery

Minor complications are:

- Minor epistaxis
- Hyposmia

- Adhesions
- Headache
- Periorbital ecchymosis
- Periorbital emphysema
- Dental/facial pain

Major complications are:

- Severe epistaxis
- Orbital hematoma
- Diplopia
- Blindness
- Decreased visual acuity
- Intracranial hemorrhage
- Anosmia
- Nasolacrimal duct trauma
- Meningitis
- Pneumocephalus
- Carotid injury
- Death

The list of complications from endoscopic sinus surgery is long and extensive [41]; however, careful understanding of the anatomy and constant visualization will help prevent the majority of these complications [26]. Most minor complications can be dealt with by careful attention during the postoperative period. Understanding that nasal polypoid disease can distort anatomy and obscure anatomy will provide the first step to avoidance of major complications. Constant visualization of instrumentation throughout the surgery will aid in prevention of inadvertent injury to the lamina papyracea or skull base. Careful dissection of mucosa and boney structures will help prevent iatrogenic injury to the normal sinus mucosa and thus prevent unpredictable scarring and surgical failure. Immediate identification of intraoperative trauma to the skull base or lamina papyracea at the time of occurrence will help prevent further damage to vital structures such as the orbital contents or dura. Once an intraoperative complication has been identified, careful planning of intraoperative management as well as postoperative management should proceed. Discussions with anesthesia and nursing staff should occur, and intraoperative or postoperative consultations with associated departments should be arranged (i.e., neurosurgical consultation or ophthalmologic consultation). Frank discussions of necessary adjunctive treatments, procedures, and hospitalizations should occur. In general, however, with careful attention to detail, proper training and visualization, major complications are a rare occurrence.

Summary

Hyperplastic rhinosinusitis with nasal polyps represents a reactive, inflammatory disease that results in nasal obstruction, hyposmia, recurrent sinus infection, recalcitrant sinus infections, headache, and asthma exacerbations. Allergies as well as conditions like cystic fibrosis and Samter's triad can all play a role in the hyperreactive disorder. Medical therapy can provide relief in some patients, but a considerable number of patients require surgical intervention to establish a patent sinonasal cavity. Surgical intervention requires careful planning and attentive surgical technique. Preservation and identification of normal anatomic structures is essential. Success rates with a single surgery and adequate postoperative medical therapy can approach between 85 and 90%.

References

1. Asero R, Bottazzi G (Mar 2001) Nasal polyposis: a study of its association with airborne allergen hypersensitivity. Annals of Allergy, Asthma, & Immunology. 86(3):283–5.
2. Batsakis JG, El-Naggar AK (Apr 1996) Cystic fibrosis and the sinonasal tract. Annals of Otology, Rhinology & Laryngology. 105(4):329–30.
3. Baumann A, Caversaccio M (Dec 2003) Hemostasis in endoscopic sinus surgery using a specific gelatin-thrombin based agent (FloSeal). Rhinology. 41(4):244–9.
4. Bhattacharyya N (Aug 2005) Symptom and disease severity differences between nasal septal deviation and chronic rhinosinusitis. Otolaryngology – Head & Neck Surgery. 133(2):173–7.
5. Bolger WE, Kuhn FA, Kennedy DW (Nov 1999) Middle turbinate stabilization after functional endoscopic sinus surgery: the controlled synechiae technique. Laryngoscope. 109(11):1852–3.
6. Chandra RK, Conley DB, Haines GK III, Kern RC (May–Jun 2005) Long-term effects of FloSeal packing after endoscopic sinus surgery. American Journal of Rhinology. 19(3):240–3.
7. Citardi MJ, Gallivan RP, Batra PS, Maurer CR Jr, Rohlfing T, Roh HJ, Lanza DC (May–Jun 2004) Quantitative computer-aided computed tomography analysis of sphenoid sinus anatomical relationships. American Journal of Rhinology. 18(3):173–8.
8. Coste A, Girodon E, Louis S, Pruliere-Escabasse V, Goossens M, Peynegre R, Escudier E (May 2004) Atypical sinusitis in adults must lead to looking for cystic fibrosis and primary ciliary dyskinesia. Laryngoscope. 114(5):839–43.
9. Damm M, Quante G, Jungehuelsing M, Stennert E (2002) Impact of functional endoscopic sinus surgery on symptoms and quality of life in chronic rhinosinusitis. Laryngoscope; 112:310–5.
10. Danielsen A, Gravningsbraten R, Olofsson J, (Oct 2003) Anaesthesia in endoscopic sinus surgery European Archives of Oto-Rhino-Laryngology. 260(9):481–6.
11. Deal RT, Kountakis SE (Nov 2004) Significance of nasal polyps in chronic rhinosinusitis: symptoms and surgical outcomes. Laryngoscope. 114(11):1932–5.
12. Dursun E, Korkmaz H, Eryilmaz A, Bayiz U, Sertkaya D, Samim E (Nov 2003) Clinical predictors of long-term success after endoscopic sinus surgery. Otolaryngology – Head & Neck Surgery. 129(5):526–31.
13. Fahmy FF, McCombe A, Mckiernan DC (Dec 2002) Sino nasal assessment questionnaire, a patient focused, rhinosinusitis specific outcome measure. Rhinology. 40(4):195–7.
14. Fokkens W, Lund V, Bachert C, Clement P, Helllings P, Holmstrom M, Jones N, Kalogjera L, Kennedy D, Kowalski M, Malmberg H, Mullol J, Passali D, Stammberger H, Stierna P (May 2005) EAACI. EAACI position paper on rhinosinusitis and nasal polyps executive summary. Allergy. 60(5):583–601.
15. Friedman M, Landsberg R, Tanyeri H (Jul 2000) Middle turbinate medialization and preservation in endoscopic sinus surgery. Otolaryngology – Head & Neck Surgery. 123(1 Pt 1):76–80.
16. Grigoreas C, Vourdas D, Petalas K., Simeonidis G, Demeroutis I, Tsioulos T (May–June 2002) Nasal polyps in patients with rhinitis and asthma. Allergy & Asthma Proceedings. 23(3):169–74.

17. Gutman M, Torres A, Keen KJ, Houser SM (May 2004) Prevalence of allergy in patients with chronic rhinosinusitis. Otolaryngology – Head & Neck Surgery. 130(5):545–52.

18. Hackman TG, Ferguson BJ (Feb 2005) Powered instrumentation and tissue effects in the nose and paranasal sinuses. Current Opinion in Otolaryngology & Head & Neck Surgery. 13(1):22–6.

19. Hadfield PJ, Rowe-Jones JM, Mackay IS (Feb 2000) The prevalence of nasal polyps in adults with cystic fibrosis. Clinical Otolaryngology & Allied Sciences. 25(1):19–22.

20. Hadley JA, Schaefer SD (Sep 1997) Clinical evaluation of rhinosinusitis: history and physical examination. Otolaryngology – Head & Neck Surgery. 117(3 Pt 2):S8–11.

21. Har-El G, Swanson RM (Mar-Apr 2001) The superior turbinectomy approach to isolated sphenoid sinus disease and to the sella turcica. American Journal of Rhinology. 15(2):149–56.

22. Hedman J, Kaprio J, Poussa T, Nieminen MM (Aug 1999) Prevalence of asthma, aspirin intolerance, nasal polyposis and chronic obstructive pulmonary disease in a population-based study. International Journal of Epidemiology. 28(4):717–22.

23. Hwang PH, McLaughlin RB, Lanza DC, Kennedy DW (May 1999) Endoscopic septoplasty: indications, technique, and results. Otolaryngology – Head & Neck Surgery. 120(5):678–82.

24. Johansson L, Bramerson A, Holmberg K, Melen I, Akerlund A, Bende M (Jan 2004) Clinical relevance of nasal polyps in individuals recruited from a general population-based study. Acta Oto-Laryngologica. 124(1):77–81.

25. Kaluskar SK,. Patil NP, Sharkey AN (Jun 1993) The role of CT in functional endoscopic sinus surgery. Rhinology. 31(2):49–52.

26. Keerl R, Stankiewicz J, Weber R, Hosemann W, Draf W (Apr 1999) Surgical experience and complications during endonasal sinus surgery. Laryngoscope. 109(4):546–50.

27. Lanza DC, Kennedy DW (1997) Adult rhinosinusitis defined. Otolaryngology – Head and Neck Surgery 117:S1–S7.

28. Liang EY, Lam WW, Woo JK, Van Hasselt CA, Metreweli C (1996) Another CT sign of sinonasal polyposis: truncation of the bony middle turbinate. European Radiology. 6(4):553–6.

29. Lynn-Macrae AG, Lynn-Macrae RA, Emani J, Kern RC, Conley DB (Aug 2004) Medicolegal analysis of injury during endoscopic sinus surgery. Laryngoscope. 114(8):1492–5.

30. Muluk NB, Oguzturk O, Ekici A, Koc C (Jun 2005) Emotional effects of nasal packing measured by the Hospital Anxiety and Depression Scale in patients following nasal surgery. Journal of Otolaryngology. 34(3):172–7.

31. Mygind N, Dahl R, Nielsen LP, Hilberg O, Bjerke T (1997) Effect of corticosteroids on nasal blockage in rhinitis measured by objective methods. Allergy. 52(40 Suppl):39–44.

32. Okuyemi KS, Tsue TT (Nov 2002) Radiologic imaging in the management of sinusitis. American Family Physician. 66(10):1882–6.

33. Olson G, Citardi MJ (Sep 2000) Image-guided functional endoscopic sinus surgery. Otolaryngology – Head & Neck Surgery. 123(3):188–94.

34. Orlandi RR, Lanza DC (Sep 2004) Is nasal packing necessary following endoscopic sinus surgery? Laryngoscope. 114(9):1541–4.

35. Pawliczak R, Lewandowska-Polak A, Kowalski ML (Nov 2005) Pathogenesis of nasal polyps: an update. Current Allergy & Asthma Reports. 5(6):463–71.

36. Polavaram R, Devaiah AK, Sakai O, Shapshay SM (Apr 2004) Anatomic variants and pearls – functional endoscopic sinus surgery. Otolaryngologic Clinics of North America. 37(2):221–42.

37. Scadding GK, Lund VJ, Darby YC, Navas-Romero J, Seymour N, Turner MW, (Mar 1994) IgG subclass levels in chronic rhinosinusitis. Rhinology. 32(1):15–9.

38. Shin SH, Ponikau JU, Sherris DA, Congdon D, Frigas E, Homburger HA, Swanson MC, Gleich GJ, Kita H (Dec 2004) Chronic rhinosinusitis: an enhanced immune response to ubiquitous airborne fungi. Journal of Allergy & Clinical Immunology. 114(6):1369–75.

39. Sipila J, Antila J, Suonpaa J (1996) Pre- and postoperative evaluation of patients with nasal obstruction undergoing endoscopic sinus surgery. European Archives of Oto-Rhino-Laryngology. 253(4–5):237–9.

40. Smith TL, Mendolia-Loffredo S, Loehrl TA, Sparapani R, Laud PW, Nattinger AB (Dec 2005) Predictive factors and outcomes in endoscopic sinus surgery for chronic rhinosinusitis. Laryngoscope. 115(12):2199–205.

41. Stankiewicz JA (Aug 1989) Complications of endoscopic sinus surgery. Otolaryngologic Clinics of North America. 22(4):749–58.

42. Stankiewicz JA, Chow JM (Feb 2005) The low skull base – is it important? Current Opinion in Otolaryngology & Head & Neck Surgery. 13(1):19–21.

43. Steinke John W PhD, Borish Larry MD (July 2003) Clarification of terminology in patients with eosinophilic and noneosinophilic hyperplastic rhinosinusitis: Journal of Allergy & Clinical Immunology. 112(1):222–3.

44. Tabaee A, Kacker A, Kassenoff TL, Anand V (Sep–Oct 2003) Outcome of computer-assisted sinus surgery: a 5-year study. American Journal of Rhinology. 17(5):291–7.

45. Taylor RJ, Chiu AG, Palmer JN, Schofield K, O'Malley BW Jr, Wolf JS (May 2005) Informed consent in sinus surgery: link between demographics and patient desires. Laryngoscope. 115(5):826–31.

46. Thakar A, Sarkar C, Dhiwakar M, Bahadur S, Dahiya S (Feb 2004) Allergic fungal sinusitis: expanding the clinicopathologic spectrum. Otolaryngology – Head & Neck Surgery. 130(2):209–16.

47. Thaler ER, Gottschalk A (Nov–Dec 1997) Samaranayake R. Lanza DC. Kennedy DW. Anesthesia in endoscopic sinus surgery. American Journal of Rhinology. 11(6):409–13.

48. Van Kessel DA, Horikx PE, Van Houte AJ, De Graaff CS, Van Velzen-Blad H, Rijkers GT (Oct 1999) Clinical and immunological evaluation of patients with mild IgG1 deficiency. Clinical & Experimental Immunology. 118(1):102–7.

49. Weber R, Hochapfel F, Draf W (Jun 2000) Packing and stents in endonasal surgery. Rhinology. 38(2):49–62.

50. Williams JW Jr, Simel DL, Roberts L, Samsa GP (1992) Clinical evaluation for sinusitis. Making the diagnosis by history and physical examination. Ann Intern Med; 117:705–10.

51. Wormald PJ (Jun 2005) Surgery of the frontal recess and frontal sinus. Rhinology. 43(2):82–5.

Chapter 11

Allergic Fungal Rhinosinusitis – Surgical Management

11

Raghu S. Athre, Bradley F. Marple

Core Messages

- Allergic fungal rhinosinusitis (AFRS) describes a clinicopathological entity characterized by nasal polyposis, crust formation, atopy, fungal sinus cultures, and lack of tissue invasion on pathological analysis.

- The pathophysiology of AFRS involves the atopic host being exposed to fungal elements, which set up a cascade of inflammation, production of allergic mucin, and self-perpetuation.

- Addressing AFRS involves combining the surgical therapy with an ongoing medical management plan that addresses the underlying inflammatory nature of AFRS.

- Despite aggressive surgical and medical management, recidivism rate of AFRS remains high.

Contents

Introduction

The term allergic fungal rhinosinusitis (AFRS) has been used to describe a clinicopathological entity characterized by:

- Nasal polyposis
- Crust formation
- Atopy
- Sinus cultures with fungus present
- Lack of tissue invasion on pathological analysis [25]

Safirstein [33] first recognized the similarity between this entity and allergic bronchopulmonary aspergillosis in 1976. Since that time, a great deal of research has been devoted to the understanding, pathophysiology, and treatment of this disease. Despite these efforts, a large number of questions still remain unanswered and serve as the nidus for future clinical research.

The presence of fungus within the paranasal sinuses has a broad range of ramifications, ranging from the benign presence of saprophytic fungal growth to invasive fungal rhinosinusitis. The presence of fungus on cultures, the AFRS hallmarks of bony expansion, and radiological evidence of invasion led many clinicians to believe that AFRS was an early stage on the spectrum of invasive fungal rhinosinusitis [12, 25]; hence, an aggressive surgical stance was adopted as the primary mode of management of AFRS. McGuirt and Harrill [30] stated in 1979, "Without question, the treatment of paranasal sinus aspergillosis is surgical – the key to successful surgical treatment is the removal of diseased mucosa and aeration and drainage of the involved sinus." Such evidence urged surgeons to perform radical surgeries such as lateral rhinotomies, craniofacial resections, and facial degloving procedures to extirpate the diseased mucosa [26]. In 1988, Sarti et al. [34] reported a case of paranasal sinus aspergillosis that exhibited expansion into the anterior cranial fossa and sella turcica. The patient was treated with a craniofacial resection, and unfortunately died secondary to a pulmonary embolus in the postoperative period. However, on final pathological examination, no evidence of tissue invasion was noted.

Numerous studies have subsequently shown AFRS to be a separate clinical entity from invasive fungal rhinosinusitis and have implicated atopy as one of the causative factors. Manning and Holman [23] showed that in vitro and in vivo allergy to fungal antigens were important to the pathophysiology of AFRS and that the predominance of eosinophil-derived inflammatory mediators in in vivo tissue specimens differentiated AFRS from other forms of chronic rhinosinusitis. These studies gave further credence to the fact that AFRS is an immunological disease rather than an entity on the spectrum of infectious/invasive fungal disease. The change in mindset from invasive disease to immunologically based disease has altered the treatment algorithms for AFRS from that of extensive surgery and antifungal therapy to mucosa-sparing surgery with adjunctive corticosteroids [25].

Pathophysiology

The exact pathophysiology of AFRS has still yet to be determined. One of the more popular theories has been proposed by Manning et al. [22] and likens AFRS to allergic bronchopulmonary aspergillosis. In this model, the atopic host is first exposed to respiratory fungus. Respiratory fungus settles on the nasal mucosa and elicits an allergic response involving eosinophilic mediators, type 1 mediated reactions, and type 3 mediated reactions, which all result in nasal mucosal edema. The inflammation and edema results in obstruction of the sinus ostial complex. Sinus outflow obstruction may be exacerbated by concomitant anatomic factors such as septal deviation and turbinate hypertrophy. Sinus stasis provides an ideal environment for fungi to proliferate and contributes to continued antigenic exposure. This cycle self-perpetuates, leading to the production of allergic mucin, which in itself blocks sinus outflow and contributes to the cycle of propagation and inflammation. Folker et. al. [11] showed that immunotherapy was effective in control and prevention of recidivism of AFRS, thereby providing some support for the aforementioned theory. Ponikau et al. [32] offered another theory for the pathophysiology of AFRS and asserted that inflammation is triggered by T-cell-mediated hypersensitivity, which subsequently triggers eosinophil chemotaxis.

Tips and Pearls
- Despite the various theories, the role of inflammation rather than infection as the basis for AFRS has become the tenet.

The difficulties associated with accurately culturing fungal specimens and the reported similarities between AFRS and allergic bronchopulmonary aspergillosis initially indicted *Aspergillus* as the causative organism in AFRS [25]. With the advent of newer culture techniques, it was found that multiple species of fungi could cause AFRS and that *Aspergillus* was not the majority causative agent [5].

A 1996 review by Manning and Holman [23] revealed that the majority of AFRS cases were caused by members of the dematiaceous family of fungi, including *Bipolaris, Curvularia, Exserohilum, Alternaria, Drechslera, Helminthosporium*, and *Fusorium*.

Clinical Presentation

AFRS is characteristically associated with nasal polyposis and allergic mucin [25] (Fig. 11.1). AFRS typically affects young adults (mean age 21.9) [23], and atopy and asthma are frequent comorbid findings [1, 6, 8, 23]. The incidence of AFRS varies geographically, with the majority of cases centered in temperate regions of the world with high humidity [8, 12]. In the USA, the majority of cases are found in the southern states [25].

The majority of patients with AFRS present with gradual progressive nasal airway obstruction, semisolid nasal crusts, and a history of chronic allergic rhinitis [25]. Occasionally, the initial symptom patients present to the physician with is gross facial dysmorphia [21, 22] or acute vision loss [27]. The facial dysmorphic features can include proptosis [4] and telecanthus [27], where orbital involvement can lead to diplopia, visual field cuts, and acute vision loss (Fig. 11.2). These features are all caused by the expansile nature of AFRS. As the sequestered allergic mucin accumulates, it exerts an outward pressure on the surrounding structures. Bony remodeling and decalcification, similar to a mucocele, may occur [14, 16, 34]. This can result in a clinical picture that mimics invasion, much like a malignant process.

Immunological testing can also be a useful diagnostic tool in the diagnosis of AFRS. Patients with AFRS can have elevated levels of immunoglobulin E [9, 17, 35], display positive radioallergosorbent test (RAST) responses to fungal and nonfungal [17, 20] antigens, and exhibit positive skin tests to fungal antigens.

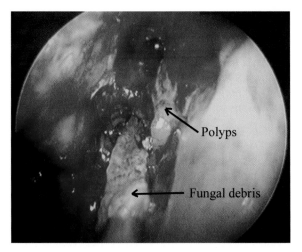

Fig. 11.1. Endoscopic picture of nasal polyps and allergic mucin in a patient with allergic fungal rhinosinusitis

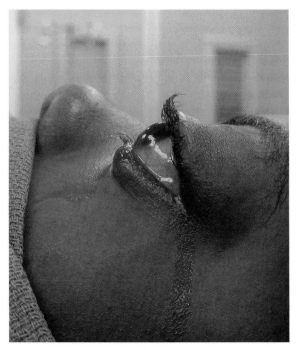

Fig. 11.2. Orbital proptosis in a patient with allergic fungal rhinosinusitis

Treatment

On the basis of the proposed pathophysiology schema presented above, treatment of AFRS is based on addressing each of the etiological entities.

Tips and Peals

- The mainstay of treatment of AFRS is surgical management.

- The primary goal of surgical management is removal of the allergenic stimulus, namely, the fungal mucin [25].

Despite aggressive and complete surgical management, the rate of recurrence is high [15, 38]. The rate of recurrence is reduced by concomitant management of the allergic portion of the AFRS cycle using immunomodulation (immunotherapy) [18–20] and/or corticosteroids [2, 35].

Preoperative Workup

Computed tomography (CT) of the sinus is an imperative part of the preoperative process. CT imaging of AFRS reveals several well-recognized findings, though these findings are not specific for AFRS (Fig. 11.3).

A recent study of CT scans of patients with AFRS revealed the following observations [31]:

- AFRS was bilateral in 51% of cases.
- Asymmetric involvement of the paranasal sinuses was noted in 78% of cases.
- Bone erosion with extension of disease into adjacent area was noted in 20% of cases.
- Thinning and remodeling of bone was common in advanced, bilateral disease.
- Areas of heterogeneous attenuation were seen in sinuses involved with AFRS.

Magnetic resonance imaging (MRI) can be a useful adjunctive study in the diagnosis of AFRS. The key useful characteristic of MRI is the preoperative identification of fungal mucin [25]. The high protein content and low water content of fungal mucin is easily identified against the backdrop of edematous nasal mucosa characterized by high water content [37]. The characteristic findings of AFRS on MRI are highly specific for AFRS in contrast to others forms of fungal rhinosinusitis as demonstrated by Manning et al. [24] These findings include hypointense central T1 signal, a central T2 signal void, and peripheral T1/T2 enhancement.

CT and MRI studies are useful tools to diagnose AFRS, but are also extremely important in preoperative surgical planning. As mentioned earlier, allergic mucin has a tendency to slowly invade into adjacent structures and intracranial/intraorbital extension is not rare. Therefore, preoperative knowledge regarding intracranial extension, erosion of the anterior cranial fossa, etc. on radiological studies can prevent costly surgical misadventures and minimize the risk

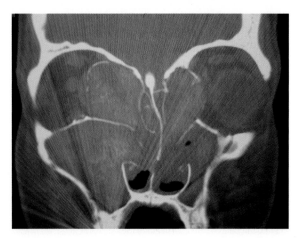

Fig. 11.3. Sinus computed tomography image of a patient with allergic fungal rhinosinusitis showing heterogeneous attenuation and orbital erosion

of complications. Another useful entity is the computerized image guidance system. The image guidance system is a valuable tool in complicated and revision cases; however, the image guidance system is not a substitute for preoperative CT planning and detailed knowledge of paranasal sinus anatomy owing to the fact that the image guidance system does not display real-time information, which can lull the inexperienced surgeon into a false state of security [26].

The senior author of this chapter advocates the use of preoperative systemic steroids to decrease intranasal inflammation.

Tips and Pearls
■ Patients with AFRS are given prednisone for 7 days at a dosage of 0.5–1.0 mg/kg/day.

It is thought that the preoperative steroids decrease overall nasal inflammation and nasal polyp volume, thereby increasing visualization and minimizing hemorrhage. Furthermore, preoperative antibiotics are also utilized because of the high incidence of postobstructive bacterial rhinosinusitis [26].

Surgery

Goals of surgery include:

■ Complete extirpation of all fungal mucin
■ Provision of a permanent drainage pathway for all involved sinuses
■ Allowing postoperative endoscopic surveillance of involved sinuses in the postoperative setting

Lack of complete extirpation of fungal mucin leads to a high rate of recidivism. Despite radiological evidence of tissue invasion, no such pathological evidence is seen; hence, radical surgeries are not necessary, and endoscopic, mucosa-sparing surgery can safely be performed.

Indications for surgery primarily include:

■ High index of suspicion for AFRS being present on the basis of history
■ Physical examination findings
■ History of atopy
■ Characteristic radiological findings
■ Possible fungal cultures in the immunocompetent host

Absolute indications for immediate surgical treatment include:

■ Vision changes
■ Diplopia
■ Mental status changes
■ A preoperative CT scan is necessary

Contraindications for AFRS surgery include the possibility of invasive fungal sinusitis in an immunocompromised host and possible sinonasal malignancy, which may both require more extensive surgery.

The surgical treatment of AFRS does not differ from other standard endoscopic techniques; hence, the following section will be dedicated to specific goals and surgical treatment algorithms unique to AFRS, rather than an in-depth discussion of endoscopic techniques.

The treatment of AFRS can be subdivided into surgical and medical therapies. Surgery has always been an integral part of the therapy plan for AFRS; however, initial hypotheses regarding the invasive nature of AFRS prompted invasive, morbid surgical procedures. Since then, surgical management for AFRS has evolved. The tenet of surgical management is to remove the allergy-/inflammation-inducing fungal mucin. Medical regimens for AFRS target the underlying inflammatory cascade. This multifaceted therapy protocol minimizes the incidence of recurrence of disease.

In the operating theater, three goals should be achieved in every AFRS case. First, complete extirpation of all allergic mucin and fungal debris is necessary to remove the inciting etiological agent in the atopically prone individual. This can be challenging, especially if fungal disease involves the frontal sinus or pneumatized portions of the pterygoid plates [25, 26].

The second goal of surgery is to provide permanent drainage of all involved sinuses without disturbing

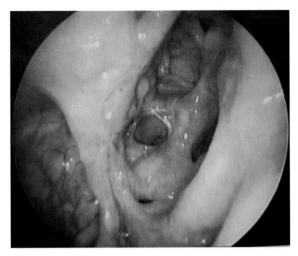

Fig. 11.4. Endoscopic picture of the right ethmoid and maxillary sinuses in a patient with a history of allergic fungal rhinosinusitis 2 years after complete surgical extirpation of fungal debris. The patient is receiving medical management for his disease

the sinonasal mucosa. Careful dissection with preservation of the mucosa ensures that underlying dura or orbital contents are not inadvertently injured. Large polyps can hamper vision; however, careful use of powered microdissection with identification of pertinent anatomic landmarks allow the surgeon to access fungal-involved sinuses [25, 26].

The final goal of surgery is to provide for easy postsurgical visualization of marsupialized sinuses in the office setting (Fig. 11.4). Despite maximum therapy, the rate of recidivism is high and identification of recurrence is important. Planning for postoperative care is important and starts intraoperatively [25, 26].

Complicating and Simplifying Factors

The progression of AFRS creates predictable clinical findings. The inflammation surrounding the sinus ostium leads to polyp formation surrounding the sinus ostium [36]. The resultant sinus outflow obstruction allows for slow accumulation of fungal mucin [25]. As the "fungal mucocele" grows and expands, it causes a pressure effect and exposes the surrounding walls of the sinus to inflammatory mediators, which subsequently cause bony remodeling and decalcification [25, 26]. This pathway is responsible for giving the appearance of invasion. The polyps that form in AFRS can traverse the spectrum of mild to severe, obscuring anatomic landmarks. The bony remodeling and presence of large polyps increase the risk of iatrogenic surgery.

However, the polyps also serve another important purpose. As described above, affected sinuses serve as the central focus of disease, as increased inflammation surrounding the sinus ostium leads to polyp formation. This allows the operating surgeon to "follow the polyps to the disease" [26]; therefore, slow careful removal of the polyps will lead to the sinus ostium, and subsequently to the affected sinus. Furthermore, the slow expansile nature of AFRS can enlarge natural sinus openings; therefore, even if fungal mucin resides in areas that are typically difficult to approach, such as the frontal sinus, the expansile tendency enlarges the natural outflow tracts, enabling greater access to the sinus [25, 29].

Once the sinus is encountered, thick tenacious fungal mucin is encountered [6, 25, 29]. This can be difficult to remove; however, patience, suction, blunt curetting instruments, and the use of forced irrigation through a 60-ml syringe attached to a curved ball-tip suction tip will aid in removal of the fungal mucin [26]. The powered microdebrider is a useful, effective tool in the removal of polyps, soft tissue, and thin bone, while simultaneous suction provides excellent visibility [25].

Complications of Surgery

The pathological features of AFRS, namely, polyps, inflammatory mucosa prone to hemorrhage, large fungal mucin accumulations, and bony remodeling, predispose the patients to increased surgical risk. These factors can all cause spatial disorientation and jeopardize security to intracranial and intraorbital compartments [25]. Therefore, the goal of complete extirpation is juxtaposed against the increased risk of iatrogenic injury.

> **Tips and Pearls**
>
> ■ Protection of the mucosa is paramount in protecting underlying structures and preventing surgical transgressions [25].

Iatrogenic injuries can result in serious complications. Intracranial injuries can result in stroke, CSF leaks, meningitis, and possible encephalocele formation. Erosion of the skull base by the expansile nature of AFRS may also theoretically cause encephalocele formation. This theory is based on the observation that dural exposure along the tegmen mastoideum secondary to otological surgery can lead to encephalocele formation in rare cases [13]. This exact correlate has not been shown in the rhinology literature, but it is a logical extension of the otological experiences. Iatrogenic penetration into the orbit can result in diplopia, blindness, and intraorbital hematomas [25].

As described in the "Pathophysiology" section, AFRS is a disease propagated by atopy in the immunocompetent patient. On the basis of available data, there is little to no evidence supporting pathological tissue invasion in AFRS patients. One case report by Tsimakas et al. [38] describes a frontal lobe *Aspergillus* abscess following treatment of AFRS that "invaded" the anterior cranial fossa. This, however, may represent fungal seeding of an inadvertent intracranial penetration during endoscopic surgery for AFRS.

Postoperative Care

Postoperative care for AFRS patients begins immediately following the operation. Patients are sent home with aggressive regimens of nasal saline irrigation and are followed up weekly for endoscopic debridement of crusts in the office setting [25]. Systemic corticosteroids are continued and tapered in the postoperative period [10]. The length of time over which the steroids are tapered is at the discretion of the treating clinician.

Recidivism

Despite complete surgical management, rates of recidivism are high and range from 10 to 100%. [28] Owing to the pathophysiology of AFRS and experience with allergic bronchopulmonary aspergillosis, a treatment protocol including systemic steroids and immunomodulation has been advocated to address the etiological and perpetuating factors of chronic inflammation [25]. A recent study by Marple and Mabry [28] showed that the two major factors in patients undergoing a complete therapy for AFRS including surgery, steroids, and immunotherapy that were associated with disease recurrence were noncompliance on the part of the patient with immunotherapy and inadequate initial surgical extirpation of disease. This study further supports the importance of complete initial surgical extirpation of disease (Fig. 11.4).

Recurrence rates of AFRS are influenced by long-term postoperative management protocols. The effect of corticosteroids in the postoperative management of AFRS patients was studied by Schubert and Goetz [35], who subsequently found that use of corticosteroids significantly increased the time to revision sinus surgery. Several studies have also shown the efficacy of immunotherapy in postoperative management of AFRS patients [11, 18–20]. Some data also exist for the postoperative usage of antifungals [3, 7, 23] and topical corticosteroids [25].

Conclusions

AFRS is a relatively new clinicopathological entity. Many studies have been performed to better characterize the disease and determine appropriate treatment strategies. AFRS is a subset of chronic rhinosinusitis potentiated by atopy to fungal antigens. The subsequent inflammatory cascade produces allergic fungal mucin that resides in affected sinuses and can cause bony remodeling and erosion of surrounding sinus walls.

Surgical therapy is an important arm in the combined treatment approach to AFRS. The goals of surgery include extirpation of disease, providing permanent drainage of involved sinuses, and creating easy access to sinuses such that they can be monitored easily in the postoperative period.

Concomitant therapies in the postoperative period include systemic corticosteroids and immunomodulation. Despite aggressive therapy regimens, the rates of recidivism are high and are affected primarily by noncompliance to immunotherapy and inadequate initial surgical extirpation.

References

1. Bent J, Kuhn F. (1994) Diagnosis of allergic fungal sinusitis. Otolaryngol Head Neck Surg; 111:580–588.
2. Bent JP III, Kuhn FA. (1996) Allergic fungal sinusitis/polyposis. Allergy Asthma Proceedings; 17:259–268.
3. Bent JP III, Kuhn FA. (1996) Antifungal activity against allergic fungal sinusitis organisms. Laryngoscope; 106:1331–1334.
4. Carter KD, Graham SM, Carpenter KM. (1999) Ophthalmologic manifefstations of allergic fungal sinusitis. Am J Ophthalmol; 127:189–195.
5. Cody D, Neel H, Gerreiro J, et al. (1994) Allergic fungal sinusitis: the Mayo Clinic experience. Laryngoscope; 104:1074–1079.
6. Corey JP. (1992) Allergic fungal sinusitis. Otolaryngol Clin North Am; 25:225–230.
7. Denning DW, Van Wye JE, Lewiston NJ. (1991) Adjunctive treatment of allergic broncho-pulmonary aspergillosis with itraconazole. Chest; 100:813–819.
8. Deshpande RB, Shaukla A, Kirtane MV. (1995) Allergic fungal sinusitis: incidence and clinical and pathological features of seven cases. J Assoc Physicians India; 43:98–100.
9. Feger T, Rupp N, Kuhn F, et al. (1997) Local and systemic eosinophil activation. Ann Allergy Asthma Immunol; 79:221–225.
10. Ferguson BJ. (1998) What role do systemic corticosteroids, immunotherapy, and antifungal drugs play in the therapy of allergic fungal rhinosinusitis? Arch Otolaryngol Head Neck Surg; 124:1174–1177.

11

11. Folker RJ, Marple BF, Mabry RL, Mabry CS. (1998) Treatment of allergic fungal sinusitis: a comparison trial of postoperative immunotherapy with specific fungal antigens. Laryngoscope; 108:1623–1627.
12. Gungor A, Adusmilli V, Corey JP. (1998) Fungal sinusitis: progression of disease in immunosuppression – a case report. Ear Nose Throat J; 77:207–215.
13. Jackson CG, Pappas DG, Manolidis S, et.al. (1997) Brain herniation into the middle ear and mastoid: concepts in diagnosis and surgical management. Am L Otol; 18:198–206.
14. Klapper SR, Lee AG, Patrinely JR, Stewart M, Alford EL. (1997) Orbital involvement in allergic fungal sinusitis. Ophthalmology; 104:2094–2100.
15. Kupferberg SB, Bent JP, Kuhn FA. (1997) The prognosis of allergic fungal sinusitis. Otolaryngol Head Neck Surgery; 117:35–41.
16. Lydiatt WM, Sobba-Higley A, Huerter JV, Leibrock LG. (1994) Allergic fungal sinusitis with intracranial extension and fromtal lobe symptoms: a case report. Ear Nose Throat J; 73:402–404.
17. Mabry R, Manning S. (1995) Radioallergosorbent microscreen and total immunoglobulin E in allergic fungal sinusitis. Otolaryngol Head Neck Surg; 113:721–723.
18. Mabry RL, Mabry CS. (1997) Immunotherapy for allergic fungal sinusitis: the second year. Otolaryngol Head Neck Surg; 117:367–371.
19. Mabry RL, Manning SC, Mabry CS. (1997) Immunotherapy in the treatment of allergic fungal sinusitis. Otolaryngol Head Neck Surg; 116:31–35.
20. Mabry RL, Marple BF, Folker RJ, Mabry CS. (1998) Immunotherapy for allergic fungal sinusitis: three years' experience. Otolaryngol Head Neck Surg; 119:648–651.
21. Manning S, Schaefer S, Close L, et al. (1991) Culture-positive allergic fungal sinusitis. Arch Otolaryngol Head Neck Surg 1991; 117:174–178.
22. Manning S, Vuitch F, Weinberg A, et al. (1989) Allergic aspergillosis: a newly recognized form of sinusitis in the pediatric population. Laryngoscope; 99:681–685.
23. Manning SC, Holman M. (1998) Further evidence for allergic fungal sinusitis. Laryngoscope; 108:1485–1496.
24. Manning SC, Merkel M, Kreisel K, Vuitch F, Marple, B. (1997) Computed tomographic and magnetic resonance diagnosis of allergic fungal sinusitis. Laryngoscope; 107:170–176.
25. Marple BF. (2001) Allergic fungal sinusitis: Current theories and management strategies. Laryngoscope 111; 1006–1019.
26. Marple BF. (2000) Allergic fungal sinusitis: surgical therapy. Otolaryngol Clin North Am; 33:409–419.
27. Marple BF, Biggs SR, Newcomer MT, Mabry RL. (1999) Allergic fungal sinusitis-induced visual loss. Am J Rhinol; 13:191–195.
28. Marple BF, Mabry RL. (2000) Allergic fungal sinusitis: learning from our failures. Am J Rhinol; 14:223–226.
29. Marple BF, Mabry RL. (1998) Comprehensive management of allergic fungal sinusitis. Am J Rhinol; 12:263–268.
30. McGuirt WF, Harrill JA. (1979) Paranasal sinus aspergillosis. Laryngoscope; 89:1563–1568.
31. Mukherji SK, Figueroa R, Ginsberg LE, et al. (1998) Allergic fungal sinusitis: CT findings. Radiology; 207:417–422.
32. Ponikau JU, Sherris DA, Kern EB, et al. (1999) The diagnosis and incidence of allergic fungal sinusitis. Mayo Clinic Proc; 74:877–884.
33. Safirstein B (1976) Allergic bronchopulmonary aspergillosis with obstruction of the upper respiratory tract. Chest; 70:788–790.
34. Sarti EJ, Blaugrund SM, Lin PT, Camins MB. (1988) Paranasal sinus disease with intracranial extension: aspergillosis versus malignancy. Laryngoscope; 98:632–635.
35. Schubert MS, Goetz DW. (1998) Evaluation and treatment of allergic fungal sinusitis. II: treatment and follow-up. J Allergy Clin Immunol; 102:395–402.
36. Schweitz LA, Gourley DS. (1992) Allergic fungal sinusitis. Allergy Proc; 13:3–6.
37. Som PM, Curtin HD. (1993) Chronic inflammatory sinonasal disease including fungal infections: the role of imaging. Radiol Clin North Am; 31:33–44.
38. Tsimakas S, Hollingsworth HM, Nash G. (1994) Aspergillus brain abscess complicating allergic aspergillus sinusitis. J Allergy Clin Immunol; 94:264–267.

Chapter 12

Endoscopic Medial Maxillectomy 12

Francis T.K. Ling, Ioannis G. Skoulas, Stilianos E. Kountakis

Core Messages

■ Endoscopic surgery avoids an external scar and allows better assessment of the tumor bed with the potential of sparing uninvolved mucosa.

■ Precise determination of the sites of tumor origin and attachment and the extent of the tumor during the operation is the key to successful treatment.

■ Tumor debulking with a powered microdebrider may be required to determine tumor origin.

■ Intraoperative endoscopy is key to determining the precise location of tumor origin and extent and may allow for mucosal sparing.

■ Long-term follow-up is required to monitor for recurrences, with biopsy of suspicious lesions as necessary.

Contents

Introduction

The surgical treatment of sinonasal tumors is constantly evolving. Lesions of the medial maxillary wall were traditionally approached through an external approach, usually a lateral rhinotomy incision. With direct visualization, en bloc resection was achieved; however, patients were left with an external scar and prolonged healing times were common. With the advent of endoscopic instrumentation in the 1980s, endonasal tumor surgery that respected oncologically correct resection was possible. The advantages of endoscopic resection included better visualization of the tumor, improved cosmesis, and faster healing times.

Inverted papilloma is a benign intranasal tumor that commonly occurs on the lateral nasal wall and middle meatus. This tumor is composed of endophytic or inverted epithelial nests within an underlying stroma [14]. It can invade surrounding structures, have a tendency to recur, and may become malignant in 10–15% of cases [16]. Surgical resection is the treatment of choice and these tumors were traditionally treated with medial maxillectomy via a transfacial or sublabial degloving approach [6]. With the improved visualization of endoscopic techniques and outcomes comparable to those of the external approach, endoscopic transnasal resection of these tumors is quickly becoming the standard of care. For inverted papilloma involving the lateral nasal wall, endoscopic medial maxillectomy is the procedure of choice.

The indications are:

1. Benign tumors such as inverted papilloma with involvement of:
   (a) Lateral nasal wall
   (b) Ostiomeatal complex
   (c) Ethmoid sinuses
   (d) Medial maxillary wall
   (e) Limited sphenoid sinus
2. Recurrent inverted papilloma
3. Malignancy confined to the medial wall of the maxillary sinus
4. Provide access to benign tumors involving:
   (a) Lateral or posterior maxillary sinus wall
   (b) Infratemporal fossa

The contraindications are:

1. Inverted papilloma with extensive involvement of:
   (a) Orbit
   (b) Intracranial invasion
   (c) Frontal sinus (endoscopic medial maxillectomy may be used in conjunction with a procedure that addresses the frontal sinus, e.g.. modified Lothrop procedure)
2. Malignant tumors with invasion to:
   (a) Bone of the posterior wall of the maxillary sinus, subcutaneous tissues, skin of cheek, floor or medial wall of orbit, infratemporal fossa, pterygoid plates
   (b) Orbital contents beyond the floor or medial wall, including any of the following: orbital apex, cribriform plate, base of skull, nasopharynx, sphenoid, frontal sinuses
3. Lack of experience by the surgeon
4. Lack of proper instrumentation
5. Presence of abundant scar tissue from previous surgery

The advantages are:

1. May provide exposure of maxillary sinus and ethmoid sinuses without the removal of the lamina papyracea, medial floor of the orbit, anterior maxillary wall and frontal process of the maxilla
2. Provides improved visualization of difficult-to-view areas such as lateral recesses of frontal, sphenoid and maxillary sinuses
3. No external scar
4. No loss of bony nasal or anterior maxillary support
5. Lower risk of infraorbital nerve paraesthesia
6. Reduced morbidity and shorter hospitalization

Preoperative Workup

The feasibility of the endoscopic medial maxillectomy is dependent upon three important factors. These are the determination of the extent of the tumor, the location and origin of tumor attachment, and the presence of malignancy [5]. In terms of location, involvement of ethmoid and maxillary sinuses occurs in the majority of cases [16].

Preoperative nasal endoscopy is important in determining the location and origin of tumor attachment as well as the extent of tumor involvement. With larger tumors, this information may be difficult to acquire by endoscopy alone and therefore imaging studies are an essential adjunct.

CT imaging of the sinuses is required in both the coronal and the axial planes as it allows the assessment of disease extent and can demonstrate the presence of bone erosion or invasion into adjacent structures such as the base of the skull or orbit. MRI further determines tumor extent by differentiating between trapped inspissated secretions from the tumor, which would otherwise appear homogeneously hyperdense on CT scans. In addition, T2-weighted images and contrast-enhanced T1-weighted images may be able to differentiate tumor from adjacent acute inflammatory changes [10]. The limitations of these studies include a reduced accuracy in distinguishing tumor from postoperative scar and/or chronic inflammatory tissue in cases of recurrent tumor.

Despite the objective information from preoperative nasal endoscopy and radiographic studies, delineation of areas of tumor origin and attachment may still be limited. This occurs especially with more extensive lesions, in which case the true extent of involvement may not be completely known until a more thorough intraoperative examination is performed.

Pathological diagnosis is essential as the presence of malignancy might preclude the endoscopic ap-

Table 12.1. Staging system for inverted papilloma [5]

Stage	Description
T1	Tumor totally confined to nasal cavity, without extension into the sinuses. The tumor can be localized to one wall or region of the nasal cavity, or can be bulky and extensive within the nasal cavity, but must not extend into the sinuses or into any extranasal compartment. There must be no concurrent malignancy
T2	Tumor involving the ostiomeatal complex and ethmoid sinuses, and/or the medial portion of the maxillary sinus, with or without involvement of the nasal cavity. There must be no concurrent malignancy
T3	Tumor involving the lateral, inferior, superior, anterior, or posterior walls of the maxillary sinus, the sphenoid sinus, and/or the frontal sinus, with or without involvement of the medial portion of the maxillary sinus, the ethmoid sinuses, or the nasal cavity. There must be no concurrent malignancy
T4	All tumor with any extranasal/extrasinus extension to involve adjacent, contiguous structures such as the orbit, the intracranial compartment, or the pterygomaxillary space. All tumors associated with malignancy

proach to tumor resection. This, however, is controversial as some authors have reported the curative effectiveness of endoscopic resection for select malignant tumors [12]. Nonetheless, biopsy should be performed in all cases of unilateral nasal mass, after the intracranial source is excluded.

Classification of inverted papilloma following preoperative workup has been advocated in order to facilitate standardization when reporting outcomes. A popular staging system has been proposed by Krouse [5] and is based on the degree of involvement of the paranasal sinuses (Table 12.1). Another classification system described by Han et al. [2] has been advocated to help guide surgical treatment.

Surgical Technique

The patient is placed under general anesthesia. The nasal cavity is decongested with 2% oxymetazoline or cocaine-soaked neurosurgical pledgets. Infiltration of 1 or 2% lidocaine in 1:100,000 epinephrine into the inferior turbinate, middle turbinate, and area of the sphenopalatine artery is performed.

The key to the success of endoscopic surgery for the management of inverted papilloma is locating the specific site of tumor origin and its attachment, defining the extension of the tumor, and completely removing all affected tissue [7]. Intraoperative endoscopic evaluation is essential in delineating the origin of attachment and the extent of the tumor. It may be determined whether the tumor has invaded tissue, or has simply "dumbbelled" into the sinus with associated retention of secretions [9]. Endoscopic evaluation is considerably better than a CT scan in its ability to differentiate between disease and normal membranes and therefore has a better specificity [13]. Normal-appearing mucous membranes found on endoscopic examination can be spared.

While en bloc resection is usually possible with smaller tumors (Krouse stage I or II), larger tumors usually require sequential segmental endoscopic surgery (Krouse stage III). Tumor debulking with a powered microdebrider may be required to determine tumor origin (Fig. 12.1). A suction trap should be used to collect the specimen for histological determination. Subsequent resections should be tailored to the extent of tumor origin and should provide an adequate margin of surrounding normal mucosa. Complete removal of the intranasal portion of the tumor is performed and the origin of the tumor is identified. A medial maxillectomy is necessary if the tumor originates from the medial maxillary wall or from within the maxillary sinus itself. This assists in the removal of the tumor and also allows easy endoscopic surveillance in the office setting. A wide middle meatal antrostomy is first performed removing the medial maxillary wall all the way up to the level of the floor of the orbit. The microdebrider or a Stammberger punch is then used to remove tissue inferiorly through the inferior middle turbinate until the nasal floor is reached (Fig. 12.2). Tumor is removed and is followed to its point of origin. The medial maxillary wall is resected posteriorly as far as needed for tumor removal until the posterior maxillary wall is reached. Bleeding from a sphenopalatine branch is handled if it occurs or the sphenopalatine artery may need clipping.

Next, backbiting forceps are used to make a cut along the floor of the orbit, and the cut is directed anteriorly until the anterior maxillary wall is reached (Fig. 12.3). Similarly, a cut is made at the floor of the nose, under the inferior turbinate, in an anterior direction until the anterior maxillary wall is encoun-

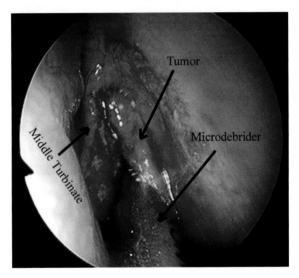

Fig. 12.1. Debulking of tumor using a microdebrider

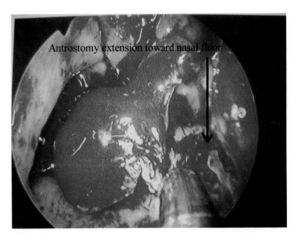

Fig. 12.2. Inferior extension of antrostomy through the inferior turbinate until the floor of the nose is reached

12

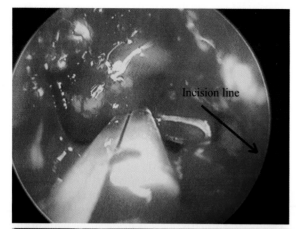

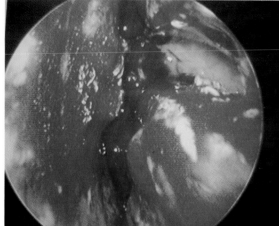

Fig. 12.3. Anterior cuts in the medial maxillary wall along the floor of the orbit until the anterior maxillary wall is reached

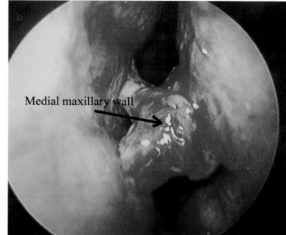

Fig. 12.4. Remnant medial maxillary wall reflected medially

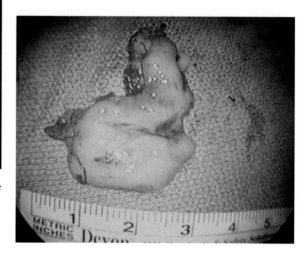

Fig. 12.5. Resected medial maxillary wall

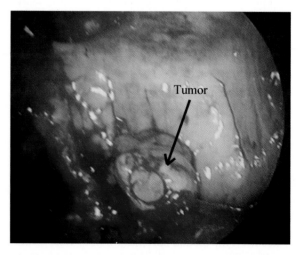

Fig. 12.6. View of tumor after medial maxillectomy. The tumor originates in the medial-inferior portion of the posterior maxillary wall

tered. In the process, the lacrimal bone with the naso-lacrimal duct is transected. All cuts can be made with an osteotome if needed. Occasionally, a lacrimal stent may be used to keep the sac open, but in our experience, most often this step is not necessary.

The freed medial maxillary wall is now only attached anteriorly at the junction between the medial and anterior maxillary walls. It is reflected medially and this anterior attachment is sharply resected (Figs. 12.4, 12.5, Video 12.1). The origin of the tumor is identified using angled endoscopes if necessary (Fig. 12.6) and the tumor is resected. The surgical margins as well as the maxillary sinus are inspected for residual tumor, through this large access to the maxillary sinus that has been created (Fig. 12.7). If needed, residual tumor can be removed from the superior, lateral, inferior, and anterior walls of the maxillary sinus through an accessory antrostomy through the canine fossa. Diseased bone can be drilled away with a cutting burr. If involved, the anterior wall of the sphenoid is resected separately. Figure 12.8 shows the

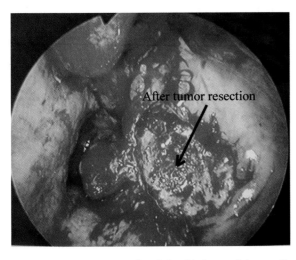

Fig. 12.7. Tumor is resected and the thin bone of the maxillary wall drilled with a diamond burr

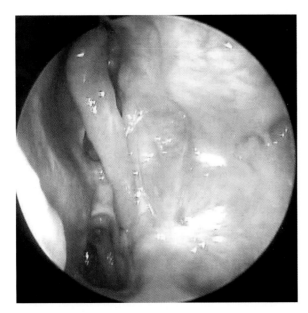

Fig. 12.8. Left nasal cavity 2 years after endoscopic medial maxillectomy for inverted papilloma

healed maxillary cavity 2 years after endoscopic medial maxillectomy.

The surgical cavity is dressed with hemostatic agents if needed or with nasal hyaluronic acid, especially in the areas of exposed bone.

Tips and Pearls

- Complete tumor resection at the site of attachment, preserving healthy tissue, is the key to successful treatment.
- Most recurrences are thought to develop because of an inadequate resection at the site of origin.

- Tumor debulking with a powered microdebrider may be required to determine tumor origin.
- The posterior limit of the resection is the posterior maxillary sinus wall. The surgeon should be mindful of the sphenopalatine artery in this area, and once it has been identified, this vessel should be clipped or cauterized to prevent hemorrhage.
- If resection involves the nasolacrimal duct, endoscopic dacryocystostomy and stenting may be necessary to prevent postoperative epiphora.

Complications and Management

Complications have been reported to be between 0 and 19.6% [1]. Minor complications include epistaxis, epiphora, temporary infraorbital hypoesthesia, minimal orbital fat exposure, and periorbital ecchymosis. Significant injury to the intraorbital contents is possible and the surgeon should be on the lookout for orbital entry. Other complications include postoperative neuralgia and temporary hypoesthesia of the upper teeth. Owing to the increased extent of surgery, blood loss may be greater. The management of these complications does not differ from that of those encountered for standard endoscopic sinus surgery.

Postoperative Care and Outcomes

Postoperative care involves prophylactic oral antibiotics for 10–14 days. Owing to the greater amount of intraoperative tissue trauma and increased bone exposure, drying and crusting of the mucosa is likely. The patient is brought back to the office for regular endoscopic debridements of the wound. Continued follow-up is required for surveillance of the surgical site for any recurrence. Most recurrences occur within the first 2 years and it is recommended that follow-up for all patients be performed for at least 5 years, as recommended for head and neck cancers [4].

With limited excision, the recurrence rate ranges from 27 to 78% [14]. With complete excision, recurrence rates vary from 0 to 33% using either endoscopic or traditional approaches [6, 14]. Lawson et al. [6] compared traditional versus endoscopic approaches in 160 patients, with an average follow-up period of 5.2 years, and found comparable recurrence rates for conservative (12%) and aggressive (18%) approaches. Pasquini et al. [11] reported a lower recurrence rate for an endoscopic approach (3%) compared with an open approach (24%). Waitz and Wigand [17] reported on 35 patients who underwent endoscopic excision with a recurrence rate of 17%. Similar results are reported by several authors [3, 4, 8, 15, 18]. It must be noted, however, that clinical staging of these tumors is unknown and therefore it can be very difficult to compare study groups. Outcomes may be biased by case selection and follow-up interval.

Cocnlusions

Treatment of inverted papilloma requires surgical excision, for which endoscopic management is becoming the approach of choice owing to its numerous advantages. The key to successful treatment is locating the specific site of tumor origin and its attachment, defining the extension of the tumor and completely removing all affected tissue. For selected tumors, endoscopic medial maxillectomy is required for complete resection. Preliminary outcomes of the endoscopic approach are comparable to those of the traditional external approach. Long-term follow-up studies which take into account the tumor stage are required, however, to accurately compare the two techniques.

12

References

1. Banhiran W, Casiano RR, (2005). Endoscopic sinus surgery for benign and malignant nasal and sinus neoplasm. Curr Opin Otolaryngol Head Neck Surg 13:50-54.
2. Han JK, Smith TL, Loehrl T, Toohill RJ, Smith MM, (2001). An evolution in the management of sinonasal inverting papilloma. Laryngoscope 111:1395-1400.
3. Kaza S, Capasso R, Casiano RR, (2003). Endoscopic resection of inverted papilloma: University of Miami experience. Am J Rhinol 17:185-190.
4. Kraft M, Simmen D, Kaufmann T, Holzmann D, (2003). Long-term results of endonasal sinus surgery in sinonasal papillomas. Laryngoscope 113:1541-1547.
5. Krouse JH, (2000). Development of a staging system for inverted papilloma. Laryngoscope 110:965-968.
6. Lawson W, Kaufman MR, Biller HF, (2003). Treatment outcomes in the management of inverted papilloma: an analysis of 160 cases. Laryngoscope 113:1548-1556.
7. Lee TJ, Huang SF, Lee LA, Huang CC, (2004). Endoscopic surgery for recurrent inverted papilloma. Laryngoscope 114:106-112.
8. Llorente JL, Deleyiannis F, Rodrigo JP et al, (2003). Minimally invasive treatment of the nasal inverted papilloma. Am J Rhinol 17:335-341.
9. Lund VJ, (2000). Optimum management of inverted papilloma. J Laryngol Otol 114:194-197.
10. Oikawa K, Furuta Y, Oridate N et al, (2003). Preoperative staging of sinonasal inverted papilloma by magnetic resonance imaging. Laryngoscope 113:1983-1987.
11. Pasquini E, Sciarretta V, Farneti G, Modugno GC, Ceroni AR, (2004). Inverted papilloma: report of 89 cases. Am J Otolaryngol 25:178-185.
12. Shipchandler TZ, Batra PS, Citardi MJ, Bolger WE, Lanza DC, (2005). Outcomes for endoscopic resection of sinonasal squamous cell carcinoma. Laryngoscope 115:1983-1987.
13. Sukenik MA, Casiano R, (2000). Endoscopic medial maxillectomy for inverted papillomas of the paranasal sinuses: value of the intraoperative endoscopic examination. Laryngoscope 110:39-42.
14. Thorp MA, Oyarzabal-Amigo MF, du Plessis JH, Sellars SL, (2001). Inverted papilloma: a review of 53 cases. Laryngoscope 111:1401-1405.
15. Tomenzoli D, Castelnuovo P, Pagella F et al, (2004). Different endoscopic surgical strategies in the management of inverted papilloma of the sinonasal tract: experience with 47 patients. Laryngoscope 114:193-200.
16. Vrabec DP, (1994). The inverted Schneiderian papilloma: a 25-year study. Laryngoscope 104:582-605.
17. Waitz G, Wigand ME, (1992). Results of endoscopic sinus surgery for the treatment of inverted papillomas. Laryngoscope 102:917-922.
18. Wormald PJ, Ooi E, van Hasselt CA, Nair S, (2003). Endoscopic removal of sinonasal inverted papilloma including endoscopic medial maxillectomy. Laryngoscope 113:867-873.

Endoscopic Management of Benign Sinonasal Tumors

Michael J. Sillers, Kris Lay

Core Messages

- With appropriate endoscopic skills and instrumentation and routine endoscopic surveillance, patients with benign sinonasal neoplasms can be treated safely and effectively.

- Certain benign neoplasms such as inverted papilloma can be locally aggressive and have a risk for malignant degeneration and should not be underestimated in treatment planning.

- Multimodality imaging with CT and MRI is important to evaluate the extent of the benign sinonasal neoplasms.

- In the management of benign sinonasal neoplasms, a successful outcome is dependent on complete tumor removal. The utilization of angled scopes can assist the surgeon in assessing the entire maxillary antrum, the frontal recess, or a laterally pneumatized sphenoid sinus for residual tumor.

- Since en bloc resection during endoscopic resection is often not possible, the location of specimens should be carefully identified to assist the pathologist.

Contents

Introduction

Endoscopic sinus surgery has been utilized as a means of treating medically refractory chronic rhinosinusitis and complicated acute rhinosinusitis for the past 20 years. In an effort to improve patient outcomes by technique refinement, improved instrumentation, and an in depth understanding of endoscopic anatomy, surgeons were able to expand minimally invasive endoscopic surgery to include the treatment of sinonasal tumors, skull base defects, and orbital pathology [1, 14]. Patients have been the beneficiary of less invasive surgery, avoiding facial scars and experiencing less morbidity. Importantly this has been accomplished without compromising long-term success in patients with benign neoplasms of the paranasal sinuses [7, 9, 15, 16]. Early concerns that tumors would be removed piecemeal rather than en bloc and would lead to unacceptable recurrence rates have not been warranted. With appropriate endoscopic skills and instrumentation and routine endoscopic surveillance, patients with benign sinonasal neoplasms can be treated safely and effectively. For many surgeons, an endoscopic approach has become the default choice. The purposes of this chapter are to outline the most commonly encountered benign neoplasms, identify unique properties of individual tumors regarding size and location, and discuss specific surgical principles for specific clinical situations.

Neoplasm is defined as an abnormal proliferation of cells, especially one that is unchecked [25]; therefore, it is not surprising that within the nasal cavity and paranasal sinuses, otolaryngologists have encountered primary tumors of epithelial, vascular, connective tissue, glandular, cartilaginous, and osseous origins (Table 13.1). Further distinction is made to differentiate benign from malignant neoplasms based on the lack of metastatic potential for benign neoplasms. It should be emphasized that, while benign, certain neoplasms such as inverted papilloma can be locally aggressive and have a risk for malignant degeneration and therefore should not be underestimated in treatment planning.

Table 13.1. Benign neoplasms of the nasal cavity and paranasal sinuses

Inverted papilloma	Squamous papilloma
Cylindrical papilloma	Fibroosseous lesions
Angiofibroma	Hemangioma/ Hemangiopericytoma
Chondroma	Pleomorphic adenoma
Neurofibroma	Fibrous histiocytoma
Meningioma	

The paranasal sinuses are lined with pseudostratified columnar epithelium, or respiratory epithelium, also referred to as Schneiderian membrane (epithelium).

The most common benign neoplasms of the paranasal sinuses are the Schneiderian papillomas, of which there are three types: squamous, inverted, and cylindrical.

Squamous papillomas typically arise in the anterior portions of the nasal cavity, often at the mucocutaneous border. These lesions generally have an exophytic, warty appearance and cause symptoms based on their size and location. They are typically associated with crusting, epistaxis, and nasal airway obstruction. Their natural history is to grow, and they respond well to simple local excision. They are not generally felt to harbor malignant potential. Inverted papilloma, the most common of the Schneiderian papillomas, classically arises from the lateral nasal wall and subsequently involves the contiguous paranasal sinuses [1]. These tumors are almost always unilateral, and patients present with nasal obstructive symptoms, bleeding, and postobstructive sinusitis. On endoscopic examination, their appearance varies from benign-appearing inflammatory polyps to a verrucous-appearing polyp. These lesions are almost always unilateral and the evaluating physician should have a high index of suspicion for neoplasm. Multimodality imaging with CT and MRI is important to evaluate the extent of the lesion, possible bone erosion which may suggest malignancy, and postobstructive sinusitis. Microscopically, one sees digitiform proliferation of squamous epithelium into the underlying stroma [1]. Complete excision is essential because of the potential for recurrence, locally aggressive spread, and the potential for malignant degeneration into squamous cell carcinoma in about 9% of patients [8, 21] (Fig. 13.1). With complete endoscopic excision, the recurrence rate for inverted papilloma compares favorably and in some cases better than in cases treated by traditional open or external approaches [6, 9, 15, 16, 21, 27] (Table 13.2). Cylindrical cell papilloma is the least common of the three types. Though it occurs rarely, similar to inverted papilloma, cylindrical papilloma

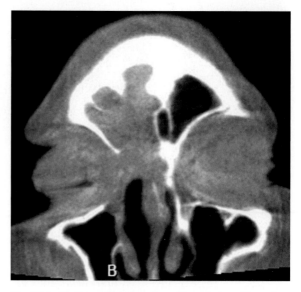

Fig. 13.1. Malignant degeneration of inverted papilloma in a patient undergoing prior "polypectomy"

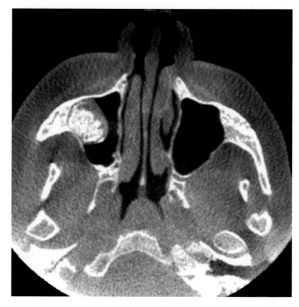

Fig. 13.2. Axial CT image of asymptomatic ossifying fibroma

should be completely excised since it also has a significant potential for malignant degeneration.

After papillomas, fibroosseous lesions represent the next most commonly encountered benign sinonasal tumor.

Fibroosseous lesions are classified into three general types: osteoma, ossifying fibroma, and fibrous dysplasia.

Each has a distinct radiographical and histological appearance and treatment options can be based on principles of cure, function, and/or cosmesis [3]. Osteomas and ossifying fibromas are generally distinct,

Table 13.2. Comparison of recurrence rate with external vs. endoscopic approaches

Authors	Year	External/endoscopic	No. of patients	Recurrence (%)
Dolgin et al. [5]	1992	External	42	25
Vrabec [24]	1994	External	101	2
Lawson et al. [14]	1995	External	112	12
Lawson et al. [15]	2003	Endoscopic	30	12
Waitz and Wigand [25]	1992	External/endoscopic	16/35	19/17
Pasquini et al. [19]	2004	External/endoscopic	50/36	24/3
Kraft et al. [13]	2003	Endoscopic	26	8
Tomenzoli et al. [23]	2004	Endoscopic	47	0

well circumscribed, and can be completely removed ("cured"), while fibrous dysplasia tends to grow along and expand the plane(s) of normal bone and therefore portions are removed to reduce functional impairment (Figs. 13.2–13.4). Furthermore, the primary histological distinction between ossifying fibroma and fibrous dysplasia is the presence of lamellar bone and peripheral osteoblasts in an ossifying fibroma and the absence thereof in fibrous dysplasia [3]. Each of these lesions can produce facial asymmetry in the absence of functional impairment and consideration can be made for intervening on the basis of improved cosmesis (Fig. 13.5). There is some controversy as to when surgical intervention is indicated. Most authors agree that symptomatic lesions should be removed [4, 8] (Figs. 13.6, 13.7). Large lesions associated with postobstructive rhinosinusitis and those in which growth is evident on serial CT scans should be considered for removal. Patients with fibrous dysplasia may have significant headaches, but unless the treating physician is certain that surgery will lead to improvement, headache alone is not a reasonable indication for intervention (Fig. 13.8). The headaches should be managed medically. Small, asymptomatic lesions, often found incidentally, can be followed by CT at intervals (3–6 months) to determine the growth rate and should be treated accordingly. Patients with small, asymptomatic lesions are also instructed to notify the treating physician if symptoms referable to the lesion arise.

Angiofibromas represent perhaps the most challenging lesions to remove endoscopically because of their potential for significant bleeding during surgery. This must be anticipated and appropriate measures taken in advance and in preparation. These tumors generally arise from the sphenopalatine artery in the pterygomaxillary space and expand to fill the nasopharynx, nasal cavity, and infratemporal fossa [22, 24]. There may be intracranial extension in some cases. It is helpful to employ classification schemes in discussing tumor size and extent.

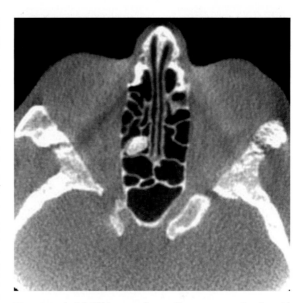

Fig. 13.3. Axial CT image of a small, asymptomatic ethmoid osteoma

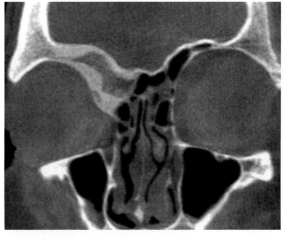

Fig. 13.4. Coronal CT image of asymptomatic fibrous dysplasia of the frontal bone

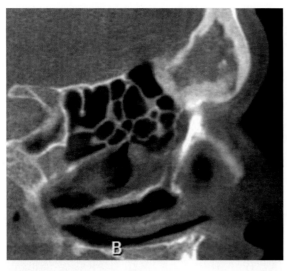

Fig. 13.5. Sagittal CT image of fibrous dysplasia in a patient with frontal bossing

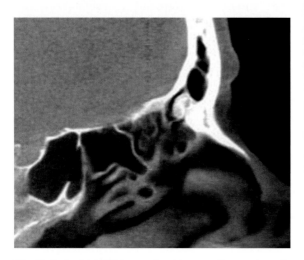

Fig. 13.6. Sagittal CT image showing a small, symptomatic frontoethmoid osteoma

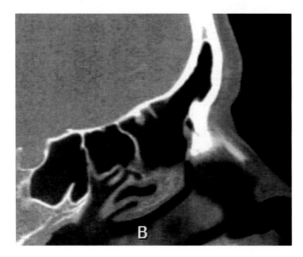

Fig. 13.7. Sagittal CT image after removal of osteoma

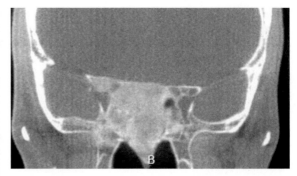

Fig. 13.8. Coronal CT image of fibrous dysplasia of the sphenoid bone without visual compromise

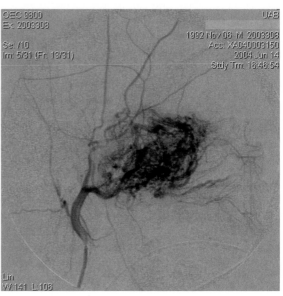

Fig. 13.9. Angiogram of angiofibroma before embolization

The Fisch classification of angiofibromas (utilized in this discussion) is:

- Stage I tumors are limited to the nasal cavity and nasopharynx, with no bone destruction.
- Stage II tumors invade the pterygomaxillary fossa and/or the paranasal sinuses with bone destruction.
- Stage III tumors invade the infratemporal fossa, orbit, and/or the parasellar region, but remain lateral to the cavernous sinus.
- Stage IV tumors invade the cavernous sinus, optic chiasm region, and/or the pituitary fossa [19].

Patients are generally adolescent white men who present with nasal airway obstruction and episodes of severe epistaxis. Because the growth rate is slow, these patients often do not have significant pain or acute postobstructive sinusitis. On endoscopic examination, the surgeon may demonstrate a benign-appearing polypoid mass, but close evaluation and valsalva maneuver may reveal pulsations. Under no circumstance should these lesions be biopsied in the office setting. Multimodality imaging with contrast-enhanced MRI and CT should lead to the diagnosis of angiofibroma in this distinct patient population [22]. Arteriography with embolization can be performed as a further diagnostic and therapeutic measure (Figs. 13.9, 13.10) [8, 18, 22].

Tips and Pearls

■ For effective potential decrease in bleeding, arteriography with embolization should be performed within 48 h of planned surgical excision [2, 5, 13, 22].

The patient's baseline hemoglobin/hematocrit and platelets as well as coagulation profile should be assessed before surgery because of prior epistaxis as well as the potential for significant intraoperative bleeding. Blood products should be made available in advance.

The surgical principles are:

■ Preoperative planning
■ Identification of the site of tumor origin
■ Complete tumor removal
■ Preservation of natural boundaries
■ Identification of the tissue site for histological orientation

Preoperative planning is an essential part of successful, uncomplicated surgery. This is true in patients operated on for medically refractory rhinosinusitis as well as those with benign sinonasal neoplasms. First and perhaps most importantly is obtaining informed consent. The risks of endoscopic surgery are well known and include bleeding, scar tissue formation, orbital and intracranial injury, and alteration/loss of sense of smell. Additional risks in tumor removal are related to the extent of surgery and may include a higher level of the aforementioned risks. There is a higher risk of epiphora, for example, in an endoscopic medial maxillectomy for inverted papilloma than in maxillary antrostomy for chronic rhinosinusitis. There is a higher risk for CSF leak during removal of a frontoethmoid osteoma than during an anterior ethmoidectomy for chronic rhinosinusitis. In fact, a CSF leak may be an anticipated occurrence and its immediate repair should be planned and discussed with the patient [4].

Patients may benefit from antibiotic treatment in cases of significant postobstructive sinusitis in an ef-

fort to decrease inflammation of the surrounding mucous membranes. This typically translates into less bleeding. Patients should be instructed against the use of aspirin, aspirin-containing products, nonsteroidal anti-inflammatory drugs, and other products which can adversely affect platelet function or coagulation for 1 week before surgery. Certain over-the-counter health aids such as gingko biloba can result in increased bleeding, and patients will often not disclose this in their medical history because it is not considered a "medication." Consultation with prescribing physicians is prudent if stopping certain medications, such as clopidogrel (Plavix) and/or warfarin sodium (Coumadin), may adversely affect other underlying medical conditions. On the day of surgery, it is help-

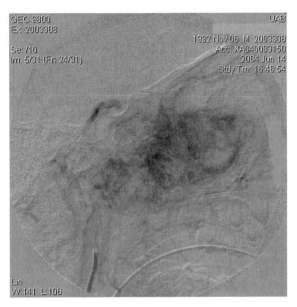

Fig. 13.10. Angiogram of angiofibroma after embolization

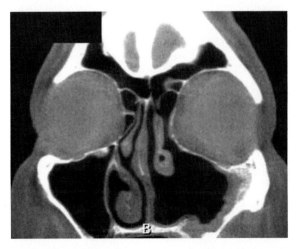

Fig. 13.11. Coronal CT image of a patient after medial maxillectomy with middle turbinate preservation for inverted papilloma

ful to apply topical decongestants to the operative side of the nasal cavity while the patient is in the holding area. Standard injection of vasoconstrictive agents along the lateral nasal wall and into the greater palatine foramen is also recommended. General anesthesia is often utilized in these patients because of the risk of sudden and severe bleeding which would make airway protection difficult in a nonintubated patient. The length of surgery may also exceed the comfort limit for a patient under conscious sedation.

Tips and Pearls

■ In general, it is imperative to recognize and identify the apparent site of origin of benign sinonasal tumors during their removal.

While inverted papilloma and angiofibroma have classic sites of origin, it may not always be so, especially in a case of recurrent/residual tumor or primary inverted papilloma in the frontal or sphenoid sinus. This has important implications in preventing recurrence, avoiding unnecessary tissue removal, and directing endoscopic surveillance. A successful outcome is dependent on complete tumor removal and the utilization of angled scopes can assist the surgeon in assessing the entire maxillary antrum, the frontal recess, or a laterally pneumatized sphenoid sinus for residual tumor. However, it may not be necessary to remove all turbinates in all cases to achieve this, and some degree of "function" can be preserved without compromising outcome (Fig. 13.11). Some tumors may expand and erode bone over time, placing the tumor against the dura of the anterior cranial cavity or the periorbita. When possible, these structures should be

preserved and not resected as they provide an excellent natural boundary to intracranial and intraorbital spread, which can become a significant treatment dilemma. The careful use of bipolar cautery in these areas is recommended over excision once all gross tumor has been removed.

Since en bloc resection is often not possible, the specimens should be carefully identified as to location for the pathologist since there may be foci of severe dysplasia, carcinoma in situ, or even malignant degeneration, particularly in inverted papilloma. This may result in several separate specimens but is essential to understanding the extent of the neoplasm and in directing future endoscopic surveillance for residual or recurrent disease.

Inverted Papilloma

Patients with inverted papilloma are taken to the operating under two different circumstances: biopsy-proven inverted papilloma or unilateral "polyposis" with a high index of suspicion. Distinctive CT and MRI characteristics can aid preoperative diagnosis [20]. In either circumstance, it is helpful to have the ability for intraoperative frozen section. Though the reported incidence of unsuspected diagnosis is less than 1% during routine histological examination of nasal polyp specimens, clinically relevant findings may be identified [12]. Frozen section diagnosis will allow the surgeon to proceed with a potentially curative procedure which would likely be more aggressive than surgery for benign inflammatory disease. It also helps avoid an unnecessary second operation. Once the patient has been appropriately anesthetized and vasoconstrictive agents have been locally infiltrated, the nasal cavity is examined with a 0° telescope (Fig. 13.12). Careful, gentle manipulation of the tumor mass often allows the surgeon to determine its origin from the lateral nasal wall. A blunt, gently curved instrument, such as the Cottle or Freer elevator, works well for this maneuver. Suction elevators are available from several vendors and are excellent tools at this point. Using a suction tip may result in abrasion of the mass and annoying bleeding. With use of a bipolar cautery the majority of the mass can be "amputated" and a more careful inspection of the middle meatus can be completed. At this point is often apparent if the middle turbinate, frontal recess, and/or ethmoid cavity are/is involved. The uncinate process may be medially displaced or destroyed from long-term tumor expansion. After any residual uncinate process is removed, the medial maxillary wall is inspected. It may be medially displaced from intraantral tumor expansion or completely replaced by tumor. When there is significant intraantral tumor, it often sits in a "dumb-

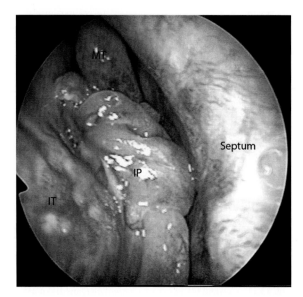

Fig. 13.12. Endoscopic view of inverted papilloma of the right nasal cavity

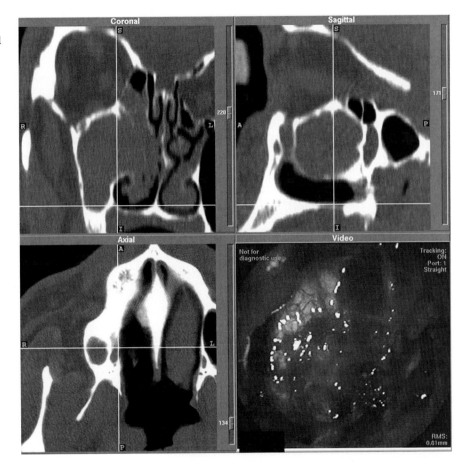

Fig. 13.13. Intraoperative view using computer-aided surgery during medial maxillectomy for removal of inverted papilloma

bell" fashion and does not demonstrate true antral mucosal involvement. When the antral mucosa is involved, the inferior turbinate is removed along with the medial maxillary wall down to the level of the nasal floor (Figs. 13.13, 13.14). Backbiting instruments and the side-biting antral punch are useful tools in this situation. Small "bites" should be taken because this bone is thick and large bites may lead to ruining expensive instruments if the surgeon is too aggressive. All tissue should all be sent to the pathology department and identified as to site. At this point, the maxillary antrum can be completely visualized and instrumented with angled scopes and instruments. It is not necessary to remove all antral mucosa in all patients. As mentioned earlier, once the site of origin has been determined, a surrounding "cuff" of grossly normal mucosa is included in the specimen.

Tips and Pearls

- If an area of hyperostosis is noted on CT, the operating surgeon should take careful note of this area. This often corresponds to the site of origin and early local extension. It is recommended to use a diamond burr to thin the bone in this area.

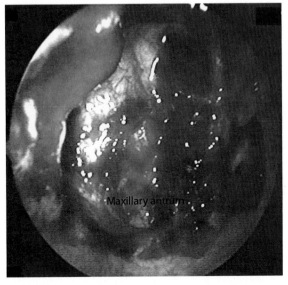

Fig. 13.14. A 30° endoscopic view of the maxillary antrum after endoscopic medial maxillectomy

If the tumor extends into the ethmoid sinus, a total ethmoidectomy should be performed and the lamina papyracea and anterior skull base should be skeletonized. Depending on the extent of tumor, it may

13

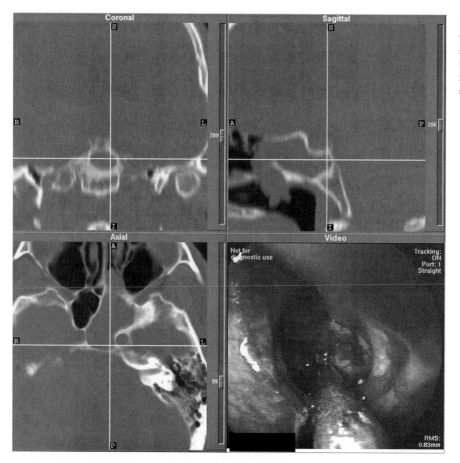

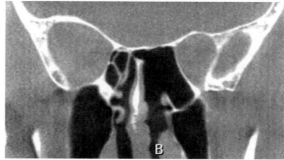

Fig. 13.15. Intraoperative view using computer-aided surgery in a patient with isolated papilloma overlying the posterior wall of the sphenoid sinus

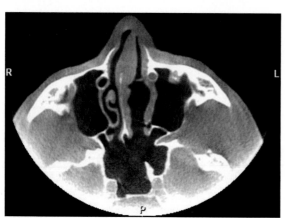

Fig. 13.16. Eight-year postoperative axial view after resection of isolated sphenoid sinus inverted papilloma

Fig. 13.17. Eight-year postoperative coronal view after resection of isolated sphenoid sinus inverted papilloma

be necessary to perform a wide sphenoidotomy[10] (Figs. 3.15–3.17). This allows for complete inspection of the sphenoid sinus and for endoscopic surveillance of that area in follow-up. If tumor extends into the frontal recess and/or frontal sinus, it is vital to distinguish pedunculated extension from true mucosal involvement. If the tumor is pedunculated, it can simply be retracted and removed. If there is mucosal involvement, a more aggressive approach such as a Draf II/III or a modified Lothrop procedure should be performed to obtain adequate exposure for tissue removal. In some cases an adjunctive "classic" approach is utilized in addition to the endoscopic approach [11, 16, 17, 26]. A Caldwell-Luc approach may be required to access the entire maxillary antrum in cases of extensive maxillary sinus involvement [16].

Fig. 13.18. Osteoplastic frontal sinusotomy in a patient with frontal sinus inverted papilloma

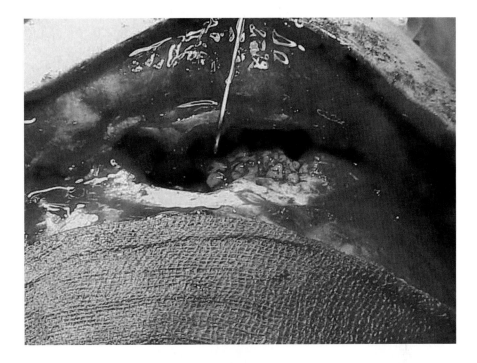

Tips and Pearls

- A frontal sinus trephination or even an osteoplastic frontal sinusotomy may be necessary to adequately visualize and remove the entire tumor from the frontal sinus (Fig. 3.18).

- If an osteoplastic frontal sinusotomy is performed, the frontal sinus should not be obliterated as this will make follow-up difficult. It is preferable to maintain a patent frontal recess and frontal sinus that can be examined with rigid and flexible nasal endoscopy rather than attempting to differentiate tumor recurrence from fat or fibrosis on CT or MRI.

Once all tumor has been removed, the cavity is irrigated with saline and inspected for bleeding. Hemostasis is obtained with bipolar cautery and temporary placement of cottonoids impregnated with vasoconstrictive agents. Packing is not routinely required but is left up to the discretion of the operating surgeon. Patients are observed for bleeding in the postanesthesia care unit and may be discharged accordingly.

Fibroosseous Lesions

Osteoma/Ossifying Fibroma

These lesions tend to be distinct and well circumscribed and therefore are amenable to complete removal. They can be classified by location as ethmoid, frontoethmoid, and frontal. Less common are primary lesions involving the maxillary or sphenoid sinuses, though these areas may become involved by extension from the ethmoid sinus. The challenge is to adequately reduce the size of the tumor so that it can be removed from the nasal cavity without damaging surrounding structures. The endoscopic removal of these lesions represents an ideal clinical situation in which computer-aided surgery may be helpful. When large lesions are encountered, the progress of tumor reduction can be compared with the patient's preoperative images (Fig. 3.19) If a large lesion is prematurely cleaved, it is very difficult to achieve further tumor reduction so that it can be safely atraumatically removed from the nasal cavity. Microdebrider technology is another advancement that allows the endoscopic surgeon to carefully reduce the bulk of these lesions with a variety of burrs.

Once the patient has been properly anesthetized and injected, the nasal cavity is inspected with a 0° telescope. The initial steps of the surgery are similar to those of a standard endoscopic ethmoidectomy. The middle turbinate is gently medialized, the uncinate process removed, and the maxillary ostium identified. Depending on the precise location of the lesion, an ethmoidectomy is also performed. Once the lesion is encountered, it can be slowly reduced in size with a cutting burr. Care should be taken not to damage surrounding mucosa as this will lead to stenosis and possible iatrogenic sinusitis. After the lesion has been adequately reduced, it should be cleaved and removed. This is perhaps the most critical step. Often the cleavage plane can be predicted from the preoperative im-

13

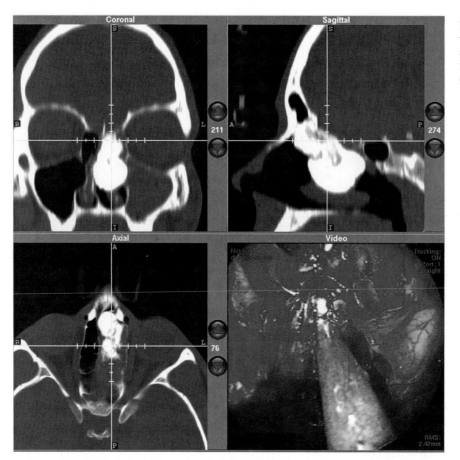

Fig. 13.19. Intraoperative view with computer-aided surgery showing reduction of osteoma prior to cleavage

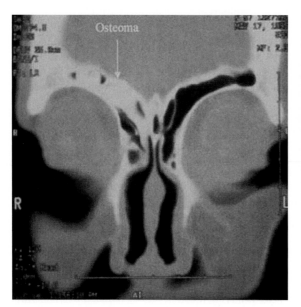

Fig. 13.20. Coronal CT image of a patient with a large symptomatic osteoma removed by combined intranasal endoscopic and osteoplastic frontal sinusotomy approaches

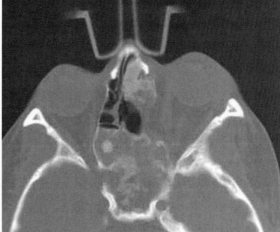

Fig. 13.21. Axial CT image demonstrating extensive fibrous dysplasia and compression of the orbital apex

Fig. 13.22. Intraoperative view with computer-aided surgery of extensive fibrous dysplasia in a patient undergoing decompression of the orbital apex for progressive visual loss

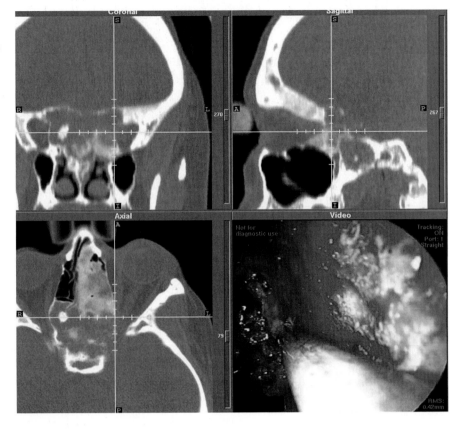

ages. Using an angled curette, the surgeon reaches behind the lesion and pulls in an anterior and inferior direction, away from the skull base. Occasionally an osteotome is required. This should be done with extreme caution as a posterior superior force may lead to fracture of the skull base and intracranial injury. If the cleavage plane involves the lateral cribriform plate lamella, the force required to achieve cleavage may exceed the resistance of the skull base, resulting in a fracture and subsequent CSF leak. This scenario should be recognized on the patient's preoperative images and discussed in advance. Following tumor removal, the skull base is carefully inspected during positive-pressure ventilation for detection of a CSF leak. If a CSF leak is suspected, it should be repaired immediately. For lesions extending into the frontal recess and frontal sinus, the use of angled burrs and scopes may enable complete transnasal removal. As with inverted papilloma, an extended Draf II/III or modified Lothrop procedure may be required. Adjunctive frontal trephination or osteoplastic frontal sinusotomy may be necessary for tumors extending superior and/or lateral in the frontal sinus (Fig. 3.20). These scenarios should be evident from the preoperative imaging studies and planned accordingly.

The operative management of fibrous dysplasia follows similar principles except that the goal is not generally complete tumor removal. The surgeon determines in advance the extent of tissue removal based on the location from the preoperative images. For example, when the orbital apex is compromised, the goal is to decompress that area by removing the posterior medial portion of the lamina papyracea and uncovering the medial portion of the optic nerve (Figs. 3.21, 3.22). The unique challenge with fibrous dysplasia is that it may vary in its consistency. When there is a significant osseous component, it can be reduced with a burr similar to osteoma/ossifying fibroma. If there is more of a fibrous component, curettage works well. Computer-aided surgery is an invaluable tool in either instance to track progress.

Angiofibroma

Complete exposure of the extent of tumor is the initial step. This is accomplished by removing the inferior portion of the middle and occasionally the superior turbinate [2]. The uncinate process is removed and a wide maxillary antrostomy is created to expose the posterior wall of the maxillary sinus. The posterior maxillary wall may have been significantly thinned from tumor pressure. The ethmoid air cells are opened and the lamina papyracea and posterior ethmoid roof are skeletonized. Tumor adherence to the nasal sep-

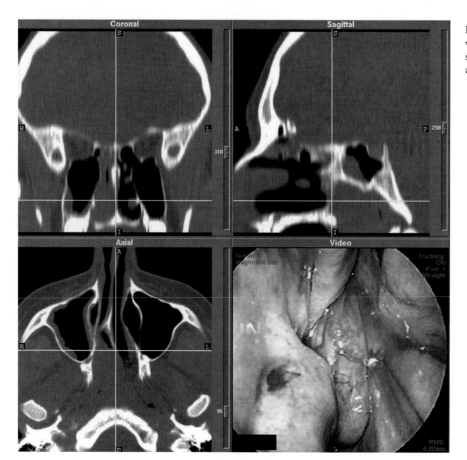

Fig. 13.23. Intraoperative view with computer-aided surgery showing a stage II angiofibroma

13

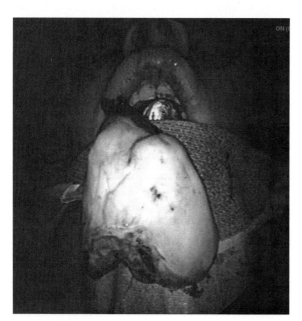

Fig. 13.24. External view of angiofibroma after endoscopic resection and transoral delivery

tum, posterior choana, and nasopharyngeal mucosa should be divided. This may be accomplished bluntly with a suction elevator or sharply depending on the tenacity of the adherence. When bleeding is encountered, tissue separation should be done with suction bipolar cautery. Once the tumor has been mobilized, the pterygomaxillary space can be dissected (Figs. 13.23, 13.24). The posterior wall of the maxillary sinus is removed with a curette. This is usually easily accomplished because the bone has been thinned or may even be absent. With blunt dissection, the tumor's vascular pedicle can be identified. The tumor is divided from its pedicle using bipolar cautery or a vascular clip. A vascular clip has the added advantage of being identified in follow-up imaging studies as the lateral boundary of surgical dissection. Depending on tumor size, it may delivered via a transoral approach through the nasopharynx. Hemostasis is obtained with bipolar cautery and packing is placed as indicated. Patients should be observed overnight for potential bleeding and can usually be discharged on the first postoperative day.

The surgical principles outlined as described for inverted papilloma, fibroosseous lesions, and angiofibroma can be applied to other less common benign neoplasms of the nasal cavity and paranasal sinuses

Fig. 13.25. Intraoperative view with computer-aided surgery during resection of a hemangiopericytoma

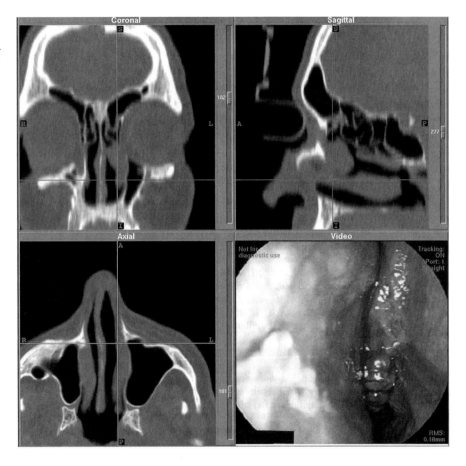

(Figs. 13.25, 13.26). With a high index of suspicion, appropriate imaging studies, careful preoperative planning, advanced endoscopic skills and tools, and endoscopic surveillance, surgeons can safely and appropriately provide care for their patients with benign neoplasms of the nasal cavity and paranasal sinuses.

Conlusion

With appropriate endoscopic skills and instrumentation and routine endoscopic surveillance, patients with benign sinonasal neoplasms can be treated endoscopically safely and effectively.

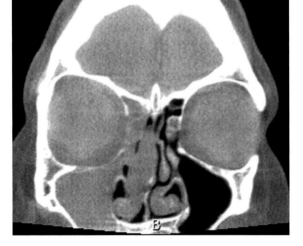

Fig. 13.26. Coronal CT image demonstrating nasal septal chondroma with postobstructive sinusitis

References

1. Banhiran, W. and R.R. Casiano, (2005) Endoscopic sinus surgery for benign and malignant nasal and sinus neoplasm. Curr Opin Otolaryngol Head Neck Surg 13(1): p. 50–4.

2. Berlucchi, M., et al., (2005), Endoscopic surgery for fibrous dysplasia of the sinonasal tract in pediatric patients. Int J Pediatr Otorhinolaryngol 69(1): p. 43–8.

3. Brodish, B.N., C.E. Morgan, and M.J. Sillers, (1999) Endoscopic resection of fibro-osseous lesions of the paranasal sinuses. Am J Rhinol 13(1): p. 11–6.

2. The ethmoid sinus
    (a) Ethmoid roof
    (b) Lateral lamella of the cribriform plate
3. The cribriform plate
4. The sphenoid sinus
    (a) Medial/planum sphenoidale
    (b) Perisellar
    (c) lateral sphenoid recess

Although most skull base defects are limited to one of these distinct sites, it is important to realize some defects encompass multiple anatomic areas. Of the different anatomic locales, skull base defects in the frontal and sphenoid sinus deserve special mention.

There are a number of specific considerations regarding endoscopic repair of frontal sinus CSF leaks and encephaloceles. Successful repair of the CSF leak is essential, but long-term patency of the frontal sinus or obliteration with meticulous removal of all mucosa in the sinus is essential and unique to this anatomic location. Endoscopic repairs of defects adjacent to the frontal recess may create iatrogenic mucoceles or frontal sinusitis if graft material, packing, or synechiae obstruct the frontal sinus outflow tract. In addition, defects located within the frontal recess are very difficult to approach surgically, because the superior extent of the defect may be difficult to reach via an endoscopic repair from below and an external approach from above. If an endoscopic repair is planned, adequate experience with angled endoscopes and frontal giraffe instruments is essential for success in this area. External approaches are certainly adequate in this area and still have a primary role for CSF leak repairs located superiorly and laterally in the frontal sinus.

Like the frontal sinus, skull base defects located in the sphenoid sinus have several important anatomical considerations. The sphenoid sinus is formed by the anterior *and* middle cranial fossae, is in close proximity of the internal carotid artery and optic nerve, and may have extreme lateral pneumatization that limits accessibility via traditional endoscopic routes. Although perisellar CSF leaks and encephaloceles are considered more common secondary to transsphenoidal pituitary resections, other sphenoid defects typically require completely different surgical and postoperative management. A thorough understanding of the underlying cause, pathophysiology, management principles, and treatment options is essential to obtain excellent outcomes.

Etiology

Most CSF leaks can be broadly classified into traumatic (including accidental and iatrogenic trauma), tumor-related, spontaneous, and congenital. These types influence the size and structure of the bony defect, the degree and nature of the dural disruption, intracranial pressure, and meningoencephalocele formation.

Trauma (Accidental and Iatrogenic)

Traumatic CSF leaks may result from blunt or penetrating trauma. Disruption of the skull base can create an obvious CSF leak or the patient may present years later with meningitis, delayed leak, or encephaloceles. Although conservative treatment is usually attempted with small CSF leaks, there is a reported 29% incidence of meningitis with long-term follow-up of CSF leaks that are managed nonsurgically [2].

Iatrogenic trauma deserves special mention. Otolaryngologists are the only surgical subspecialty trained to perform sinus surgery. In the age of endoscopic sinus surgery and powered instrumentation, iatrogenic skull base injuries are all too frequent. Otolaryngologists should have the ability to repair a CSF leak that results as a complication of sinus surgery.

Idiopathic/Spontaneous

Patients with spontaneous CSF leaks likely have a variant of benign intracranial hypertension with evidence of an empty sella on an MRI scan [13, 15]. Elevated CSF pressure increases hydrostatic force at the weakest sites of the skull base. Spontaneous leaks rarely occur in the frontal sinus, but are more likely to occur immediately adjacent to the frontal recess in the ethmoid roof or anterior cribriform plate. Another common area for spontaneous CSF leaks and encephaloceles is in the lateral recess of the sphenoid sinus. These latter areas were relatively undocumented until recently [4, 5, 9]. In these cases, temporal-lobe tissue herniates through a middle cranial fossa defect lateral to the foramen rotundum and vidian canal. These patients have excessive pneumatization of the pterygoid process with an attenuated sphenoid sinus recess roof and skull base. This increases the likelihood of defects developing in the floor of the middle fossa [11]. Elevated CSF pressures may contribute to the development of these CSF leaks. The elevated CSF pressures seen in this subset of patients leads to the highest rate (50–100%) of encephalocele formation, and the highest recurrence rate following surgical repair of the leak (25–87%), compared with less than 10% for most other causes [7, 8, 12]. Underlay bone grafts in these patients may help prevent encephalocele herniation and disruption of the repair. In addition, we recommend lumbar drains perioperatively and acetazolamide postoperatively to lower elevated intracranial pressure.

Neoplasms

Sinonasal tumors and skull base neoplasms can create CSF leaks directly through erosion of the anterior cranial fossa or middle cranial fossa, or indirectly secondary to therapeutic treatments for the tumor. Repair of a skull base defect following endoscopic tumor resection is a routine part of operative planning. (Fig. 14.1) Persistent malignant tumor following resection and repair will continue to erode the skull base and create a CSF leak. Prior chemotherapy or radiation creates significant difficulties with healing.

Congenital

Congenital encephaloceles were initially divided into sincipital (also referred to as anterior or frontoethmoidal) and basal encephaloceles. The basal-type encephaloceles are intranasal in location and have been variously described as transethmoidal, sphenoethmoidal, sphenomaxillary, sphenoorbital, transsphenoidal, and transtemporal [6]. In reality, congenital dehiscence can likely occur through any point in the skull base. Although these defects are present since birth, they may not be diagnosed clinically until the patient presents with nasal obstruction, CSF leak, meningitis, or facial deformity. With appropriate instrumentation and experience, many of these defects can be repaired endoscopically in patients as young as 2 years of age [17, 18].

Diagnosis and Preoperative Tests

An ideal test that detects the presence of a CSF leak while also identifying the location of the skull base

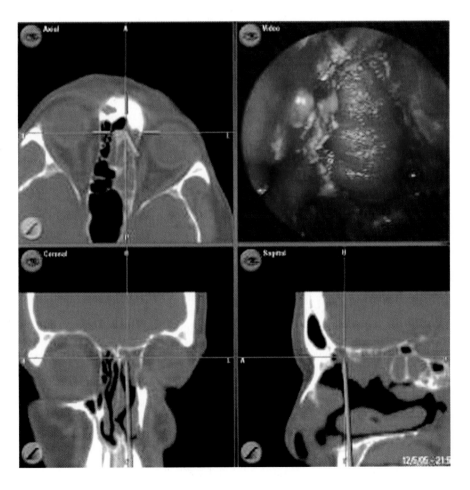

Fig. 14.1. CT scan triplanar imaging of an esthesioneuroblastoma with an endoscopic view (*upper right*) of the large skull base defect following endoscopic resection. A soft-tissue underlay graft using Duragen® (Integra NeuroSciences, Plainsboro, NJ, USA) was tucked into the epidural space

defect with 100% accuracy is not currently available; therefore, a combination of preoperative tests is often necessary to establish the diagnosis and localize the defect. The tests should be chosen on the basis of the clinical picture and the precise information needed, rather than following a rigid algorithm. The invasiveness of the test and the risks to the patient should always be considered.

The following are techniques for diagnosing and localizing CSF leaks:

1. β_2-Transferrin
   Advantages: Accurate, noninvasive, low incidence of false positives and negatives [14, 16]
   Disadvantages: Nonlocalizing
   Comments: Beta-trace protein is another marker used primarily in Europe [1]

2. High-resolution coronal and axial CT scans
   Advantages: Excellent bony detail
   Disadvantages: Inability to distinguish CSF from other soft tissue; bony dehiscences may be present without a leak
   Comments: Performed in every patient for operative planning

3. Radioactive cisternograms
   Advantages: Localizes side of the leak, identifies low volume or intermittent leaks
   Disadvantages: Invasive, localization imprecise
   Comments: Imaging technique – more information obtained than with a radionucleotide cisternogram

4. MRI/magnetic resonance cisternography
   Advantages: Excellent soft-tissue (CSF/brain vs. secretions) detail, noninvasive
   Disadvantage: Poor bony detail
   Comments: Imaging useful for lateral sphenoid opacities and suspected encephaloceles

5. Intrathecal fluorescein
   Advantages: Precise localization, blue-light filter improves sensitivity
   Disadvantages: Invasive; skull base exposure required for precision localization
   Comments: See below

One of the most useful advancements in diagnosing and localizing CSF leaks has been the use of intrathecal fluorescein with a thorough endoscopic examination. For those patients with an unclear diagnosis, a thorough endoscopic examination following the administration of intrathecal fluorescein can be particularly helpful in establishing the preoperative diagnosis. This test is more useful in individuals who have had prior sinus surgery and have an exposed, skeletonized skull base. For this reason, fluorescein is more commonly administered intraoperatively, so that complete skeletonization of the skull base may permit accurate diagnosis and localization. We typi-

cally use this intraoperatively in all cases, since it poses little risk, is useful in localizing the defect, and ensures a watertight closure. The fluorescein may be significantly diluted or excreted by the time skull base exposure is attained depending upon the rate of the leak, the rate of CSF turnover, and the timing of the intrathecal injection. The addition of a blue-light filter can improve the detection of dilute fluorescein.

Fluorescein is not FDA-approved for intrathecal injection, because seizures and neurotoxicity have been reported when using higher concentrations or more rapid injections. We have had no complications using a mixture of 0.1 ml of preservative-free 10% fluorescein diluted in 10 ml of the patient's CSF slowly injected over 10–15 min. We obtain informed written consent regarding the risks and benefits of intrathecal fluorescein and its lack of FDA approval in all patients.

Operative Technique

Each case begins with rapid sequence intubation, in order to minimize the risk of pneumocephalus from bag mask ventilation. For almost all cases, our neurosurgical service then places a lumbar drain. This can be useful in cases that demonstrate elevated CSF pressures or when a repair is somewhat tenuous. We then inject intrathecal fluorescein as previously described [14], which is extremely useful for localizing the exact site of the skull base defect. If the lumbar drain is not needed postoperatively, it is easily removed at the end of the case.

The appropriate surgical approach varies depending upon the exact site and size of the defect, the equipment available, and the experience of the surgeon.

The Frontal Sinus

Repairing frontal sinus CSF leaks via an endoscopic approach requires a thorough knowledge of frontal recess anatomy and its variants. All air cells encroaching on the frontal sinus outflow tract, such as agger nasi cells anterolaterally or suprabullar cells posteriorly, must be removed in their entirety to increase the chance of long-term frontal patency. At the same time, careful attention to preserving the mucosa surrounding the outflow tract will also increase long-term patency. Stripping the mucosa will ultimately lead to scar tissue formation and osteitic bone and increase failure rates. Therefore, expertise with angled scopes and frontal giraffe instruments is indispensable for adequate visualization and operating efficiency.

After wide exposure of the skull base defect through a wide frontal sinusotomy, an intraoperative judgment must be made regarding the ability to perform a successful CSF leak repair while maintaining patency of the frontal recess. (Fig. 14.2) Attempting endoscopic repair initially does not burn any bridges, since an open procedure can be performed at a later time if failure or outflow tract obstruction ensues. When the defect approaches the midline, a modified endoscopic Lothrop procedure can increase surgical access and provide bilateral frontal sinus drainage if ipsilateral stenosis of the duct is expected from the repair. Likewise, a frontal trephine can provide access to the superior limits of a defect and endoscopes may be utilized through the trephine as well as from below.

Although we discourage the use of hard stents to maintain frontal sinus patency secondary to an increased probability of reactive scar formation and osteitic bone formation, we have found soft silastic stents useful in maintaining patency, if the mucosa is preserved and the stent is gently placed in the frontal sinus outflow tract. This stent has the added advantage of helping maintain placement of the soft-tissue overlay graft, especially when the skull base defect is located in the vertical plane of the posterior table.

Although the limits of endoscopic approaches continue to expand with improved equipment and experience, posterior table defects located beyond the reach of frontal sinus instruments superiorly or laterally to the sinus outflow tract still require an open approach [19]. We feel that this is the only area in the anterior skull base not amenable to endoscopic techniques. The method most often used is an osteoplastic flap with thorough removal of all mucosa and unilateral or bilateral obliteration (depending upon the size of the frontal sinus). Repairing a posterior table defect via an osteoplastic flap can be performed without obliteration if the defect is sufficiently superior or lateral to avoid compromising the sinus outflow tract. A well pneumatized frontal sinus with a defect in the lateral recess can be repaired via an osteoplastic flap or trephine without compromising the frontal recess. Since the potential for mucocele formation is significant regardless of the surgical approach, close follow-up is essential and must be emphasized to the patient.

The Ethmoid Roof/Cribriform Plate

The posterior ethmoid roof and lateral lamella of the cribriform plate are two of the most common areas for iatrogenic CSF leaks [14]. In general, these are the easiest areas to repair because they only require an ethmoidectomy for exposure of the defect. The mucosa is easily elevated around the defect for preparation of the graft. However, CSF leaks and encephaloceles originating in the olfactory cleft/cribriform plate are much more difficult to repair. Unlike other areas, such as the ethmoid roof, sphenoid sinus, and posterior table of the frontal sinus, the bone is not smooth. Elevating the mucosa on the defect is extremely difficult because the cleft is very narrow and often has multiple perforations where the olfactory filaments exit the cribriform plate. Placing an underlay graft in the epidural space in this area is almost impossible. Instead of elevating mucosa here, we typically cauterize it with a bipolar device to try to ablate the mucosa, and then use a simple overlay graft with cadaveric fascia, alloderm, or mucosa. We typically resect the middle turbinate up to skull base to gain access to this area, but leave the septum intact to provide support for packing materials. Although, this repair does not seem as structurally sound as those repairs with an underlay graft, we have not noticed a drop in success rate when compared with that for other areas.

The Sphenoid Sinus

Simple defects in the central sphenoid or perisellar regions can be approached either through a direct parasagittal endoscopic approach or transethmoid approach. The middle turbinate is gently lateralized and the inferior portion of the superior turbinate is resected following topical and injected vasoconstriction. Just medial to the superior turbinate within the sphenoethmoid recess, the natural ostium of the sphenoid is identified and a wide sphenoidotomy performed using straight mushroom and Kerrison punches. Additional midline exposure is gained by resecting the posterior portion of the nasal septum and the intersinus septum. If the defect is located more laterally, a complete endoscopic ethmoidectomy is performed with perforation of the basal lamella, resection of the inferior third of the superior turbinate, and identification of the natural ostium of the sphenoid. The sphenoidotomy is extended laterally to the medial orbital wall and the lateral wall of the sphenoid sinus as needed.

Skull base defects of the middle cranial fossa in the lateral recess of the sphenoid sinus are difficult to access by the midline transeptal/parasaggital or transethmoid approaches and ultimately require an endoscopic transpterygoid approach [3]. A complete ethmoidectomy, wide maxillary antrostomy, and wide sphenoidotomy are performed first. The posterior wall of the maxillary sinus is removed to gain access to the pterygopalatine fossa. The internal maxillary artery

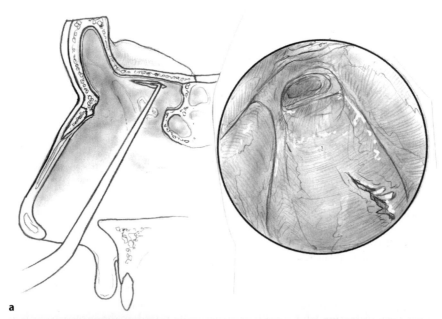

Fig. 14.2. a This skull base defect is located in the ethmoid roof posterior to the frontal recess. The ethmoid roof is skeletonized for exposure of the defect and the frontal recess is meticulously dissected with mucosal sparing technique. A frontal sinusotomy is necessary for exposure and prevention of iatrogenic frontal sinusitis or mucocele from packing material. b Triplanar CT imaging of a patient with a similar defect just posterior to the frontal recess

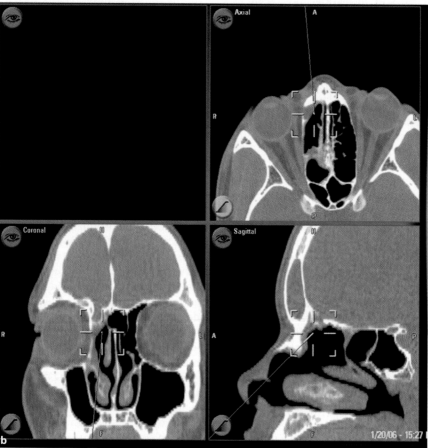

and its branches are identified and reflected inferiorly or clipped and divided. The vidian and the maxillary nerve are meticulously dissected within the pterygopalatine fossa to avoid the unnecessary morbidities of cheek anesthesia and problems with lacrimation. The anterior face of the sphenoid sinus that has pneumatized into the pterygoid plates is drilled away for exposure of the lateral recess of the sphenoid sinus.

14

Repair of Skull Base Defect

Once adequate identification and exposure of the skull base defect has been obtained using one of the surgical approaches described in the preceding sections, the recipient bed is prepared by removal of several millimeters of mucosa around the bony defect (Fig. 14.3). Malleable suction elevators are particularly helpful, since these can be molded to the appropriate angle for defects located almost anywhere on the anterior skull base. Encephaloceles are ablated using bipolar cautery as much as possible. Malleable suction monopolar cautery devices can reach difficult areas in the anterior and lateral skull base, but should be avoided near the optic nerve or carotid artery. Meticulous hemostasis is mandatory while ablating the encephalocele to avoid retraction of the sac and possible intracranial hemorrhage. After reduction of the encephalocele, if a lumbar drain has been placed preoperatively, the drain is opened and 10–15 ml of CSF is shunted into the collection bag. The bag is then positioned to establish a flow rate of 5–10 ml/h. This will decrease intracranial pressure and aid in the reduction of the encephalocele base, thereby facilitating graft placement.

A multilayer repair technique of CSF leaks that consists of an underlay graft placed in the epidural space and an overlay graft placed intranasally beneath the bony skull base is preferred. Ball-tipped probes are useful for tucking the graft inside the bony edges of the skull base into the epidural space. As stated previously, the placement of an underlay graft in the olfactory cleft/cribriform area is very difficult, so an overlay graft only is placed in this area. Underlay grafts are also unnecessary for linear cracks in the skull base, since attempted placement may increase the size of the defect (Fig. 14.4). If the patient has elevated CSF pressures, a rigid underlay graft, such as bone, in the epidural space can provide support for the repair. Leaks with other causes where there are normal intracranial pressures probably do not require rigid grafting and can be repaired successfully by using soft-tissue grafts.

Options for rigid grafting include bone grafts from the nasal septum, turbinates, or mastoid. Septal bone provides significant strength and is easily trimmed to shape using through-cutting sinus instruments. Turbinate bone is often thin and may have a shape that does not conform to the native skull base. Mastoid bone can be sculpted to the precise shape needed, but requires additional time to harvest. Cartilage has a tendency to fracture, is very thick, and has a lower structural strength than bone grafts.

A variety of soft-tissue materials may be used for underlay or overlay grafts, including:

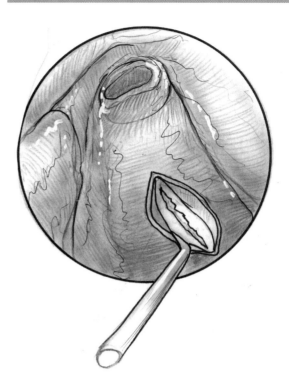

Fig. 14.3. The mucosa is gently elevated around the defect for several millimeters

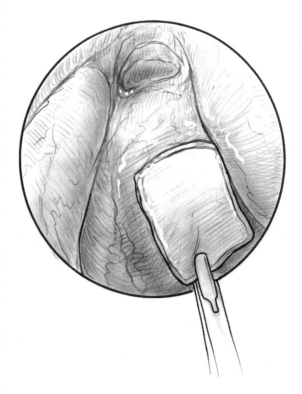

Fig. 14.4. An overlay graft is placed against the defect

- Temporalis fascia
- Fascia lata
- Cadaveric dermis or fascia
- Commercially available animal collagen, fascia, or pericardium
- Mucosa or mucoperichondrium (overlay only)

Mucosal grafts placed in the epidural space are unacceptable, because mucoceles, meningitis, and other intracranial complications can occur when contaminated mucosa is placed intracranially. In most cases, fibrin glue or other tissue glue is rarely necessary after placement of the graft. Blood is often present around the wound bed and likely contributes its own fibrin matrix to help seal the repair. Proper placement of the graft with tight packing for structural support is the most important aspect of the repair. We place multiple layers of gelfoam or other absorbable packing underneath the graft (Fig. 14.5). A removable finger cot can be placed under the packing material for additional support.

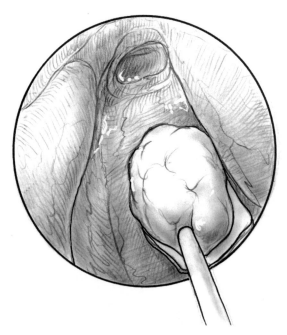

Fig. 14.5. Multiple layers of gelfoam are placed under the graft for support. Placement of a soft silastic stent (1 week) through the frontal sinusotomy to prevent placement of packing material in the frontal recess may be necessary

Adjuvant Treatment and Postoperative Care

Lumbar drains are very useful in the repair of CSF leaks for a variety of reasons. Preoperative injection of intrathecal fluorescein can help identify the location of the CSF leak. In patients with spontaneous CSF leaks and possibly elevated intracranial pressure, they aid the placement of graft materials by temporarily lowering that pressure. Increased pressure can occur postoperatively owing to overproduction of CSF in the absence of a release-valve mechanism. Increased CSF pressure against a closed defect can dislodge the graft materials and lower the chance of success. Maintaining a lumbar drain in these individuals for 2–3 days postoperatively will increase the chance of successful repair. However, we have noticed no difference in our success rates with immediate removal of lumbar drains in those individuals with normal CSF pressure.

Acetazolamide is a carbonic anhydrase inhibitor diuretic that is a useful adjunct in patients with elevated CSF pressure. It decreases CSF production in these individuals and may decrease CSF leak recurrence. We prescribe 500 mg of sustained-release acetazolamide administered twice daily. As with any diuretic, periodic electrolyte monitoring is absolutely necessary to correct imbalances that develop. Patients who develop multiple CSF leaks in the presence of high intracranial pressure not alleviated by acetazolamide should be referred to a neurosurgeon for the placement of a ventriculoperitoneal shunt.

Patients are limited to light activity for 6 weeks postoperatively. All patients are placed on a stool softener and are seen every 1–2 weeks postoperatively for a conservative endoscopic debridement. Debridements are performed to maintain patency of the paranasal sinuses on the side of the repair, avoid stasis of secretions, and help prevent bacterial infections. An antistaphylococcal antibiotic is appropriate until the finger cots are removed at the first postoperative visit, usually 5–7 days after the surgical repair. Patients return to normal activity at around 6 weeks postoperatively.

Conclusion

The underlying cause and pathogenesis of anterior skull base defects and CSF leaks greatly affects the subsequent repair. A thorough understanding of the management principles and treatment options available is important to achieve excellent outcomes. A careful preoperative evaluation and localization of the CSF leak will aid in the selection of the surgical approach and the options for skull base reconstruction. Meticulous operative technique, appropriate adjuvant treatment, and thorough postoperative care ultimately generate the most successful results.

References

1. Bachmann G (2005) Beta-trace protein: an unknown marker for cerebrospinal fluid leaks. Laryngoscope; 115(4):756; author reply 756–7.

2. Bernal-Sprekelsen M, Bleda-Vazquez C, Carrau RL (2000) Ascending meningitis secondary to traumatic cerebrospinal fluid leaks. Am J Rhinol; 14:257–9.

3. Bolger WE (2005) Endoscopic transpterygoid approach to the lateral sphenoid recess: surgical approach and clinical experience. Otolaryngol Head Neck Surg 2005; 133(1):20–6.

4. Buchfelder M, Fahlbusch R, Huk JW, Thierauf P (1987) Intraspehenoidal encephaloceles: a clinical entity. Acta Neurochir; 89:0–15.

5. Daniilidis J, Vlachtsis K, Ferekidis E, Dimitriadis A (1999) Intrasphenoidal encephalocele and spontaneous CSF rhinorrhea. Rhinology; 37:186–189.

6. David DJ (1993) Cephaloceles: classification, pathology, and management – a review. J Craniofac Surg; 4:192–202.

7. Gassner HG, Ponikau JU, Sherris DA, Kern EB (1999) CSF Rhinorrhea: 95 consecutive surgical cases with long term follow-up at the Mayo Clinic. Am J Rhinol; 13:439–447.

8. Hubbard JL, McDonald TJ, Pearson BW, Laws, ER Jr (1985) Spontaneous cerebrospinal fluid rhinorrhea: Evolving concepts in diagnosis and surgical management based on the Mayo Clinic experience from 1970 through 1981. Neurosurgery; 16:314–21.

9. Landreneau FE, Mickey B, Coimbra C (1998) Surgical treatment of cerebrospinal fluid fistulae involving lateral extension of the sphenoid sinus. Neurosurgery; 42:1101–1105

10. Mattox DE, Kennedy DW (1990) Endoscopic management of cerebrospinal fluid leaks and cephaloceles. Laryngoscope; 100:857–62.

11. Reynolds JM, Tomkinson A, Grigg RG, Perry CF (1998) A LeFort I osteotomy approach to lateral sphenoid sinus encephaloceles. J Laryngol Otol; 112:679–681.

12. Schick B, Ibing R, Brors D, Draf W (2001) Long-term study of endonasal duraplasty and review of the literature. Ann Otol Rhinol Laryngol; 110:142–7.

13. Schlosser RJ, Bolger WE (2003) Significance of empty sella in cerebrospinal fluid leaks. Otolaryngol Head Neck Surg. Jan; 128(1):32–8.

14. Schlosser RJ, Bolger WE (2004) Nasal cerebrospinal fluid leaks: critical review and surgical considerations. Laryngoscope; 114(2):255–65.

15. Schlosser RJ, Woodworth BA, Wilensky EM, Grady MS, Bolger WE. Spontaneous cerebrospinal fluid (CSF) leaks: A variant of benign intracranial hypertension (BIH). Annals of Otol Laryngol. (in press)

16. Skedros DG, Cass SP, Hirsch BE, Kelly RH (1993) Sources of error in use of beta-2 transferrin analysis for diagnosing perilymphatic and cerebral spinal fluid leaks. Otolaryngol Head Neck Surg; 109:861–4.

17. Woodworth BA, Schlosser RJ (2005). Endoscopic repair of a congenital intranasal encephalocele in a 23 months old infant. Int J Pediatr Otorhinolaryngol; 69(7):1007–1009.

18. Woodworth BA, Schlosser RJ, Faust RA, Bolger WE (2004) Evolutions in the management of congenital intranasal skull base defects. Arch Otolaryngol Head Neck Surg; 130:1283–1288.

19. Woodworth BA, Schlosser RJ, Palmer JN (2005) Endoscopic repair of frontal sinus cerebrospinal fluid leaks. J Laryngol Otol; 119(9):709–13.

Chapter 15

The Management of Frontal Sinus Fractures

Andrew A. Winkler, Timothy L. Smith, Tanya K. Meyer, Thomas T. Le

15

Core Messages

- Frontal sinus fractures may be divided into those involving the anterior table and posterior table, with and without nasofrontal outflow tract involvement.

- Options for surgical management of frontal sinus fractures include reduction and fixation of anterior table fragments, frontal sinus obliteration and frontal sinus cranialization.

- With good technique, early and late complications can be kept to a minimum.

Contents

Introduction

Frontal sinus fractures offer significant challenges to surgeons and the treatment paradigm has been debated for many years. Acute concerns include protection of intracranial structures, identification of associated injuries and control of cerebrospinal fluid (CSF) leakage. The aesthetic forehead contour is an important consideration in repair. Past surgical modalities that removed the anterior bony frontal surface left life-long disfiguring defects and have been largely replaced by techniques that leave a smooth contour without visible scars. Concerns about aesthetic deformity, however, must yield to practices that will provide a "safe" sinus resistant to late complications. Long-term issues revolve around surveillance and management of late complications that can occur decades after the inciting injury. Traditional treatment paradigms were conceived before the advent of modern endoscopic and advanced imaging techniques, and focus on open techniques for fracture reduction and sinus management. Newer modified algorithms incorporate these technologic advancements with improved functional and cosmetic results.

Anatomy

The frontal sinus is formed by pneumatization of anterior ethmoid air cells into the frontal bone during the fourth fetal month. The sinus begins its predominant phase of expansion from 5 years of age until adolescence, and is usually characterized by two asymmetric sinuses separated by a thin, bony septal plate. The frontal sinus often demonstrates variable pneumatization, with 4–15% of people showing developmental failure of one of the sinuses. The frontal sinus is in close proximity to several intracranial structures. The posterior wall forms the anterior wall of the cranial vault, and the floor of the frontal sinus contributes to the anterior superior roof of the orbit. The skull base abutting the posterior aspect of the frontal sinus is the cribriform plate. The nasofrontal outflow tract is an hour-glass-shaped structure that drains secretions from the frontal sinus mucosa into the frontal recess. The frontal recess is bounded by the agger nasi anteriorly, the middle turbinate medially, the skull base posterosuperiorly, the ethmoid bulla posteroinferiorly, and the lamina papyracea laterally. The agger nasi cells are important landmarks for identifying this drainage tract. These cells are anterior ethmoid cells at the anterior aspect of the middle meatus that form the floor of the frontal sinus. To functionally enlarge the natural frontal sinus ostium, the surgeon must remove the posteromedial and superior walls of the agger nasi cell [6].

Tips and Pearls

- The frontal sinus fails to develop in 4–15% of people.
- The frontal sinus is in close proximity to several intracranial structures.
- The frontal sinus drains into the nasofrontal outflow tract, which is bounded by the agger nasi anteriorly, an important surgical landmark.

Epidemiology

Frontal sinus fractures are rare and occur in only 5–12% of maxillofacial traumas [16, 27, 28]. A study conducted at four separate level 1 trauma centers including 892 patients demonstrated that in patients with frontal sinus fractures the median age is 32 years and 88% are male [26]. Approximately 58% of frontal sinus fractures are associated with other facial trauma, including nasoorbital ethmoid fractures (34%), zygomaticomaxillary complex fractures (17%) and orbital wall fractures (27.5%) [12–14]. Forty-three percent of all frontal sinus fractures are isolated anterior table fractures, 7% are isolated posterior table fractures and 49% are combined anterior and posterior table fractures. Motor vehicle accidents account for most fractures (62%), with assaults (12%) and falls (11%) also having a fairly high incidence.

The extent of sinus pneumatization, direction of impact, and collision force influence the degree of injury. Nahum [33] reported the force required to fracture the frontal sinus to be 800–1600 lb, which is significantly higher than that of any other area of the skull. The forces required to produce frontal sinus fractures will often cause multiple craniofacial injuries. Posterior table fractures indicate severe injury and result in pneumocephalus in 25% of patients, CSF leak in 25% and extradural hematoma in 10% [14]. In addition, up to 59% of patients with frontal sinus trauma may present with concomitant orbital trauma [22, 35].

Diagnosis

The hallmark of frontal sinus fracture is frontal depression, often accompanied by forehead lacerations. A neurosurgical consultation is necessary if there is any concern for intracranial injury or suspicion of CSF leak [1]. Fractures involving the supraorbital foramen will result in hypoesthesia in the V_1 distribution. Often periorbital ecchymosis and edema is present. Abnormal vision or extraocular movement restriction warrants an ophthalmologic evaluation.

Although plain films have been used in the past to diagnose fractures of the frontal sinus, high-resolution thin-cut computed tomography (CT) is essential to the diagnosis and treatment of frontal sinus injuries in the modern era (Fig. 15.1) [27]. In addition to the standard axial and coronal images, sagittal reconstructions of the paranasal sinuses can enhance visualization of the nasofrontal outflow tract [20]. Although sagittal reformats can assist in further characterization of the drainage pathway (Fig. 15.2), their prognostic accuracy for eventual normal ventilation of the frontal sinus in the trauma setting is unknown. Certain findings on CT, such as nasoorbital ethmoid complex fractures and anterior skull base injury near the junction of the posterior table and the cribriform plate strongly suggest injury to the nasofrontal outflow [17].

Tips and Pearls

- High-resolution thin-cut CT is essential to the diagnosis of frontal sinus injuries.
- Sagittal reconstructions of the paranasal sinuses enhance visualization of the nasofrontal outflow tract.

Current Management Techniques

The main goals in the treatment of frontal sinus fractures are (1) protection of intracranial structures and control of CSF leakage, (2) prevention of late complications and (3) correction of aesthetic deformity. Frontal sinus fractures can be classified into fractures of the anterior table or the posterior table with or without associated nasofrontal outflow tract injury:

1. Anterior table fracture
   (a) With or without displacement
   (b) With or without outflow tract injury
2. Posterior table fracture
   (a) With or without displacement
   (b) With or without dural injury/CSF leak
   (c) With or without outflow tract injury

15

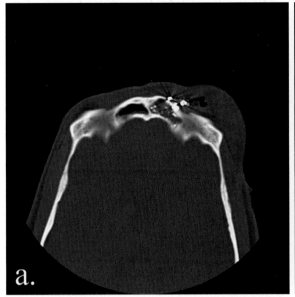

a.

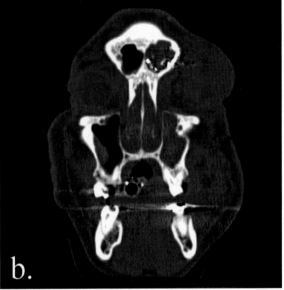

b.

Fig. 15.1. Axial (**a**) and coronal (**b**) computed tomography (*CT*) images demonstrating opacification and metallic foreign bodies in the left frontal sinus in a patient who sustained a gunshot wound to the frontal sinus

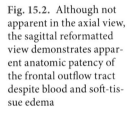

Fig. 15.2. Although not apparent in the axial view, the sagittal reformatted view demonstrates apparent anatomic patency of the frontal outflow tract despite blood and soft-tissue edema

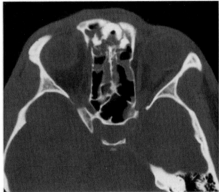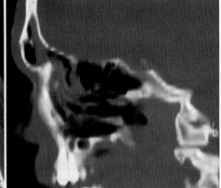

Displacement is defined as greater than one table width. Posterior table fractures commonly occur in combination with anterior table fractures, and are frequently associated with dural or intracranial injury. Management of CSF leaks and dural tears will often dictate acute treatment. Surgical intervention of this high-risk region must provide a "safe" sinus that will resist future infectious complications.

Anterior Table Fractures

Low-energy frontal sinus trauma results in isolated, nondisplaced anterior table fractures. The treatment options can be summarized as follows:

1. Nondisplaced or minimally displaced: no treatment necessary

2. Displaced: open reduction and internal fixation for cosmesis
3. Involvement of the nasofrontal outflow tract
   (a) Open reduction and internal fixation of anterior table and osteoplastic flap with obliteration
   (b) Outflow tract reconstruction (not highly recommended)
   (c) Observation and medical management with future endoscopic ventilation if necessary

The risk of mucosal entrapment and mucocele formation in this type of fracture is low and the aesthetic deformity is generally minimal. Surgical intervention is therefore often avoidable. However, depressed fractures of the anterior table must be reduced and fixed. Care should be taken to prevent entrapment of the mucosa within the fracture line. Access to the depressed bony fragments can often be gained using an overlying laceration. Alternatively, brow or coronal incisions provide adequate exposure and are well camouflaged by the eyebrows and hair. The use of titanium miniplates in frontal sinus fracture fixation is a durable method of repair and has a very low complication rate [18]. Titanium is a high strength, corrosion-resistant material with low tissue reactivity that produces minimal artifacts on MRI and CT scanning [21, 44]. Recently, research has been directed at increasing the biointegration of titanium alloys using chemical and heat treatments [42]. A bony precipitate strongly adheres to the heat-treated titanium substrate and promotes living bone bonding.

Patients with isolated and minimally displaced anterior table fractures may be addressed endoscopically using a brow lift incision and subperiosteal dissection [43]. To assist with fracture reduction and plate fixation, additional small stab incisions are made in the brow and along forehead mimetic lines [34]. If exposure is suboptimal, the endoscopic approach can be converted to a traditional coronal incision. A study of endoscopic-assisted reduction of both simple and comminuted anterior table fractures found no complications at up to 28 months follow-up [3].

Repair of the comminuted anterior table requires additional fixation to restore the original contour. Titanium mesh is used to reapproximate and secure bone fragments. Infection rates with mesh implants are low [21]. Large defects can be reconstructed using split calvarial grafts taken from the parietal calvarium. If bone fragments within the sinus are of moderate size but contaminated, they are cleansed and soaked in povidone–iodine solution before further use [8, 32]; however, in the setting of extensive fragmentation with gross contamination or infection, a better option may be to obliterate the sinus.

Tips and Pearls

- Frontal sinus fractures depressed more than one table width must be reduced.
- Titanium miniplates are durable and are associated with a very low complication rate.
- Comminuted anterior table repair requires titanium mesh to reapproximate bone fragments.

Posterior Table Fractures

Fractures of the posterior table commonly occur in conjunction with anterior table fractures and require a separate treatment algorithm. The treatment options can be summarized as follows:

- Nondisplaced without CSF leak: observation
- Nondisplaced with CSF leak: conservative management of CSF leak with progression to sinus exploration if no resolution in 4–7 days
- Displaced (more than one table width): Sinus exploration, repair of dura, obliteration or cranialization depending on involvement of the posterior table
- Involvement of the nasofrontal outflow tract: obliteration or cranialization

Most surgeons advocate observation in those patients with uncomplicated (without nasofrontal outflow tract involvement, CSF leak or dural exposure), nondisplaced posterior table fractures [11]; however, nondisplaced posterior table fractures that result in significant CSF leakage require immediate repair. In addition, surgery is recommended for all displaced posterior table fractures (defined as displacement greater than one posterior table width) because the risk of dural injury is unacceptably high. Though direct dural repair may be considered in experienced hands, the majority of these sinuses should be cranialized.

Cranialization involves removal of the posterior table to create a common intracranial and frontal sinus cavity. Typically a coronal incision is used and a bifrontal craniotomy is made to obtain wide exposure of the area. The frontal lobe is gently retracted to isolate the posterior table. The posterior wall of the frontal sinus is resected and the mucosa lining the anterior wall is meticulously removed with a high-speed diamond burr to prevent mucocele formation. To separate the cranium from the nasal cavity, the nasofrontal outflow tracts are plugged using autogenous material such as fat, bone or muscle plugs. In patients with extensive comminution or cribriform injury, a pericranial flap can be used to augment the skull base and dural repair. Large concomitant defects of the anterior skull base and cribriform area may necessitate reconstruction with calvarial bone graft or titanium mesh in conjunction with an overlying pericranial flap. Anterior or posterior ethmoidectomies to remove traumatized cell partitions may be necessary to ensure sinonasal drainage to prevent cephalad infection.

Tips and Pearls

- Nondisplaced posterior table fractures may be observed, but in those with CSF leaks or displacement more than one posterior table width, cranialization should be strongly considered.
- Cranialization involves removal of the posterior table to create a common intracranial and frontal sinus cavity.

■ A pericranial flap can be used to augment the skull base and dural repair.

Nasofrontal Outflow Tract Fractures

For decades controversy has surrounded management of fractures that involve the nasofrontal outflow tract. Unrecognized injury to the outflow tract can occur in one third or more frontal sinus fractures and commonly results in long-term sequelae [8, 27]. Treatment options include reconstruction of the drainage system, obliteration of the sinus or observation with medical management.

Prolonged stenting of the outflow tract has been advocated by Luce [24], but is associated with stenosis and is considered by many to have an unacceptable failure rate (30%) [39]. Alternatively, the Sewall–Boyden reconstruction may be attempted, which involves enlarging the nasofrontal outflow tract and relining the tract with a septal mucoperiosteal flap.

Most authors recommend obliteration of the sinus when injury to the nasofrontal outflow tract is suspected [14, 22, 27, 33, 35, 38] because this has traditionally been considered the safer long-term option [46]. Although most nasofrontal outflow tract reconstruction attempts have historically been plagued by stenosis, new endoscopic techniques may allow delayed nasofrontal outflow tract recanalization (endoscopic frontal sinusotomy) after a trial of medical management in highly selected patients (see "Endoscopic Management") [40].

Tips and Pearls
■ Unrecognized injury to the outflow tract can occur in one third of frontal sinus fractures and results in long-term sequelae.

Endoscopic Management

Advances in endoscopic equipment and modern imaging over the last two decades have allowed for an endoscopic treatment alternative to sinus ablation. Anterior table fractures involving the nasofrontal outflow tract have traditionally been treated by sinus obliteration. Historically, attempts at outflow tract reconstruction have been disappointing secondary to stenosis and subsequent sinus obstruction [39]. Recent endoscopic developments, however, may allow for delayed nasofrontal outflow tract recanalization through endoscopic frontal sinusotomy. A cohort of reliable and responsible patients may be offered surgery to restore the anterior table with expectant man-

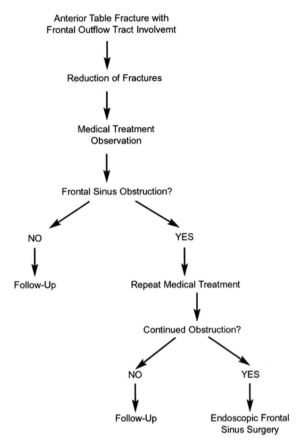

Fig. 15.3. Modified treatment algorithm for highly selected patients

agement of the outflow tract (Fig. 15.3). In these select, responsible patients, a trial of medical management may be undertaken. It should be emphasized that only patients who will dependably return for follow up appointments and periodic CT scans should be considered for conservative management, as delay in the recognition of complications may result in life-threatening consequences. These patients are treated with a prolonged course of broad-spectrum antibiotics (4 weeks) and oral steroids if there are no medical contraindications. Serial sinus CT scans at 1, 2, 4 and 6 months, and yearly thereafter are used to assess the frontal sinus for ventilation and restoration of mucociliary clearance [40]. Individuals failing two courses of antibiotics or those who suffer an infectious complication are considered for an extended endoscopic frontal sinusotomy procedure, including either the extended endoscopic frontal sinusotomy (Draf type II) or the endoscopic modified Lothrop procedure (Draf type III or frontal sinus drill-out) [10]. Often these individuals require computer-assisted image guidance for the surgeon to safely proceed with surgery. If the frontal sinus should fail after endoscopic frontal sinusotomy, or if the patient wishes to forego endoscopic treatments, the time-honored ablative procedures may be undertaken.

In 2002, Smith et al. [40] reported a series of seven patients with displaced anterior table fractures and potential nasofrontal outflow tract injury by multi-planar CT scanning. Five of the seven patients experienced spontaneous sinus ventilation with conservative treatment. The two patients that did not ventilate had concomitant nasoorbital ethmoid fractures and were successfully treated with endoscopic frontal sinus surgery with 2 years follow-up. Chandra et al. [2] confirmed these findings in patients who presented with complications several years after conservative management of frontal sinus fractures. These complications included mucoceles in nine patients, chronic sinusitis in three patients and osteomyelitis in one patient. All patients underwent endoscopic frontal sinusotomy with image guidance and had no evidence of disease up to 3 years postoperatively. In experienced hands, the combination of medical therapy and endoscopic sinusotomy appears to be a safe and effective alternative to traditional ablative procedures.

Tips and Pearls

- Recent endoscopic developments allow for delayed nasofrontal outflow tract recanalization through endoscopic frontal sinusotomy.
- Reliable patients with outflow tract injuries may be managed expectantly.
- Responsible patients with nasofrontal outflow tract injury are treated with a prolonged course of antibiotics and oral steroids.
- Serial sinus CT scans are used to assess the frontal sinus for ventilation.
- If the frontal sinus fails to ventilate or if the patient wishes to forego endoscopic treatments, the time-honored procedures may be undertaken.

Frontal Sinus Obliteration

The most common method of frontal sinus obliteration today is the osteoplastic flap procedure. This method exposes the interior of the frontal sinus by elevating a flap of the anterior table hinged inferiorly on pericranium (osteoplastic flap) [15]. The mucosa of the frontal sinus is removed with a burr, and the duct is plugged with one of several different materials and sealed with fibrin glue. The ducts may be obdurated with autogenous bone graft, temporalis muscle plugs [15, 24] or pericranial or galeal flaps [25]. Complications of remucosalization and mucocele formation are reduced when the nasofrontal duct mucosa is inverted into the nasal cavity [50]. The demucosalized sinus space is then obliterated with a choice of several materials to promote osteoneogenesis (see discussion below) [45] and the osteoplastic flap is then reduced and fixated.

A great deal has been written about the ideal frontal sinus obliteration material. Samoilenko discovered that the frontal sinus cavity becomes filled with serous fluid and is later replaced by osseofibrous ingrowth, a process termed osteoneogenesis. It is now commonplace to fill the denuded frontal space in order to provide a matrix that encourages osteoneogenesis. Numerous autogenous graft materials, including fat, pericranial fascia, muscle, cancellous bone and lyophilized cartilage, have been successfully used [36, 37]. Abdominal fat graft is the most commonly used material because it is autogenous, easily obtainable at the time of surgery and efficacious with a low complication rate [15]. Studies using MRI to follow patients treated with osteoplastic flap sinus obliteration using adipose revealed a mucocele recurrence rate of approximately 10% [19, 23, 48]. In 1963, Montgomery [31] questioned the ability of the fat graft to persist in a bony cavity. In a cat model, he reported that a variable amount of fat persisted 1 year after implantation and that the amount of fibrosis or osteoneogenesis was negligible. The clinical result appears to be independent of the viability of the implanted fat [49].

Recently, alloplastic materials such as hydroxyapatite, cellulose, silicone and methyl methacrylate have also found use in frontal sinus obliteration. Hydroxyapatite cement is perhaps the most promising alloplastic material used for this purpose and has been shown to be effective, with no reported complications at a range of follow-up from 1 to 54 months [4, 41]. The multitude of materials for sinus obliteration attests to the fact that all have been used with some success. Indeed, the material placed in the sinus is not as important as the steps used to prepare the sinus cavity with the graft [30].

Although obliteration has been touted as the gold standard and safest method to treat the injured frontal sinus, there are many disadvantages, including facial scarring, frontal bone embossment, frontal neuralgia due to surgical injury of the supraorbital and supratrochlear sensory nerves, and donor site morbidity. In addition, the loss of physiologic ventilation of the sinuses hampers the use of radiographic studies in the evaluation of sinus disease. Patients may also complain of chronic frontal headache, which presents a diagnostic dilemma owing to limitations in radiographic evaluation of the sinus. Patients undergoing osteoplastic flap with autogenous adipose tissue obliteration display partial replacement of the fat graft with soft tissue (granulation and fibrosis) in most cases, and there are no consistent MRI features to distinguish recurrent sinusitis or early mucopyocele formation from expected adipose graft remodeling [23].

Tips and Pearls

- To avoid the late complication of mucocele formation, the sinus mucosa must be meticulously removed.
- It is equally important to invert the nasofrontal duct mucosa into the nasal cavity.
- Although abdominal fat is commonly used today, numerous graft materials, including pericranial fascia, muscle, cancellous bone, lyophilized cartilage, hydroxyapatite, cellulose, silicone and methyl methacrylate, have been successfully used.

Complications

The early complications occurring within the first few weeks include forehead pain, numbness and incisional tenderness [29, 51]. A CSF leak occurs in the early postoperative period in 3–10% of patients [5, 8, 9, 25, 47]. Clinically, CSF has a distinctively salty taste and if mixed with blood will form a "halo" when placed on absorbent cloth owing to the higher protein content [45]. Biochemical analysis of the fluid revealing β2-transferrin confirms the diagnosis. Most CSF leaks will resolve with conservative management of antibiotics and a lumbar drain. If the leak persists, an exploratory surgery is warranted to prevent meningitis. Gerbino et al. [14] reported on two patients who suffered fatal meningitis in the immediate postoperative period. It is critical to recognize and treat this complication promptly.

Late complications occur months to years after the initial operation and include chronic sinusitis, osteomyelitis, subdural empyema, meningitis and mucoceles. Mucoceles are encapsulated collections of mucus that cause bony erosion and remodeling as they enlarge. They can erode into the nasal sinuses, orbit, and soft tissue of the forehead or even the anterior cranial fossa. They are generally asymptomatic until they are extensive and involving surrounding structures. Xie et al. [51] described their experience with frontal sinus trauma over a 30-year period. The authors found the rate of mucocele formation to be the highest when anterior table (6%), posterior table (14%) and both anterior and posterior table (11%) without evidence of outflow tract injury were treated by observation. Chronic headache is also a common complaint after frontal sinus surgery [12]. A retrospective study of 11 patients who underwent cranialization for posterior table fractures demonstrated no major complications, but three of the 11 patients complained of headache [7].

Case Reports

Case 1

A 22-year-old woman presented following a motor vehicle crash in which she sustained an open, displaced anterior table frontal sinus fracture with associated nasoorbital ethmoid fracture. Fine-cut CT demonstrated these fractures and was highly suspicious for frontal sinus outflow tract fracture (Fig. 15.2). The patient underwent open reduction and internal fixation of the frontal sinus and NOE fractures using a forehead laceration for exposure. There was extensive comminution of the anterior table with small areas of bone loss. The bone fragments were meticulously reduced and fixated with miniplates. She was discharged home with a 4-week course of broad-spectrum antibiotics, nasal spray and close follow-up.

At the 4-week follow-up visit, she described pressure over the frontal region. Follow-up CT demonstrated opacification of the frontal sinuses with evidence of frontal outflow obstruction. Endoscopic evaluation revealed no purulence or significant inflammation in the middle meatus. Topical nasal steroid spray, prednisone taper and empiric antibiotic treatment was initiated for an additional 4 weeks. Follow-up CT demonstrated no improvement.

The patient was prepared for endoscopic frontal sinus surgery. High-resolution thin-cut multiplanar CT scanning was repeated to enable use of computer guidance. A modified endoscopic Lothrop procedure was performed (Fig. 15.4). Clinical follow-up with endoscopic examination and debridement was performed at day 6, day 13, and then weekly for 6 weeks. Medical therapy was maximized during the initial 6-week postoperative period, which included nasal saline irrigations, topical nasal steroid sprays, perioperative tapering dose of prednisone and culture-directed antibiotics. Endoscopic examination at 6 months revealed a widely patent nasofrontal communication. At 2 years follow-up, CT demonstrated excellent ventilation of the sinus with return of mucociliary clearance (Fig. 15.5). At 5 years follow-up, no clinical evidence of frontal disease is apparent.

Case 2

A 58-year-old man presented to the trauma center after sustaining massive head trauma in a motor vehicle accident. His injuries included a left comminuted depressed frontal bone and frontal sinus fractures with comminution of the left posterior table into the frontal lobe of the brain with associated intracerebral hemorrhage. He also had associated anterior cranial

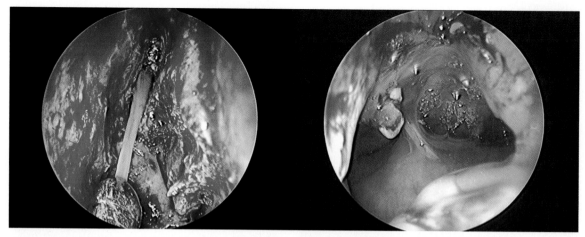

Fig. 15.4. Intraoperative view of the right frontal sinusotomy (with retained secretions) and the completed modified Lothrop procedure. The tips of the screws used in fixation of the ante- rior table fracture can be seen penetrating the anterior wall of the frontal sinus

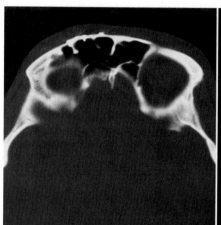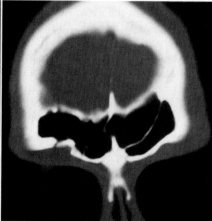

Fig. 15.5. CT views of the frontal sinus 2 years postoperatively, which is widely patent

fossa fractures of the left supraorbit and left ethmoid roof. At presentation, this patient was noted to have CSF which was emanating from the nostrils.

Once stabilized, the patient underwent a bilateral frontal sinus cranialization and skull base reconstruction for repair of his injuries. After bifrontal craniotomy using a standard coronal incision by the neurosurgical team, a 1.5 cm × 2 cm dural tear in the region of the midethmoid roof on the left side was identified and repaired in a watertight manner. A significant comminution of the left anterior cranial fossa was discovered in the posterior table of the left frontal sinus as well as in the left anterior and posterior ethmoid roofs (Fig. 15.6). A left partial ethmoidectomy was performed to ensure sinonasal drainage. The fractures had violated the frontal intrasinus septum, and therefore a bilateral frontal sinus cranialization was undertaken. The contiguous left cranialized frontal sinus and ethmoid defects resulted in a 2 cm × 5 cm skull base defect, which was repaired using onlay titanium mesh followed by a pericranial flap and fibrin glue over the entirety of the bilaterally cranialized frontal sinus and left ethmoid roof defect. Next, the comminuted fragments of the frontal bone and anterior frontal sinus were reapproximated and fixated using titanium metal plates.

The patient did well postoperatively and was discharged on postoperative day 18. After 8 months, CT of the sinuses reveals an intact anterior skull base reconstruction with good ventilation of the remaining left ethmoid cells.

References

1. Adkins, W.Y., R.D. Cassone, and F.J. Putney, (1979) *Solitary frontal sinus fracture.* Laryngoscope 89(7 Pt 1): p. 1099–104.
2. Chandra, R.K., D.W. Kennedy, and J.N. Palmer, (2004) *Endoscopic management of failed frontal sinus obliteration.* Am J Rhinol 18(5): p. 279–84.

15

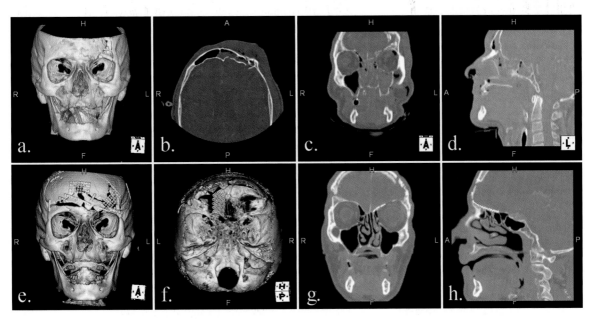

Fig. 15.6. a–d Preoperative frontal, axial, coronal, and sagittal views. e–h Postoperative frontal, posterior, coronal, and sagittal views. Note significant comminution of the left anterior skull base and ethmoid roof in association with left frontal sinus fractures of the anterior and posterior tables. After bilateral frontal sinus cranialization and left partial ethmoidectomy, reconstruction was achieved with titanium mesh and a pericranial flap

3. Chen, D.J., et al., (2003) *Endoscopically assisted repair of frontal sinus fracture.* J Trauma 55(2): p. 378–82.

4. Chen, T.M., et al., (2004) *Reconstruction of post-traumatic frontal-bone depression using hydroxyapatite cement.* Ann Plast Surg 52(3): p. 303–8; discussion 309.

5. Correa, A.J., et al., (1999) *Osteoplastic flap for obliteration of the frontal sinus: five years' experience.* Otolaryngol Head Neck Surg 121(6): p. 731–5.

6. Davis, W.E., J. Templer, and D.S. Parsons, (1996) *Anatomy of the paranasal sinuses.* Otolaryngol Clin North Am 29(1): p. 57–74.

7. Day, T.A., et al., (1998) *Management of frontal sinus fractures with posterior table involvement: a retrospective study.* J Craniomaxillofac Trauma 4(3): p. 6–9.

8. Donald, P.J., (1982) *Frontal sinus ablation by cranialization. Report of 21 cases.* Arch Otolaryngol 108(3): p. 142–6.

9. Donald, P.J. and L. Bernstein, (1978) *Compound frontal sinus injuries with intracranial penetration.* Laryngoscope 88(2 Pt 1): p. 225–32.

10. Draf, W., (1991) *Endonasal micro-endoscopic frontal sinus surgery: the Fulda concept.* Op Tech Otolaryngol Head Neck Surg. Vol. 2. 234–240.

11. Duvall, A.J., 3rd, et al.,)1987) *Frontal sinus fractures. Analysis of treatment results.* Arch Otolaryngol Head Neck Surg 113(9): p. 933–5.

12. El Khatib, K., A. Danino, and G. Malka, (2004) *The frontal sinus: a culprit or a victim? A review of 40 cases.* J Craniomaxillofac Surg 32(5): p. 314–7.

13. Gabrielli, M.F., et al., (2004) *Immediate reconstruction of frontal sinus fractures: review of 26 cases.* J Oral Maxillofac Surg 62(5): p. 582–6.

14. Gerbino, G., et al., (2000) *Analysis of 158 frontal sinus fractures: current surgical management and complications.* J Craniomaxillofac Surg 28(3): p. 133–9.

15. Goodale, R.L. and W.W. Montgomery, (1958) *Experiences with the osteoplastic anterior wall approach to the frontal sinus; case histories and recommendations.* AMA Arch Otolaryngol 68(3): p. 271–83.

16. Gonty, A.A., R.D. Marciani, and D.C. Adornato, (1999) *Management of frontal sinus fractures: a review of 33 cases.* J Oral Maxillofac Surg 57(4): p. 372–9; discussion 380–1.

17. Harris, L., G.D. Marano, and D. McCorkle, (1987) *Nasofrontal duct: CT in frontal sinus trauma.* Radiology 165(1): p. 195–8.

18. Islamoglu, K., et al., (2002) *Complications and removal rates of miniplates and screws used for maxillofacial fractures.* Ann Plast Surg 48(3): p. 265–8.

19. Keerl, R., et al., (1995) *Magnetic resonance imaging after frontal sinus surgery with fat obliteration.* J Laryngol Otol 109(11): p. 1115–9.

20. Kim, K.S., et al., (2001) *Surgical anatomy of the nasofrontal duct: anatomical and computed tomographic analysis.* Laryngoscope 111(4 Pt 1): p. 603–8.

21. Lakhani, R.S., et al., (2001) *Titanium mesh repair of the severely comminuted frontal sinus fracture.* Arch Otolaryngol Head Neck Surg 127(6): p. 665–9.

22. Levine, S.B., et al., (1986) *Evaluation and treatment of frontal sinus fractures.* Otolaryngol Head Neck Surg 95(1): p. 19–22.

23. Loevner, L.A., et al., (1995) *MR evaluation of frontal sinus osteoplastic flaps with autogenous fat grafts.* AJNR Am J Neuroradiol 16(8): p. 1721–6.

24. Luce, E.A., (1987) *Frontal sinus fractures: guidelines to management.* Plast Reconstr Surg 80(4): p. 500–10.

25. Manolidis, S., (2004) *Frontal sinus injuries: associated injuries and surgical management of 93 patients.* J Oral Maxillofac Surg 62(7): p. 882–91.

26. Martin, M., et al., *The Influence of Hospital- and Patient-Level Characteristics on Outcomes of Frontal Sinus Frac-*

ture Treatment: A Multi-Institutional Study of 892 Frontal Sinus Fractures. Presented at the 84th Annual Meeting of the American Association of Plastic Surgeons. Scottsdale, AZ, 2005.

27. May, M., J.H. Ogura, and V. Schramm, (1970) Nasofrontal duct in frontal sinus fractures. Arch Otolaryngol 92(6): p. 534–8.

28. McGraw-Wall, B., (1998) Frontal sinus fractures. Facial Plast Surg 14(1): p. 59–66.

29. Mendians, A.E. and S.C. Marks, (1999) Outcome of frontal sinus obliteration. Laryngoscope 109(9): p. 1495–8.

30. Mickel, T.J., R.J. Rohrich, and J.B. Robinson, Jr., (1995) Frontal sinus obliteration: a comparison of fat, muscle, bone, and spontaneous osteoneogenesis in the cat model. Plast Reconstr Surg 95(3): p. 586–92.

31. Montgomery, W.W., (1964) The Fate Of Adipose Implants In A Bony Cavity. Laryngoscope 74: p. 816–27.

32. Nadell, J. and D.G. Kline, (1974) Primary reconstruction of depressed frontal skull fractures including those involving the sinus, orbit, and cribriform plate. J Neurosurg 41(2): p. 200–7.

33. Nahum, A.M., (1975) The biomechanics of maxillofacial trauma. Clin Plast Surg 2(1): p. 59–64.

34. Onishi, K., M. Osaki, and Y. Maruyama, (1998) Endoscopic osteosynthesis for frontal bone fracture. Ann Plast Surg 40(6): p. 650–4.

35. Rohrich, R.J. and L.H. Hollier, (1992) Management of frontal sinus fractures. Changing concepts. Clin Plast Surg 19(1): p. 219–32.

36. Rohrich, R.J. and T.J. Mickel, (1995) Frontal sinus obliteration: in search of the ideal autogenous material. Plast Reconstr Surg 95(3): p. 580–5.

37. Samoilenko, A., (1913) Obliteration post-operatoire des sinus frontaux. Arch. Int. Laryngol 35: p. 337.

38. Shockley, W.W., et al., (1988) Frontal sinus fractures: some problems and some solutions. Laryngoscope 98(1): p. 18–22.

39. Shumrick, K.A. and C.P. Smith, (1994) The use of cancellous bone for frontal sinus obliteration and reconstruction of frontal bony defects. Arch Otolaryngol Head Neck Surg 120(9): p. 1003–9.

40. Smith, T.L., et al., (2002) Endoscopic management of the frontal recess in frontal sinus fractures: a shift in the paradigm? Laryngoscope 112(5): p. 784–90.

41. Snyderman, C.H., et al., (2001) Hydroxyapatite: an alternative method of frontal sinus obliteration. Otolaryngol Clin North Am 34(1): p. 179–91.

42. Spriano, S., et al., (2005) New chemical treatment for bioactive titanium alloy with high corrosion resistance. J Mater Sci Mater Med 16(3): p. 203–11.

43. Strong, E.B., G.M. Buchalter, and T.H. Moulthrop, (2003) Endoscopic repair of isolated anterior table frontal sinus fractures. Arch Facial Plast Surg 5(6): p. 514–21.

44. Sullivan, P.K., J.F. Smith, and A.A. Rozzelle, (1994) Cranio-orbital reconstruction: safety and image quality of metallic implants on CT and MRI scanning. Plast Reconstr Surg 94(5): p. 589–96.

45. Swinson, B.D., W. Jerjes, and G. Thompson, (2004) Current practice in the management of frontal sinus fractures. J Laryngol Otol 118(12): p. 927–32.

46. Thaller, S.R. and P. Donald, (1994) The use of pericranial flaps in frontal sinus fractures. Ann Plast Surg 32(3): p. 284–7.

47. Wallis, A. and P.J. Donald, (1988) Frontal sinus fractures: a review of 72 cases. Laryngoscope 98(6 Pt 1): p. 593–8.

48. Weber, R., et al., (1995) [Behavior of fatty tissue in frontal sinus obliteration]. Laryngorhinootologie 74(7): p. 423–7.

49. Weber, R., et al., (1999) Obliteration of the frontal sinus--state of the art and reflections on new materials. Rhinology 37(1): p. 1-15.

50. Woods, R.R., (1995) Operation for chronic frontal sinusitis. AMA Arch Otolaryngol 61(1): p. 54–60.

51. Xie, C., et al., (2000) 30-year retrospective review of frontal sinus fractures: The Charity Hospital experience. J Craniomaxillofac Trauma 6(1): p. 7–15; discussion 16–8.

15

Chapter 16

Paranasal Sinus Mucoceles

16

Benjamin Bleier, Satish Govindaraj, James N. Palmer

Core Messages

- The most common location of paranasal sinus mucoceles is the frontal sinus.

- The incidence of intracranial extension of paranasal sinus mucoceles is reported as high as 55%.

- The development of a mucocele results from retained mucus with loss of a normal sinus outflow tract.

- Although uncommon, sphenoid sinus mucoceles have the potential for catastrophic sequelae owing to their close proximity to the internal carotid artery, optic nerves, and sella turcica.

- Marsupialization is an effective method of mucocele management as studies demonstrate essentially normal mucociliary transport mechanisms within previously marsupialized cavities.

- Current surgical management of these lesions is largely dictated by the sinus involved and the degree of extrasinus extension noted on preoperative imaging.

- During endoscopic management of frontal sinus mucoceles, the first steps involve identification of the medial orbital wall and skull base.

- Occasionally, during the surgical management of frontal mucoceles, clear, serous fluid may be expressed from the mucocele cavity which resembles cerebrospinal fluid (CSF). The key differentiating factor is that this fluid should *not* flow continuously. This finding would be suspicious for a CSF leak.

- Mucoceles within the sphenoid sinus occur secondary to circumferential scarring of the sphenoid ostium as a result of chronic sinusitis or postsurgical scarring.

- The initial step in the surgical management of sphenoid mucoceles involves the identification of the natural ostium of the sphenoid sinus when feasible.

- The differential diagnosis of isolated mucoceles along the ethmoid skull base includes the presence of an encephalocele.

Contents

Introduction

Paranasal sinus mucoceles represent an interesting clinical entity whose workup and management have evolved significantly in the past 30 years. Mucoceles typically occur as an indolent, expansile cyst containing mucus lined with respiratory epithelium. These lesions may be locally destructive and may become infected, resulting in a mucopyocele. Classically, these lesions were treated by complete surgical resection often with obliteration of the involved sinus cavities. With the advent of transnasal endoscopic surgical techniques, management of mucoceles has shifted towards more conservative drainage and marsupialization techniques which preserve native mucociliary function and have yielded excellent results.

Epidemiology

Mucoceles have no sex predilection and can occur at any age although most are diagnosed in patients between the ages of 40 to 60 years old [1]. Those occurring in children are usually idiopathic although many may be associated with cystic fibrosis and some authors have even advocated cystic fibrosis screening in any child found to have a mucocele [5, 7]. While mucoceles can form within any sinus cavity, the first series of 14 patients noted the frontal sinus to be the most common location [12]. This finding has been supported by subsequent larger series which report incidences of 60–90% in the frontal sinus and 8–30% within the ethmoid sinus. Mucoceles of the maxillary and sphenoid sinus are rare although some authors report an incidence of up to 5 and 10% respectively [1, 9, 13].

Local complications result from the expansile nature of these slow-growing lesions and include intraorbital extension with eye displacement or frank proptosis as well as skull base erosion. Incidence of intracranial extension has been reported as high as 55%, with half of the patients having a larger intracranial than sinus component [9].

Secondary infection of the stagnant mucus within the cyst can also occur, resulting in a mucopyocele. This may lead to rapid expansion of the lesion with an increased incidence of local complications.

Common culture isolates from mucopyoceles include:

- *Staphylococcus aureus*
- α-hemolytic streptococci
- *Haemophilus influenzae*
- *Pseudomonas aeruginosa*
- Anaerobes including *Propionibacterium acnes*, *Prevotella*, and *Fusobacterium* [3, 5]

Pathophysiology

The rationale for the current management of mucoceles may be derived from an understanding of the pathophysiology of this disease. Studies by Lund et al. demonstrated that the mucocele lining is composed of normal respiratory mucosa, namely, ciliated pseudostratified columnar epithelium. Thus, the development of a mucocele can be extrapolated to an event resulting in retained mucus with loss of a normal outflow tract. One proposed mechanism implicates the cystic degeneration of a seromucinous gland with formation of a retention cyst [2]. Sinus outflow obstruction resulting from benign or malignant intranasal neoplasm may also contribute to mucocele formation. Iatrogenic mucocele formation was demonstrated in the setting of both external and endoscopic sinus surgery secondary to trapped mucosa or scarring of a paranasal sinus ostium. One series reported a 9.3% incidence of frontal sinus mucocele following osteoplastic flap [8]. Other etiologic factors include a history of chronic rhinosinusitis, allergic rhinitis, and previous maxillofacial trauma.

Once formed, mucoceles may effect bony remodeling via an inflammatory cascade focused at the bone–mucocele interface. Inflammatory mediators including IL-1 and IL-2 as well as fibroblast-derived prostaglandin E2 and collagenase act to promote bone resorption, which in conjunction with the mass effect of the lesion itself can result in local bony destruction and displacement of adjacent soft-tissue structures [14–16].

Tips and Pearls
- Common causes of paranasal sinus mucoceles are chronic rhinosinusitis, prior sinus surgery (external or endoscopic), maxillofacial trauma, allergy, neoplasm, and idiopathic

Presentation and Preoperative Evaluation

Presentation

The presentation of an enlarging mucocele is intrinsically linked to its cause and location. The general symptoms patients present with echo those of any obstructive abnormality within the sinonasal cavity and the extent of mucocele expansion.

Symptoms associated with paranasal sinus mucoceles that patients present with include:

- Congestion
- Headache
- Rhinorrhea
- Pressure
- Eye pain
- Diplopia
- Decreased visual acuity
- Epiphora
- Proptosis

16

In severe cases, patients may present with:

- Exposure keratopathy and central retinal block secondary to profound exophthalmos [6]
- Forehead mass secondary to erosion of the anterior table
- Cerebrospinal fluid (CSF) leak or with meningitis secondary to posterior table erosion and subsequent intracranial extension

Although uncommon, sphenoid sinus mucoceles have the potential for catastrophic sequelae owing to their close proximity to the internal carotid artery, optic nerves, and sella turcica. Many times these structures will be exposed after mucocele marsupialization.

Preoperative Evaluation

The diagnosis and preoperative evaluation relies primarily on history and physical examination coupled with radiographic evaluation. The aforementioned symptoms that patients present with along with nasal endoscopy provide clues to the location and the extent of the mucocele. While plain films have been utilized in the past, computed tomography (CT) has become the modality of choice to evaluate these lesions. Mucoceles appear as well-circumscribed cysts within the paranasal sinus with homogenous mucoid contents whose attenuation increases with chronicity of the lesion secondary to increasing protein content (10–40 HU). High-resolution images in both axial and coronal planes provide valuable information regarding integrity of surrounding bony structural elements and help to plan surgical intervention.

Magnetic resonance imaging (MRI) is also a useful adjunct when assessing intracranial extent or attempting to differentiate a mucocele from other sinonasal soft-tissue findings such as neoplasm. In most situations, a mucocele will have low signal intensity on T1 and gadolinium-enhanced images while having high signal intensity on T2 imaging [13]. MRI findings, similar to those of CT, also will evolve as the protein content within the mucocele increases. In general, as the protein concentration increases (associated with an old or long-standing mucocele), T1 signal intensity will increase and T2 intensity will decrease to the point that the signal may drop out, causing the reader to confuse these lesions for fungus or inspissated secretions.

Tips and Pearls

Imaging characteristics of mucoceles:
1. CT:
   (a) Well-circumscribed with homogenous mucoid content
      - New lesions 10–18 HU
      - Chronic lesions 20–40 HU
   (b) Expansion of surrounding bone
   (c) Bony dehiscence seen late
   (d) Evidence of prior trauma or chronic sinusitis
2. MRI:
   (a) Early
      - T1-dark
      - T2-bright
      - Gadolinium enhanced-none
   (b) Late
      - T1-bright
      - T2-dark or signal void
      - Gadolinium enhanced-none

Tips and Pearls

Preoperative evaluation checklist:
1. Perform a complete history and physical examination, including nasal endoscopy
2. Obtain a high-resolution CT scan with axial and coronal cuts
3. Carefully review the CT scan with specific attention to the site of involvement, the presence of bony erosion, and the degree of intraorbital and/or intracranial extension
4. Obtain an MRI scan with any significant intracranial involvement or concern over sinonasal neoplasm

Surgical Technique

The treatment of the paranasal sinus mucocele is primarily surgical. Traditionally, surgical intervention was directed towards effecting a complete resection of the lesion, which typically involved an open approach such as a Lynch–Howarth frontoethmoidectomy or osteoplastic flap with subsequent sinus obliteration. These techniques were associated with significant morbidity and cosmetic deformity as well as a relatively high recurrence rate [17]. Marsupialization is an effective method of mucocele management as studies demonstrate essentially normal mucociliary transport mechanisms within previously marsupialized cavities [11]. In addition, with the advent of endoscopic surgery, transnasal approaches have been established as the procedure of choice for the management of paranasal sinus mucoceles [10].

Current surgical management of these lesions is largely dictated by the sinus involved and the degree of extrasinus extension noted on preoperative imaging. The use of stereotactic computer-assisted navigation is determined on a case-by-case basis. In general, those mucoceles that are present in revision cases or possess extrasinus extension may benefit from the use of image guidance. These systems are not a substitute for knowledge of the anatomy.

General surgical principles include the use of general anesthesia, topical decongestion of the sinonasal cavity with oxymetazoline-impregnated pledgets, and the local infiltration of 1% lidocaine with epinephrine at a concentration of 1:100,000 into the lateral nasal wall (at the anterior attachment of the middle turbinate). In those cases involving the sphenoid sinus, a transoral or transnasal sphenopalatine artery injection may be formed. Multiple aspirations should be performed while injecting to ensure the absence of an intravascular injection, and a maximum of 1.5 ml of 1% lidocaine with epinephrine (1:100,000) should be used.

Frontal Sinus

The first steps involve identification of the medial orbital wall and skull base. The medial orbital wall is identified first. A 0° endoscope is adequate to accomplish this. In those cases with significant osteoneogenesis of the medial orbital wall, drilling of the diseased bone is necessary to create an adequate ostium as well as to avoid dissection too medially and risk intracranial entry. One clue to medial orbital wall location is utilization of the maxillary sinus ostium as a reference point. The lamina papyracea will be in line with the medial wall of the maxillary sinus, so removal of residual bony partitions or removal of osteoneogenic bone can be safely done to that level.

The skull base is identified either in the posterior ethmoid cavity or within the sphenoid sinus. The use of a reverse 30° scope facilitates this portion of the procedure. The light cables exit the scope from above, so instruments can easily be passed from below without difficulty. Keys to this portion of the procedure are palpating behind residual skull base bony partitions and working laterally. Through-cutting instruments are used on the skull base to avoid undue torque on critical bony boundaries (i.e., fovea ethmoidalis). This is done to the level of the frontal recess. At that point a more angled scope (45° or 70°) will be required to perform an adequate frontal recess dissection. Once again, reverse scopes are used to facilitate instrument passage.

In cases of frontal sinus mucoceles, the cause of outflow obstruction is determined and dealt with ac-

cordingly. In general, frontal recess obstruction is secondary to soft or hard tissue. Soft tissue can consist of polyps, edematous allergic mucosa, or epithelial benign or malignant tumors. This discussion will focus on nonneoplastic causes since the presence of tumor may alter the ultimate management and is beyond the scope of this chapter. In cases of frontal recess stenosis from nonneoplastic soft tissue, through-cutting giraffe instruments or a curved microdebrider are used to remove only excess tissue and leave a fully mucosalized frontal recess. The key is mucosal preservation within the frontal recess, as mucosal violation can convert a soft-tissue obstruction into a one that is bony.

Hard-tissue obstruction consists of residual bony partitions within the frontal recess, the presence of osteoneogenesis obliterating frontal sinus outflow, or rarely the presence of a fibroosseous tumor. In cases where residual bony partitions are left behind, once again through-cutting instruments are utilized to preserve mucosa. In cases where these cell walls are too dense, gentle fracture of the segment with an angled curette in an anterior-lateral direction is performed, and then the fragment is teased away from overlying mucosa with giraffe forceps. Redundant mucosa may then be reduced with a microdebrider. The presence of osteoneogenesis is a problem that will require drilling and inevitable mucosal devitalization. As a result, postoperative care must be diligent until this area is resurfaced with adjacent mucosa. A self-irrigating, angled drill is used. This portion of the procedure may require hours of drilling depending on the extent of new bone growth (Fig. 16.1). Once the sac is entered, the mucocele is widely marsupialized using giraffe forceps. Careful dissec-

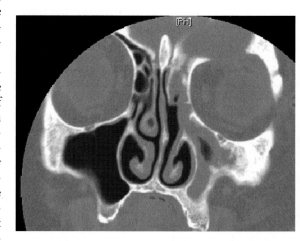

Fig. 16.1. Note the degree of osteoneogenesis within the frontal recess which resulted in mucocele formation with secondary erosion of the roof of the frontal sinus and orbit. This patient underwent successful endoscopic frontal sinusotomy using an angled drill to remove this osteitic bone without the need for an adjunctive open procedure

tion is imperative in those cases with posterior table or orbital roof dehiscence, where the mucocele lining in these areas is not manipulated. Occasionally, clear, serous fluid may be expressed from the mucocele cavity which resembles CSF (Fig. 16.2, Video 16.1). The key differentiating factor is that this fluid should *not* flow continuously. This finding would be suspicious for a CSF leak.

The mucocele cavity is completely suctioned and cultured. A frontal sinus stent formulated from silas-

tic sheeting may be inserted at the conclusion of the procedure. This is kept in place for 1 week, and it is important to note if the surgeon decides to use stenting, it should be made from a soft, conformable material and be removed within 2–4 weeks to prevent biofilm formation on the stent itself, as it might create a nidus for inflammation. Figure 16.3 demonstrates a patient after marsupialization of a frontal sinus mucocele.

Tips and Pearls

- Early identification of the medial orbital wall and then the skull base
- Mucosal preservation within the frontal recess
- Self-irrigating drill reserved for cases with osteoneogenesis
- Short-term stenting of frontal sinus ostium

Sphenoid Sinus

Mucoceles within the sphenoid sinus occur secondary to circumferential scarring of the sphenoid ostium as a result of chronic sinusitis or postsurgical scarring. Obstruction to sinus outflow may also be the result of extrinsic tumors or polyps. Rarely, fibroosseous tumors such as fibrous dysplasia can lead to secondary development of sphenoid mucoceles (Fig. 16.4). In these cases, marsupialization of a sphenoid mucocele will require either subtotal or complete resection of the obstructing tumor and then enlargement of the sphenoid ostium (Video 16.2). If circumferential scarring is the underlying cause, the use of a self-irrigating diamond burr drill may be needed to remove osteoneogenic bone.

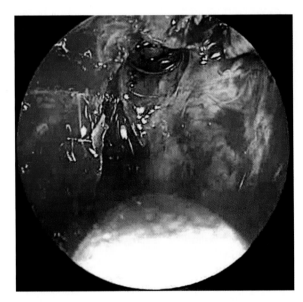

Fig. 16.2. Note the serous drainage draining from the right frontal sinus after removal of an obstructing neoplasm. This fluid can easily be misconstrued as cerebrospinal fluid, and is secondary to marked hypersecretion from the mucosa of the mucocele. Video 16.1 demonstrates this phenomenon

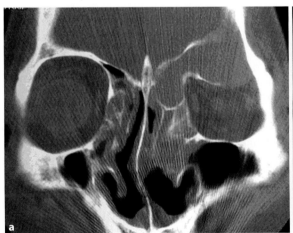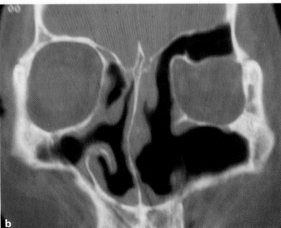

Fig. 16.3. a Preoperative computed tomography (*CT*) scan of a patient with a left frontal sinus mucocele eroding into the orbit. **b** Postoperative CT scan showing a wide-open frontal recess and mucocele evacuation. Note the return of the orbit to its anatomic position

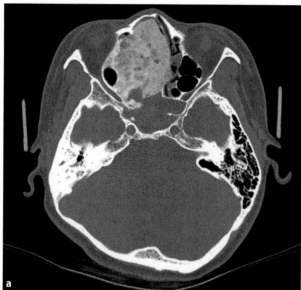

Fig. 16.4. **a** Axial noncontrast CT image demonstrating a large right sinonasal fibroosseous tumor with ground-glass appearance. Posterior to the tumor is a mass with decreased attenuation within the sphenoid sinus. This represents a muco-cele of the sphenoid sinus. The bone over the carotid arteries is intact on this view. **b** MRI (T2) demonstrating a postobstructive mucocele within the sphenoid sinus. The high-signal intensity represents an early mucocele with low protein content

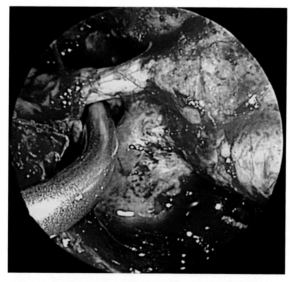

Fig. 16.5. Postoperative endoscopic view into the right sphenoid sinus of the patient shown in Fig. 16.3 demonstrating complete exposure of the right optic nerve and internal carotid artery. The suction lies within the opticocarotid recess. This patient did not have a cerebrospinal fluid leak. Video 16.2 shows resection of the tumor and drainage of the sphenoid mucocele

The initial step calls for identification of the natural ostium of the sphenoid sinus when feasible. If circumferential scarring has occurred and an ostium is not visualized, careful palpation with an image-guidance straight suction or a J curette may permit initial entry into the sinus. At times, a self-irrigating drill will be necessary for entry. As with frontal sinus mucoceles, initial entry may result in the expression of thin, clear fluid that resembles CSF. There may even be a pulsatile evacuation of this fluid secondary to the pressure within the sinus. Once entry has been established, the superior and lateral walls are taken flush with the skull base and the medial orbital wall, respectively. A combination of a straight mushroom and a rotating sphenoid punch does this quite nicely. The sinus is then examined endoscopically using angled endoscopes to assess the presence of carotid artery, optic nerve, or brain parenchymal exposure (Fig. 16.5).

Ethmoid Sinus

The numerous bony partitions within the ethmoid sinus are at risk of mucocele development in the postsurgical cavity as scarring and secondary obstruction may develop. In isolated mucoceles along the ethmoid skull base, another entity that should be entertained especially in patients with prior sinus surgery is an encephalocele (Fig. 16.6). Review of prior operative reports should be performed to determine if there was any violation of the ethmoid roof. A MRI scan is recommended in the preoperative evaluation as well.

Once the presence of a mucocele is confirmed, endoscopic marsupialization of these lesions is performed by initial entry into the lesion followed by removal of surrounding osteitic bony partitions. In cases where there is significant scarring along the eth-

16

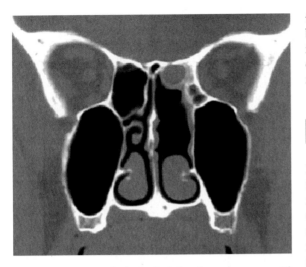

Fig. 16.6. A patient who had prior left endoscopic surgery with a well-circumscribed lesion of the ethmoid skull base with low attenuation. MRI of this lesion demonstrated no intracranial communication and increased T2 signal intensity consistent with a mucocele. This lesion underwent endoscopic marsupialization

moid roof, identification of the skull base may be difficult. In these cases, the skull base is identified within the sphenoid sinus at its lowest point, and is then skeletonized in a posterior to anterior direction. The dissection progresses to the region of the mucocele. As mentioned earlier, the use of through-cutting instruments along the skull base cannot be emphasized enough in order to avoid inadvertent skull base injury.

Maxillary Sinus

Maxillary mucoceles are approached endoscopically as well. Residual uncinate process is removed in order to identify the natural ostium. A wide maxillary antrostomy is then created by resection of the posterior fontanelle flush with the posterior wall of the sinus. A 30°, 45°, or 70° endoscope can assist in visualization into the sinus after entry into the sinus.

Postoperative Care

Postoperatively, packing is rarely required. Nasal saline irrigation and topical nasal steroids are critical in helping to clear the operative site of debris and maintain patent ostia. Endoscopic debridements may be performed at 1, 2, and 4 weeks after surgery to ensure a well-healed sinus ostium free of synechiae. In the setting of a mucopyocele or positive intranasal cultures, patients are placed on a culture-directed antibiotic regimen, and consideration should be given for intravenous therapy. Patients are monitored postoperatively until healing and reestablishment of normal mucociliary clearance pathways are complete.

Results

In 1989, Kennedy et al. reported a series of 18 patients treated with endoscopic marsupialization with a 0% recurrence at an 18-month average follow-up period. This success was replicated in several subsequent studies and in 2000 Har-El [9] reported the largest series to date of 103 patients with 108 paranasal sinus mucoceles with a 0.9% recurrence rate with a median follow-up of 4.6 years. In this series, only one major complication was reported, and this consisted of a CSF leak in the setting of marsupialization of a large frontoethmoidal mucocele with intracranial extension.

Conclusion

Mucoceles of the paranasal sinus are benign, expansile lesions which most often occur in the frontal and ethmoid sinus and can result in local bony destruction with subsequent intraorbital and intracranial extension. Traditional open approaches with the goal of complete resection have been largely replaced by less morbid endoscopic transnasal marsupialization techniques which have yielded excellent results in multiple reported series.

References

1. Arrue P, Thorn Kany M, Serrano E et al. (1998) Mucoceles of the paranasal sinuses: Uncommon location. J Laryngol Otol, 112:840–844
2. Batsakis JG (1980) Tumours of the head and neck. Williams and Wilkins, Baltimore
3. Brook I, Frazier EH (2001) The microbiology of mucopyocele. Laryngoscope, 111:1771–1773
4. Delfini R, Missori P, Ianetti G, Ciappetta P, Cantore G 1993) Mucoceles of the paranasal sinuses with intracranial and intraorbital extension: report of 28 cases. Neurosurgery, 32: 901–906
5. al-Dousary S, al-Kaharashi S (1996) Maxillary sinus mucopyocele in children: a case report and review of literature. Int J Pediatr Otol, 36:53–60

6. Garston JB (1968) Frontal sinus mucocele. Proc R Soc Med, 61:549–551

7. Guttenplan MD, Wetmore RF (1989) Paranasal sinus mucoceles in cystic fibrosis. Clin Pediatr, 28:429–430

8. Hardy JM, Montgomery WW (1976) Osteoplastic frontal sinusotomy: An analysis of 250 operations. Ann Otol Rhinol Laryngol, 85:523–532

9. Har-El G (2000) Endoscopic management of 108 sinus mucoceles. Laryngoscope, 111:2131–2143

10. Har-El G (2001) Transnasal endoscopic management of frontal mucoceles. Otolaryngol Clin North Am, 34:243–251

11. Har-El G (2000) Dimaio. Histologic and physiologic studies of marsupialized sinus mucoceles. J Otolaryngol, 29:195–198

12. Howarth, WG (1921) Mucocele and pyocele of the nasal accessory sinuses. Lancet, 2:744–746

13. Lloyd G, Lund VJ, Savy L, Howard D (2000) Optimum imaging for mucoceles. J Laryngol Otol, 114:233–236

14. Lund VJ (1991) Fronto-ethmoidal mucoceles: a histopathologic analysis. J Laryngol Otol, 105:921–923

15. Lund VJ, Harvey W, Meghji S, Harris M (1988) Prostoglandin synthesis in the pathogenesis of fronto-ethmoidal mucoceles. Acta Otolaryngol, 106:145–151

16. Lund VJ, Henderson B, Song Y (1993) Involvement of cytokines and vascular adhesion receptors in the pathology of fronto-ethmoidal mucoceles. Acta Otolaryngol, 113:540–546

17. Rubin JS, Lund VJ, Salmon B (1986) Frontoethmoidectomy in the treatment of mucoceles. A neglected operation. Arch Otolaryngol Head Neck Surg, 112:434–436

16

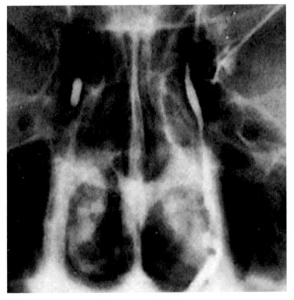

Fig. 17.3. A normal dacryocystogram demonstrating complete filling and evacuation of the lacrimal drainage system on the *left* and revealing obstruction at the lower end of the lacrimal sac on the *right*. Dacryocystography may be useful in demonstrating localized stricture, partial obstruction, lacrimal diverticuli, fistulae, dacryoliths, extrinsic and intrinsic tumors of the lacrimal drainage system

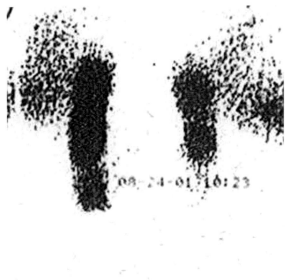

Fig. 17.4. Dacryoscintigraphy in a bilateral functioning nasolacrimal system. Both lacrimal drainage systems fill normally, with tracer concentrated in the canaliculi, sac and duct. Dacryoscintigraphy may provide functional information about physiological function.

- ■ Dye (fluorescein) disappearance test
- ■ Primary Jones dye test (Jones I and Jones II)
- ■ Lacrimal irrigation
- ■ Ultrasonography
- ■ Dacryocystography
- ■ Radionuclide dacryoscintigraphy
- ■ Computed tomography
- ■ Computed tomography dacryocystography
- ■ MRI
- ■ Magnetic resonance dacryocystography
- ■ Lacrimal endoscopy

Although clinical evaluation of gross lacrimal function is not difficult and can be made on the basis of history, determination of the cause may be extremely difficult and requires a variety of diagnostic procedures [11].

The routine preoperative evaluation includes dacryoscintigraphy or dacryocystography. Dacryocystography is a safe, quick, and easy procedure using a radio-opaque material. It is widely established for demonstration of stenosis. This procedure should not be performed in the presence of active dacryocystitis. The disadvantage of dacryocystography is that it provides restricted functional information as in dysfunction of the canalicular muscle pump, slight narrowing of the ductal lumen, and mucous membranes, since intubation of canaliculi and active injection of the contrast material may overcome stenosis. Dacryoscintigraphy (Fig. 17.3) is also a simple noninvasive physiologic test.

Limiting factors are methodologically inherent minimal morphologic information and relatively large variations of normal transit times. Dacryocystography gives finer anatomic detail; however, dacryoscintigraphy (Fig. 17.4) is a more physiologic assessment since no instrumentation is necessary [18].

Surgical Technique

The surgical technique is demonstrated in Video 17.1. The indications and contraindications for surgery are:

1. Indications
   (a) Distal obstruction of nasolacrimal system
   (b) Dacryocystorhinostomy failure
   (c) Mucocele of the lacrimal sac
2. Contraindications
   (a) Benign or malignant lesion in the lacrimal system or the surrounding tissues
   (b) Children less than 1 year of age (obstruction should be treated by probing)
   (c) Active Wegener's granulomatosis
   (d) Canalicular obstruction[1]
   (e) A functional sac

---

[1] If distal nasolacrimal obstruction is accompanied by canalicular obstruction, surgery for proximal obstruction may be done together with DCR.

The surgical approaches to the nasolacrimal sac are:
1. Endocanalicular
   (a) Lacrimal endoscopy
   (b) Balloon dacryocystoplasty
   (c) Endocanalicular laser-assisted dacryocystorhinostomy
2. Endonasal approach
   (a) Transseptal approach
   (b) Transnasal (classical) approach
   (c) Transnasal (endoscopic or microscopic) approach
   (d) Endonasal laser-assisted dacryocystorhinostomy
3. Paranasal approach
   (a) Transantral approach
   (b) Paranasal approach
4. External approach
   (a) Dacryoethmoidostomy
   (b) Falk's operation
   (c) Toti operation
   (d) Modifications of Toti operations

The following instruments are used:
A punctual dilator and lacrimal probes of all sizes
1. A Kerrison punch
2. A Suction elevator
3. A long-shanked nasal drill
4. A 4-mm chisel (optional)
5. Through-cutting forceps and other functional endoscopic sinus surgery instruments
6. Microscopic surgical instruments
   (a) Alligator forceps
   (b) Bellucci scissors
   (c) A canal knife
   (d) No. 6 ear suctions
7. Microdebrider (optional)

Endonasal Endoscopic or Microscopic Dacryocystorhinostomy

This procedure can be done under local or general anesthesia and on an outpatient basis [10]. If it is done under general anesthesia, hypotensive anesthesia is preferred. The inside of the nose is decongested. The head is elevated by bringing the table 20° or 30° in a reverse Trendelenburg position. The mucosa anterior to the middle turbinate may be infiltrated with 1 ml lidocaine with 1:100,000 adrenaline. The disadvantage of this infiltration is that it may obscure the bulging of the nasolacrimal sac. It is important not to traumatize the nasal mucosa since bleeding prevents visualization. At this stage any septal deviation, concha bullosa, or paradoxical middle turbinate obstructing the view must be corrected. Occasionally the head of the middle turbinate needs to be removed to expose the sac area. Chronic maxillary sinusitis or pansinusitis should be addressed simultaneously by the same endonasal route [19, 26, 27, 33].

Localization of the Lacrimal Sac and Duct

The key initial landmark is the posterior border of the frontal process of the maxilla, which is usually identifiable as a ridge or an indentation into the nasal airway just anterior to the middle turbinate [47]. This ridge extends from the highest point of the inferior turbinate upwards and ends immediately in front of the middle turbinate attachment. The nasolacrimal duct and sac lie immediately lateral and posterior to this ridge. Superiorly the duct joins the sac halfway between the attachments of the middle and inferior turbinates. The superior border of the lacrimal sac is above the middle turbinate anterior attachment. The average position of the apex of the lacrimal sac is 6.10±2.02 mm (range, 2–12) above the opercule of the middle turbinate [13]. The anterior attachment of the uncinate process is at the junction of the lacrimal fossa and the orbital plate of the lacrimal bone (Fig. 17.5).

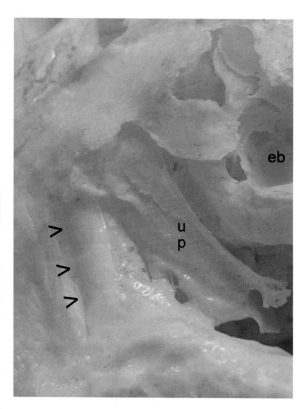

Fig. 17.5. The nasolacrimal sac is always situated immediately anterior to the uncinate process and makes the uncinate process a good landmark in dacryocystorhinostomy operations. *up* uncinate process, *eb* ethmoid bulla, *arrowheads* the bulge over the nasal wall of the nasolacrimal sac and duct

17

It is important not to enter beyond this point in a lateral direction since it may cause orbital penetration [27]. A 20-gauge fiberoptic light pipe may also be used to identify the location of the sac and inserted into the lacrimal sac through either of the lacrimal canaliculi into contact with the medial wall of the lacrimal sac. The light is visualized endonasally with a rigid endoscope [34].

Mucosal Incision

A rectangular cut is made in the mucosa anterior to the middle turbinate and superior to the inferior turbinate. Wong et al. [48] advise an oval cut 2 cm × 1 cm into the mucosa. Indeed removal of nasal mucosa 7–8 mm in diameter might be enough. A canal knife as used in ear surgery can be used for this procedure. Since bleeding mainly occurs from the edge of the cut mucosa, it is important to make a complete cut, and not to pull and tear the mucosa [34]. After the cut is completed through the mucoperiosteum all the way down to the bone, the mucosa is elevated off the bone and removed or can be used as a posteriorly based flap. It does not appear to be necessary to apply special mucosal flaps [17]. If needed, through-cutting forceps may be used instead of Blakesley forceps to avoid tearing of the mucosa. Cautery may also be used to excise the mucosa.

Bone Removal

The medial side of the bone of the maxillary portion of the lacrimal fossa can be removed either from posterior to anterior or from anterior to posterior. Since it is thinner in the posterior part, it makes sense to start from posterior. However it is really challenging to remove the bone with conventional endoscopic sinus instruments alone. There are currently no bone-removing instruments specifically designed for this location. Kerrison forceps or backbiting forceps may be used for this purpose [49]. The surgeon may feel safer if he/she starts from the anteromedial part of the bony sac, identifies the sac, and continues posteriorly. The use of a laser takes more time and may cause thermal injury. The laser can only ablate the much thinner lacrimal bone. Removal of part of the frontal process of the maxilla gives better access and visualization of the lacrimal sac, but a laser cannot ablate this thick bone. Drills specifically designed for intranasal use make it easier to remove the bone but may be associated with thermal injury and damage to surrounding mucosa. Drills may spray bone and blood and may obscure the endoscopic view, slowing down

the procedure [48]. Use of cutting instruments, rather than drills or lasers, may reduce the degree of burning; however, these instruments are as yet unavailable [12]. A 4-mm chisel may be used to remove the bone. If the chisel is located correctly, less time is needed and the medial half of the bone is removed completely [9]. However, there is a learning curve and it needs skill in this surgery. If the chisel is placed too anteriorly, the surgeon will encounter the thick maxillary bone, will cause bleeding and will be unable to remove the bone. If the chisel is located too posteriorly, there is the danger of sliding of the chisel and entry into the orbit. Ethmoid sinuses may be entered. The marked distinction between ethmoid and nasal mucosa (nasal mucosa is 2 or 3 times thicker than ethmoid sinus mucosa) may help location during surgery [38]. In approximately 8% of patients there is an agger nasi cell in this area. In such situations, it will be necessary to open the agger nasi cell up and go through it before going through the lateral wall and the lacrimal bone into the sac [35]. Under endoscopic or microscopic control, the entire medial bony covering of the sac can be removed. In the case of interference from blood or secretions, a special suction irrigation hand piece may be attached to the endoscope [44]. If a chisel is used, attention should be given not to leave any bony fragments, since they may cause obstruction later. Previously irradiated patients should be handled carefully owing to healing problems and anatomic derangements [8].

How Big Should the Bony Osteotomy Be?

Inadequate bone removal is a common cause of failure in dacryocystorhinostomy and it is important to decide how large the bony opening should be [47]. Weidenbecher et al. [44] suggest removing the entire medial bony covering of the sac. Whittet et al. [47] insert a Leibrich lacrimal probe into the inferior canaliculus, direct it against the medial wall of the lacrimal sac in order to tent, and decide how much bone to remove after this procedure. They advocate leaving approximately 5 mm free of bone around the canaliculus, especially at the junction of attachment of the middle turbinate and the lateral nasal wall, a point that demarcates the floor of the lacrimal fossa. Welham and Wulc [46] think that the ideal osteotomy should remove all the bone between the medial wall of the sac and the nose. Thus, following dacryocystorhinostomy, the sac and the duct should coexist as anatomic structures and be incorporated instead into the nose. Lindberg et al. [25] have shown that the healed ostium does not remain as large as the initial bony opening. In their study, the healed intranasal ostium in successful cases measured 1–4 mm (average 1.4mm)

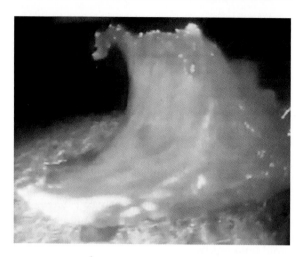

Fig. 17.6. The medial half of the bony nasolacrimal canal removed

in diameter after the surgical bony opening ranging from 10 to 17 mm (average 11.75 mm) and a functional result was achieved with a fistula of 6 mm². No statistical correlation was found between the size of the ostium at the surgery and after healing. Iliff removed a 10-mm diameter piece of bone with one failure out of 87 cases. The mean diameter of the healed ostium was 1.8 mm, representing an area only 2% of that of the initial anastomosis. So the aim is not to create a very large bony osteotomy, but a functioning osteotomy of efficient size (Fig. 17.6).

The sac should not be opened very high up without opening it inferiorly in order to prevent sump syndrome. Preservation of as much mucosa as possible will inhibit new bone formation and therefore the surrounding mucosa should not be disturbed. The bony osteotomy should be as big as the mucosal opening (7–10 mm) and the periosteum should be removed with mucosa (since new bone formation requires the presence of periosteum).

Removal of the Medial Mucosal Wall of the Sac

After the bone has been removed, the sac is identified. The vascularized white color of the sac is characteristic and can easily be identified. A lacrimal probe may be used to identify the lacrimal sac. A lacrimal probe is passed through a canaliculus and directed medially into the obstructed sac. The tenting of medial sac wall by the probe is visualized endonasally. While it is tented by the lacrimal probe, the sac mucosa is incised by a sickle knife. Mucopus, residual contrast material may drain from the sac, or dacryoliths may be seen in the interior of the sac. Once the sac

has been entered, the lacrimal probe may be seen. Using Bellucci scissors, one can extend the incision and use through-cutting instruments to enlarge the intranasal opening. Blakesley forceps are not through-cutting and may tear the sac mucosa; for this reason, through-cutting forceps are preferred. A carbon dioxide laser can also be used. As much of the medial wall of the sac should be removed as possible. Metson [28] advises enlarging of intranasal opening to a diameter of approximately 10 mm, allowing free passage of the lacrimal probes into the nose from both superior and inferior canaliculi.

A silicone tube is placed through the upper and lower canaliculi into the nasal cavity, the ends of the tubing are grasped with forceps, guided out of the nose, and are tied and trimmed so that the knot lies within the nasal cavity. The tubing thus forms a continuous loop, which passes through the intranasal ostium and is unlikely to become dislodged [28]. The knot may be fixed by a suture or a vessel clip. Wong et al. [48] use a black silk suture to tie round the silicone tubes. According to Allen and Berlin [1] and Bartley [2], silk sutures can produce pyogenic and giant cell granulomas. Packing of the nose is unnecessary unless bleeding is a problem.

■ High and small rhinostomy may cause sump syndrome

Is Silicone Tubing Necessary in All Cases?

Silicone tubing may serve to dilate constricted passages in patients with canalicular or common internal punctual stenosis and marks the site of the intranasal ostium [7]. Kohn [21] believes that silicone tubing keeps the anterior and posterior flaps separate, and also discourages cicatricial closure of the bony ostium. Some reports [1, 22, 32] give less favorable results when tubes are inserted. Allen and Berlin [1] believe intubation may be the reason for failure. Tubes may cause inflammation, granulation, and slit the canaliculus. Silicone tubing may incite granulamatous inflammation at the internal ostium, chronic infection, or canalicular laceration. Walland and Rose [41] did not find any difference in failure rates or inflammation with or without silicone intubation. Bolger et al. [5] stated that silastic tubing or Merocel sponge may be a cause of failure.

However insertion of silicone tubes is generally encouraged [3]. Snead et al. [37] showed that silicone intubation did not increase canalicular inflammation in animals. Walland and Rose [42] found no significant difference in the rate of failure or soft-tissue infection between silicone intubated and nonintubated cases. Silicone intubation may be recommended in cases with canalicular stenosis, a small scarred lacrimal sac, a tight upper nasal cavity, and in reoperations, and if the flaps of the lacrimal sac and nasal mucosa are not sutured. In other cases it is the surgeons' preference to use silicone tubes or not.

How Long Should the Silicone Tubes Be Kept in Place?

It is advised to keep silicone stents in place for 2–6 months; however, tubes kept in place for over 3 months are associated with inflammation and granulation. Wong et al. [48] and Weidenbecher et al. [44] advise removing the tubes in 6 weeks. El Guindy et al. [12] keep the tubes for only 2 months and recommend early removal (at 2 months) because silicone tubing may incite a granulomatous reaction. Hartikainen et al. [14] keep the tubes in place for 6 months. Hausler and Caversaccio [15] use the tubes for the long term and they have several cases where silicone tubes have been used for over 3 years without any complications. They even suggest leaving the tubes permanently in persistent cases and think that the silicone tubing produces a maximal dilatation of the canaliculi and a natural aspiration of tear liquid by capillary force.

Mitomycin C

Mitomycin C, an antiproliferative agent, which is widely used in pterygium excision and trabulectomy with favorable results, was also used to inhibit fibrous tissue growth and scarring at the osteotomy site and to decrease the failure rate. Cottonoids soaked with 0.2 mg/ml mitomycin C are applied to the osteotomy site. Kao et al. [20] and Liao et al. [23] reported that mytomicin C improved success rates; Zilelioğlu et al. [50] found no benefit in using mitomycin C. Use of mitomycin C needs further investigation.

Revision Dacryocystorhinostomy

Failure of dacryocystorhinostomy is attributable to a variety of causes. The majority of cases were found to be related to internal nasal problems. Endonasal endoscopic or microscopic dacryocystorhinostomy is generally the preference of many authors in instances of failed dacryocystorhinostomies. An endonasal approach allows the intranasal ostium to be opened in the presence of fibrosis from prior surgery. Under direct endoscopic or microscopic visualization,

the ostium can be enlarged and properly positioned to increase the likelihood of continued patency [28]. Adjacent deviated nasal septum, adhesions, and granulomas can be addressed through an endonasal approach.

Complications

Soft-tissue infection after open lacrimal surgery occurs in 8% of patients. It is reduced fivefold with routine administration of antibiotics [42]. Vardy and Rose [40] demonstrated that intraoperative or postoperative broad-spectrum antibiotics reduced the incidence of cellulitis after open primary lacrimal surgery.

Tsirbas and McNab [39] reported 3.8% of cases with secondary hemorrhage after dacryocystorhinostomy. The incidence of bleeding was higher in patients taking nonsteroidal anti-inflammatory drugs (NSAID). Severe nasal hemorrhage requiring nasal packing was also reported [31, 45]. Orbital complications were also mentioned [36, 43]. Prolapsed tubes, punctal widening, corneal irritation, and intranasal discomfort are the complications related to silicone tubing [6]. There are rare reports of cerebrospinal fluid leaks and meningitis [4, 16, 29].

The complications can be summarized as follows:

- Hemorrhage
- Soft-tissue infection may be prevented by postoperative antibiotics
- Intranasal adhesions
- Extensive nasofrontal drainage pathway obstruction. Surgery in the frontal recess area owing to wrong localization of the sac may cause obstruction
- Orbital emphysema. The patients should not blow the nose for at least 2 weeks following surgery

Conclusion

Endonasal dacryocystorhinostomy has become popular in the last 15 years since it allows preservation of the pump function of the sac and avoids an external scar. In addition, it allows sinus surgery to be performed in the same sitting if needed. The endonasal technique allows the surgeon to localize the sac accurately in the nasal cavity and create a fistula from the lacrimal sac into the nose under direct vision with minimal trauma. The success of the surgery depends on accurate diagnosis ruling out canalicular obstruction and meticulous surgical technique with appropriate instruments.

References

1. Allen K, Berlin AJ (1989) Dacryocystorhinostomy failure: Association with nasolacrimal silicon intubation. Ophthalmol Surg, 20:486–489.

2. Bartley GB (1992) Acquired lacrimal drainage obstruction. Part 1. Ophthal Plast Reconstr Surg, 8:237–242.

3. Beigi B, Westlake W, Chang B, Marsh C, Jacob J, Chatfield J (1998) Dacryocystorhinostomy in South West England. Eye, 12:358–362.

4. Beiran I, Pikkel J, Gilboa M, Miller B (1994) Meningitis as a complication of dacryocystorhinostomy. Br J Ophthalmol, 78:417–418

5. Bolger WE, Crawford J, Cockerham KP (1998) Retained stenting material. Ophthalmology, 106:1306–1309.

6. Brookes JL, Oliver JM (1999) Endoscopic endonasal management of prolapsed silicone tubes after dacryocystorhinostomy. Ophthalmology, 106:2101–2105.

7. Burns JA, Cahill KV (1985) Modified Kinosian Dacryocystorhinostomy. Ophthal Surg, 16:710–716.

8. Civantos FJ, Yoskovitch A, Casiano RR (2001) Endoscopic sinus surgery in previously irradiated patients. Am J Otolaryngol, 22:100–106.

9. Çokkeser Y, Evereklioğlu C, Er H (2000) Comparative external versus endoscopic dacryocystorhinostomy. Otolaryngol Head Neck Surg, 123:488–491.

10. Dresner SC, Klussman KG, Meyer DR, Linberg JV (1991) Outpatient dacryocystorhinostomy. Ophthal Surg, 22:222–224.

11. Dutton JJ (1988) Diagnostic tests and imaging techniques. In: Linberg JV (Ed) Lacrimal Surgery. Churchill Livingstone, New York, pp 19–48.

12. El-Guindy A, Dorgham A, Ghoraba M (2000) Endoscopic revision surgery for recurrent epiphora occurring after external dacryocystorhinostomy. Ann Otol Rhinol Laryngol, 109:425–430.

13. Fayet B, Racy E, Assouline M, Zerbib M (2005) Surgical anatomy of the lacrimal fossa. A prospective computed tomodensitometry scan analysis. Ophthalmology, 112:1119–1128.

14. Hartikainen J, Antila j, Varpula M, Puukka P, Seppa H, Grenman R (1998) Prospective randomized comparison of endonasal endoscopic dacryocystorhinostomy and external dacryocystorhinostomy. Laryngoscope, 108:1861–1866.

15. Hauslaer R, Caversaccio M (1998) Microsurgical endonasal dacryocystorhinostomy with long term insertion of bicanalicular silicone tubes. Arch Otolaryngol Head Neck Surg, 124:188–191.

16. Heerman J Jr (1991) Rhinologische Aspekte bei Traenenwegstenosen. Otorhinolaryngol Nova, 1:227–232.

17. Hosemann WG, Weber RK, Keerl RE, Lund VJ (2002) Minimally Invasive Endonasal Sinus Surgery. Georg Thieme Verlag, Stuttgart, pp 66–70.

18. Hurwitz JJ (1996) The Lacrimal System. Lippincott Raven, Philadelphia

19. Jokinen K, Karja J (1974) Endonasal dacryocystorhinostomy. Arch Otolaryngol, 100:41–44.

20. Kao SCS, Liao CL, Tseng JHS, Chen MS, Hou PK (1996) dacryocystorhinostomy with intraoperative mitomycin C. Ophthalmology, 104:86–91.

21. Kohn R (1988) Ophthalmic Plastic and Reconstructive Surgery. Lea & Feabiger, Philadelphia.

22. Kunavisarut S, Phonglertnapagorn S, (1990) Dacryocystorhinostomy at Rhamathibodi Hospital. J Med Assoc Thailand, 73:47–52.

23. Liao SL, Kao CS, Tseng JHS, Chen MS, Hou PK (2000) Results of intraoperative mytomicin C application in dacryocystorhinostomy. Br J Ophthalmol, 84:903–906.

24. Linberg JV (1988) surgical anatomy of the lacrimal system. In: Linberg JV (Ed) Lacrimal Surgery. Churchill Livingstone, New York, pp 1–18.

25. Lindberg JV, Anderson RL, Bumsted RM, Barreras R (1982) Study of intranasal ostium external dacryocystorhinostomy. Arch Ophthalmol, 100:1758–1762.

26. Mantynen J, Yoshitsugu M, Rautiaınen (1997) Results of dacryocystorhinostomy in 96 patients. Acta Otolaryngol (Stockh) Suppl 529:187–189.

27. McDonogh M, Meiring JH (1989) Endoscopic transnasal dacryocystorhinostomy. J Laryngol Otol, 103:585–587.

28. Metson R (1990) The endoscopic approach for revision dacryocystorhinostomy. Laryngoscope, 100:1344–1347.

29. Neuhaus RW, Baylis HI (1983) Cerebrospinal fluid leakage after dacryocystorhinostomy. Ophthalmology, 90:1091–1095.

30. Onerci M (2002) Dacryocystorhinostomy. Rhinology, 40:49–65.

31. Orcutt JC, Hillel A, Weymuller EA Jr (1990) Endoscopic repair of failed dacryocystorhinostomy. Ophthal Plast Reconstr Surg, 6:197–202.

32. Psilas K, Eftaxias V, Kastaniondakis J, Kalogeropoulos C (1993) Silicon intubation as an alternative to dacryocystorhinostomy for nasolacrimal drainage obstruction in adults. Eur J Ophthalmol, 3:71–76.

33. Rice DH (1990) Endoscopic intranasal dacryocystorhinostomy. Arch Otolaryngol Head Neck Surg, 116:1061.

34. Shun-Shin GA (1998) Endoscopic dacryocystorhinostomy. Eye, 12:467–470.

35. Simmen D, Jones N (2005) Manual of Endoscopic Sinus Surgery. Georg Thieme Verlag, Stuttgart, pp 194–203.

36. Slonim CB, Older JJ, Jones PL (1984) Orbital hemorrhage with proptosis following a dacryocystorhinostomy. Ophthalmic Surg, 15:774–775.

37. Snead JW, Rathbun JE, Crawford JB (1980) Effects of silicone tube on the canaliculus. An animal experiment. Ophthalmology, 87:1031–1036.

38. Talks SJ, Hopkisson B (1996) The frequency of entry into an ethmoidal sinus when performing a dacryocystorhinostomy. Eye, 10:742–743.

39. Tsirbas A, McNab AA (2000) Secondary hemorrhage after dacryocystorhinostomy. Clin Exp Ophthalmol, 28:22–25.

40. Vardy SJ, Rose GE (1999) prevention of cellulitis after open lacrimal surgery. Ophthalmology, 107:315–317.

41. Walland MJ, Rose GE (1994) The effect of silicone intubation on failure and infection rates after dacryocystorhinostomy. Ophthal Surg, 25: 597–600.

42. Walland MJ, Rose GE (1994) Soft tissue infections after open lacrimal surgery. Ophthalmology, 101:608–611.

17

43. Weber R, Draf W, Kolb P (1993) Die endonasale mikro-chirurgische Behandlung von Traenenwegsstenosen. HNO, 41:11–18.
44. Weidenbecher M, Hosemann W, Buhr W (1994) Endoscopic endonasal dacryocystorhinostomy. Ann Otol Rhinol Laryngol, 103:363–367.
45. Welham RA, Hughes SM (1985) Lacrimal surgery in children. Am J Ophthalmol, 99:27–34.
46. Welham RAN, Wulc AE (1987) Management of unsuccessful lacrimal surgery. Br J Ophthalmol, 71:152–157
47. Whittet HB, Shun-Shin GA, Awdry P (1993) Functional endoscopic transnasal dacryocystorhinostomy. Eye, 7:545–549.
48. Wong RJ, Glicklich RE, Rubin PAD, Goodman M (1998) Bilateral nasolacrimal duct obstruction managed with endoscopic techniques. Arch Otolaryngol Head Neck Surg, 124:703–706.
49. Yung MW, Logan BM (1999) The anatomy of the lacrimal bone at the lacrimal bone at the lateral wall of the nose. Clin Otolaryngol, 24:262–265.
50. Zilelioğlu G, Uğurbaş SH, Anadolu Y, Akıner M, Aktürk T (1998) Adjunctive use of mytomicin C on endoscopic lacrimal surgery. Br J Ophthalmol, 82:63–66.

Endoscopic Transsphenoidal Hypophysectomy

18

Adam M. Zanation, Brent A. Senior

Core Messages

■ The three most common pituitary tumors are pituitary adenomas, craniopharyngiomas, and meningiomas. The most common pituitary tumors in children are craniopharyngiomas.

■ Pituitary apoplexy is a surgical emergency that results from parasellar compression of the cavernous sinus and cortical brain secondary to infarction or hemorrhage of a pituitary adenoma. Prompt surgical decompression is required.

■ Endoscopic transsphenoidal hypophysectomy is preferred over the traditional transseptal approach since it results in less postoperative epistaxis, lower rates of lip anesthesia and septal perforation. It also has been shown to allow for shorter postoperative hospitalization.

■ Endoscopic transsphenoidal hypophysectomy with hydroscopy allows for visualization of the tumor bed and completeness of the resection.

■ Absolute contraindications in performing an endoscopic transsphenoidal hypophysectomy include inadequate surgical training and lack of proper instrumentation.

Contents

Introduction

Interest in pituitary surgery began in 1893 when Caton and Paul operated on an acromegalic patient via a temporal approach; that tumor was never reached and the patient subsequently died. Between 1904 and 1906, Horsley operated on ten patients using a combination of subfrontal and middle cranial fossa approaches with a 20% mortality rate. A transfacial approach via transglabellar incision with excision of the frontal sinuses and the superior nose was described in 1897. This laid the framework for Schloffer in 1907 to perform the first transsphenoidal approach via a superior rhinectomy incision. In 1909, Kocher added resection of the septum submucosally; while Kanavel described an inferior nasal approach reflecting the external nose superiorly. In 1910, Hirsch described his classic endonasal transseptal approach. Hirsch's approach avoided a lateral rhinotomy incision, but his visualization was limited by the diameter of the external nares. Finally in 1910, Halstead added a sublabial incision to Hirsch's transseptal approach. This avoided external scarring, while improving the breadth of the operative field. Cushing, utilizing a combination of these transsphenoidal techniques between 1910 and 1925, had a mortality rate of 5.6% in 231 cases. With morbidity usually from infection, Cushing began developing and using more transcranial approaches in order to reduce infectious complications, and by 1931 he had abandoned the transsphenoidal approach. This resulted in a dominance of frontal approaches for pituitary tumors during the 1930s to 1960s [2, 4, 7].

In 1956, Dott (one of Cushing's understudies) performed 80 consecutive transseptal transsphenoidal operations with no mortality. Dott introduced this technique to Guiot in 1956. Guiot improved the surgical access to the sella by utilizing radiofluoroscopic control, while also advocating the use of postoperative radiation to achieve the best results. As a fellow under Guiot, Hardy learned the transsphenoidal approaches and in 1967 introduced the use of the operating microscope to this procedure. This allowed for brighter lighting and improved sellar visualization, resulting in more aggressive resection of pituitary and parasellar lesions. These technical advances along with the development of antibiotics in the 1950s lowered the mortality rates to well below the reported rates for transcranial approaches at the time [2, 4, 7]. The sublabial transseptal transsphenoidal approach is still utilized in many medical practices today.

Endoscopic assistance in transsphenoidal surgery was described by Bushe and Halves in 1978, but it was not until otolaryngologists had gained significant experience using the endoscope for management of inflammatory sinus disease that it gained acceptance in management of pituitary tumors. In 1996, Carrau et al. [3] reported a series of 50 patients who underwent endoscopic endonasal transsphenoidal pituitary surgery. This landmark paper became a springboard for further advances in minimally invasive endoscopic transsphenoidal hypophysectomy. Endoscopic transsphenoidal hypophysectomy (also known as minimally invasive pituitary surgery, MIPS) offers several advantages over transseptal approaches and is becoming the procedure of choice for many otolaryngologists and neurosurgeons for management of pituitary adenoma.

Pituitary Gland Anatomy

The pituitary gland is a reddish-gray body, measuring approximately 10 mm in diameter, attached to the brain through the infundibulum and resting in the sella turcica. The gland is composed of two lobes. The anterior lobe derives from the ectoderm, and starts developing around the fourth week of gestation when an evagination of the stomodeum enlarges dorsally, forming Rathke's pouch. This then gradually becomes sealed off from the aerodigestive tract, forming a cyst that is then invaded by mesodermal tissue to form the anterior lobe of the pituitary. A diverticulum arising from the floor of the third ventricle then abuts this lobe and eventually develops into the infundibulum and posterior lobe of the pituitary [8, 10, 11].

The anterior lobe of the pituitary is composed of epithelial cells surrounded by vascular sinusoids. Three distinct cell types are identified on hematoxylin and eosin staining. Acidophils include somato-

tropes (growth hormone) and lactotropes (prolactin); basophils include thyrotropes (thyroid-stimulating hormone), gonadotropes (luteinizing hormone and follicle stimulating hormone), and corticotropes (adrenocorticotrophic hormone); while chromophobes are essentially nonsecretory. The posterior lobe is composed largely of nonmyelinated axons whose cell bodies are located in hypothalamic nuclei. These neurons secrete antidiuretic hormone and oxytocin [8, 10, 11].

Sella Turcica Anatomy

The pituitary gland sits in the sella turcica, a deep depression on the superior aspect of the body of the sphenoid bone. The posterior boundary of the sella is defined by the dorsum sellae and the posterior clinoid processes. Below the dorsum sellae is the clivus, which slopes inferiorly and is continuous with the occipital bone. The roof of the fossa is formed by the diaphragm, which is a dural fold traversed by the pituitary stalk. The lateral extension of the diaphragm forms the roof of the cavernous sinus [8, 10, 11].

Vital structures in proximity to the pituitary include:

- Optic chiasm and nerve
- Carotid arteries
- Third, fourth, fifth, and sixth cranial nerves in the cavernous sinus
- The basilar artery and brainstem posteriorly (Figs. 18.1, 18.2) [8, 10, 11].

Proper knowledge of this anatomy is therefore essential during these approaches.

Sphenoid Sinus and Sinonasal Anatomy

The sphenoid sinus starts developing at about the 12th week of gestation. The sinus is not present at birth, with pneumatization beginning at about 5–7 years of age, while the adult size is usually reached by 15–18 years. [8]

The sphenoid sinus is variably pneumatized into the sphenoid bone.

Three types of sphenoid sinuses are described according to the degree of pneumatization in relation to the sella:

1. Conchal sphenoid is one which has pneumatized only to a small degree with thick bone still over the face of the sella.

18

Fig. 18.1. The anatomy of the sphenoid, sella, and cavernous sinus

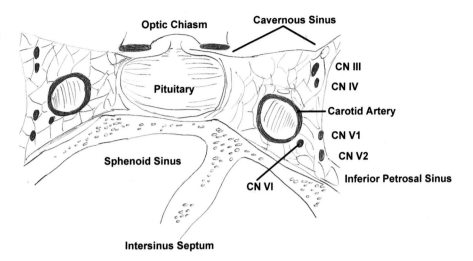

2. Sellar pneumatization occurs when pneumatization has occurred to the face of the sella.
3. Postsellar describes a sinus that has pneumatized beyond the face of the sella.

The majority of sinuses are of the sellar type and postsellar type [11].

The two sphenoid sinuses are separated by a septum that is off the midline in 60–70% of cases; the two cavities are therefore rarely symmetrical. The septum often inserts on or near the bony covering of the carotid artery and/or the optic nerve.

Multiple structures can be seen running along the walls of the sphenoid sinuses (Figs. 18.1, 18.2):

- The vidian canal runs laterally along the floor, while the carotid arteries and optic nerves run along the lateral walls.
- The optic-carotid recess is located between the bulges of the more superiorly located optic nerve and inferiorly located carotid and may extend into the anterior clinoid process (Fig. 18.3b) [8, 10, 11].

Indications and Patient Selection

Indications for endoscopic transsphenoidal hypophysectomy include:

- Hormone-excreting pituitary adenomas that do not respond to medical therapy
- Nonsecreting adenomas or pituitary tumors that cause hypopituitarism or visual impairment

- Pituitary apoplexy
- Tumors that show progressive growth with serial imaging

The differential diagnosis for sellar masses includes:

- Pituitary adenomas and carcinomas
- Craniopharyngiomas
- Meningiomas
- Chordomas
- Gliomas
- Germoid tumors
- Benign cysts such as Rathke's cleft cysts or arachnoid cysts
- Inflammatory lesions such as lymphocytic hypophysitis or Langerhans' cell histiocytosis
- Infectious abscesses
- Vascular aneurysms of the cavernous carotid

Pituitary Adenomas

The most common sellar neoplasm is a pituitary adenoma. This accounts for 15% of all intracranial tumors [5, 11]. The annual incidence of operative lesions is 15 per 100,000 patients; however, the lifetime prevalence of pituitary adenomas is much higher [5, 11]. Studies suggest 17–22% of unselected autopsies reveal a pituitary adenoma [5]. The highest incidence is between the third and sixth decades of life, with higher incidence in postmenopausal women. Pituitary lesions are classified as secreting/nonsecreting, with or without extrasellar extension, and microadenomas (less than or equal to 10 mm) or macroadenomas (greater than 10 mm). Pituitary carcinoma is ex-

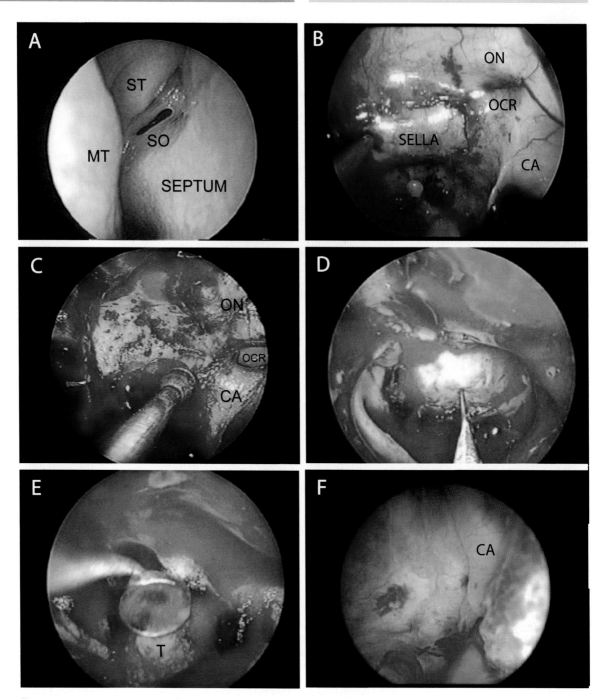

Fig. 18.2. Intraoperative series of photographs. **A** Sphenoid ostium. **B** Posterior–superior sphenoid sinus. **C** Resecting the bony sella. **D** Opening the dura with a sickle knife. **E** Pituitary tumor resection with a ring curette. **F** Hydroscopy of the tumor bed with visualization of the surrounding dura and carotid artery laterally. *SO* sphenoid ostium, *MT* middle turbinate, *ST* superior turbinate, *ON* optic nerve, *OCR* optic-carotid recess, *CA* carotid artery, *T* tumor

tremely rare. It is thought to arise from benign pituitary adenomas, and is defined by distant spread of disease and is not based solely on histologic grading. Lesions of the neurohypophysis (posterior lobe of pituitary) are also extremely rare. The most common of these is the granular cell tumor.

Craniopharyngiomas

Craniopharyngiomas are remnants of Rathke's pouch. They comprise less than 3% of all intracranial tumors, but are the most common parasellar tumor of children and the second most common adult sellar lesion [11].

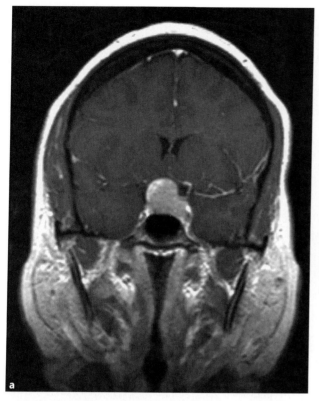

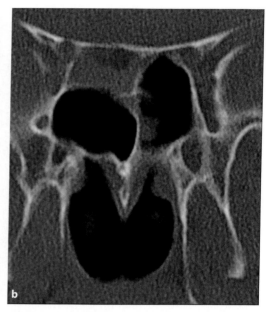

Fig. 18.3. Radiology of the sella/sphenoid. **a** Coronal MRI (T1 with gadolinium) showing a pituitary tumor. **b** Noncontrasted coronal sinus CT illustrating Onodi (sphenoethmoid) cells

Meningiomas

Meningiomas are the third most common sellar tumor, comprising between 1 and 3% of parasellar lesions. Pure intrasellar meningiomas are exceedingly rare and almost all arise from the meninges of the frontal lobes, sphenoid wings, or cavernous sinus [11].

Pituitary Apoplexy

Pituitary apoplexy is a rare clinical syndrome that must be recognized and treated emergently. Apoplexy arises from a hemorrhage or infarction of a pituitary adenoma resulting in compression of parasellar structures such as the optic nerves, cavernous sinus, and brain. The clinical presentation is usually a severe headache with accompanied emesis and meningeal signs. Complete or partial ophthalmoplegia and loss of consciousness may also occur. Rapid diagnosis by MRI and prompt decompression of the sella is required.

Preoperative Evaluation

Patients present with pituitary tumor evaluation most commonly with visual impairment and secondly pituitary hormonal dysfunction. Less common symptoms that patients present with include other cranial neuropathies from cavernous sinus involvement, headaches from stretching of the parasellar dura, hydrocephalus, and cortical brain involvement/symptoms. MRI is the mainstay for assessing pituitary lesions (Fig. 18.4a).

Tips and Pearls

- Patients with pituitary adenomas are best evaluated by a multidisciplinary team including an endocrinologist, a neurosurgeon, an otolaryngologist, and an ophthalmologist.

During the preoperative visit with the otolaryngologist, a complete history and head and neck examination is performed. Nasal endoscopy is essential for evaluating the sinonasal anatomy and ruling out any concurrent infectious process that may mandate a delay in surgery. The CT scan is reviewed for further an-

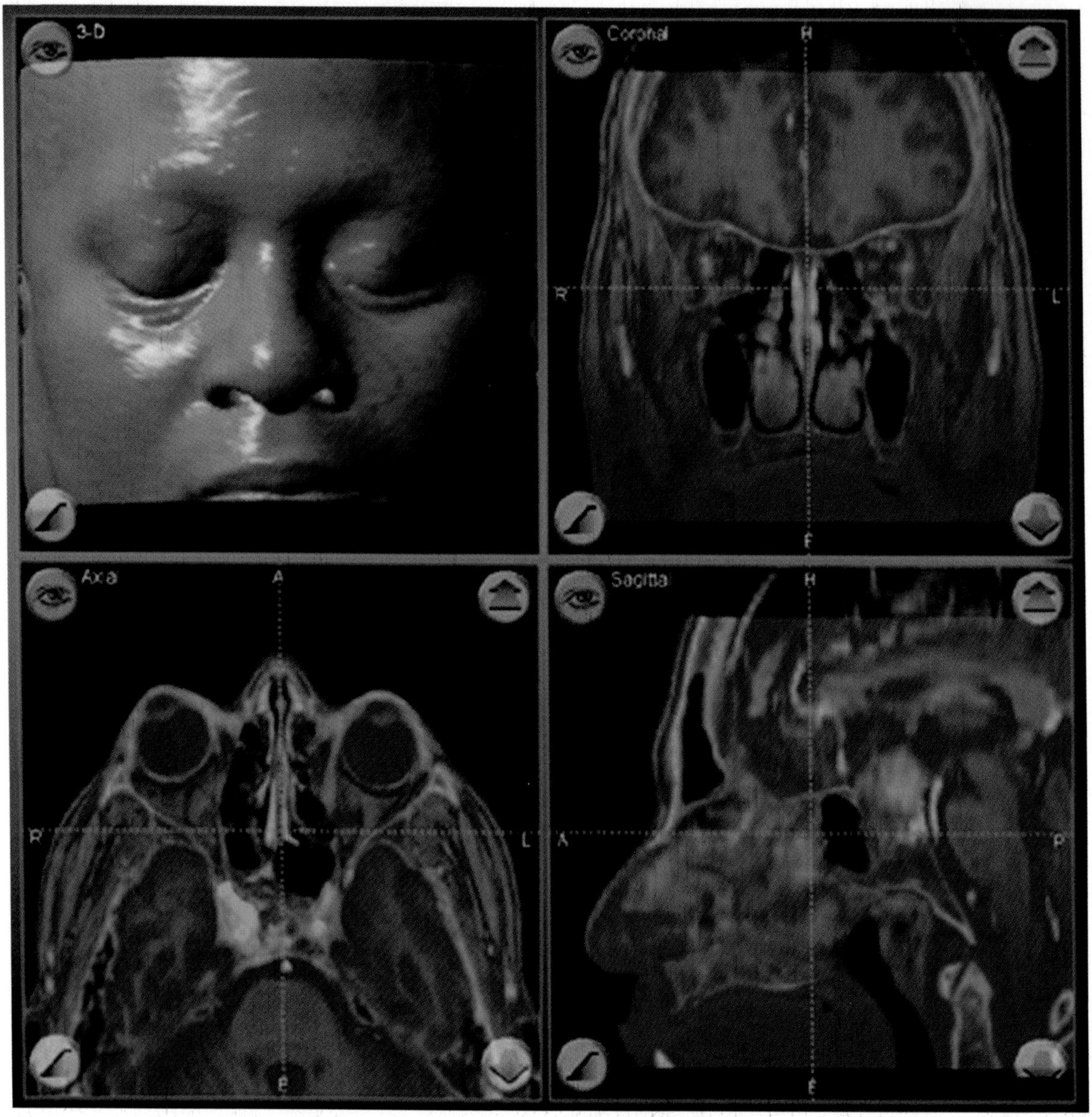

Fig. 18.4. MRI/CT fusion image for intraoperative stereotactic image guidance

18

atomic details such as the presence of Onodi (sphenoethmoid) cells, asymmetry of the sphenoid sinuses, or possible dehiscence of the carotid arteries and/or optic nerves (Fig. 18.4b). The operative plan and potential variations are discussed by the two operative teams. At our institution, all patients have a fine-cut CT scan for use with the computer-guided navigation system. In the setting of revision surgery, the preoperative MRI and CT scans are fused together on the navigational system, allowing for improved intraoperative orientation (Fig. 18.5). The risks and benefits of the procedure are discussed at length and all questions are answered, while the expected postoperative course is also explained to the patient and family. Preoperative evaluation by an ophthalmologist is essential. This includes visual acuity and visual fields as well as retinal examination, and serves as a baseline for postoperative comparisons to determine improvement, or possibly degeneration in vision. A significant number of patients with pituitary tumors will usually present themselves to the surgical team referred by an endocrinologist, sometimes after unsuccessful medical management. Preoperative medications are usually continued; hyperthyroidism is ideally well controlled, and stress doses of steroids are given preoperatively as necessary.

Fig. 18.5. Intraoperative photograph showing the fixed pneumatic endoscope holder

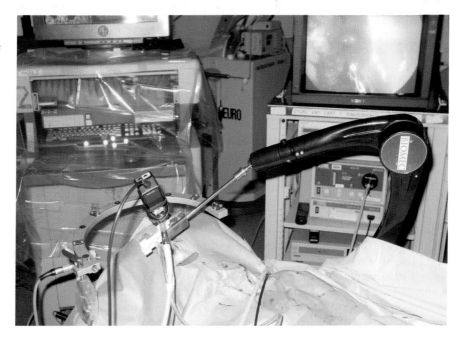

Surgical Technique

The surgical technique is demonstrated in Video 18.1.

Many of the surgical instruments used by otolaryngologists in functional endoscopic sinus surgery are used in MIPS. The standard-length 0°, 4-mm endoscope with attached scope irrigation provides the best illumination and visualization for approaching the sella, while a longer scope may be used to assist with tumor resection. Forty-five degree (and occasionally 70°) scopes are usually used later in the procedure after the sella is entered and the tumor removed to facilitate exploration.

The patient is positioned in the reverse Trendeleburg position, with the torso elevated at approximately 30° and the knees slightly bent for comfort. The head is rotated approximately 15° towards the surgeon. In our earlier cases, we used a three-point pin holder, such as a Mayfield head holder, but we have found this to be unnecessary and time-consuming. Instead, the patient's head rests on a foam donut, which allows the degree of flexion and rotation to be optimized for exposure during different parts of the procedure.

Tips and Pearls

■ We routinely use computer-guided navigation to facilitate identification of sellar landmarks and tumor orientation, while negating the need for fluoroscopy. The latest navigation systems allow for rapid, simple registration in addition to easy integration and tracking of the surgeon's own instrumentation.

The patient's face is not sterilely prepared as the instruments will be passing through the contaminated nasal cavity. The abdomen is always prepped with Betadine, in case a fat graft is needed at the end of the procedure. Care is taken to maintain sterility of the abdominal region, with the nasal field being kept distinct throughout the procedure.

Hemostasis is aided by performing greater palatine blocks by injecting approximately 1.5 ml of a solution of 1% lidocaine with 1:100,000 epinephrine transorally into each greater palatine canal. The nasal cavities are decongested with pledgets soaked in a solution of 0.05% oxymetazoline hydrochloride. Under endoscopic guidance, more lidocaine with epinephrine is injected at the junction of the horizontal portion of the basal lamella and lateral nasal wall in the region of the sphenopalatine foramen to obtain a sphenopalatine artery block. See Chap. 4 on local anesthesia by Das and Senior for more details.

Most neurosurgeons are trained to perform pituitary surgery via the midline, transseptal route. The endoscopic transnasal approach, however, is an extra-axial approach and will result in a slightly different perspective for sellar visualization. The side of approach to the tumor is determined by several factors, including, most notably, the degree of obstruction of the nasal cavity. The preoperative endoscopic examination following maximal decongesting of the nose along with review of preoperative CT aids in this assessment. For patients without significant nasal obstruction with smaller pituitary lesions that are off the midline, and for those larger tumors extending laterally into the cavernous sinus, the contralateral nasal cavity presents a better angle of approach to result in complete resection. Occasionally, an approach using both nasal cavities has been used, with the endoscope in one side and the instruments in the other. This can be the case in patients with unusually narrow nasal cavities and is usually reserved for the tumor resection part of the procedure where more than one instrument has to be inserted in addition to the endoscope.

The approach to the anterior face of the sphenoid follows the paraseptal corridor, medial to the middle turbinate. This approach allows the remaining sinuses lateral to the middle turbinate to be left undisturbed, minimizing the risk of postoperative sinusitis and long-term problems. When necessary, gentle lateralization of the middle turbinate is done with the soft end of a Hurd tonsil retractor. Occasionally, a concha bullosa is encountered which may need to be resected to provide good access.

Tips and Pearls

- Key to the identification of the sphenoid sinus ostium is the identification of the superior turbinate and the region of the sphenoethmoid recess (Fig. 18.2a).

The recess is bounded by the skull base superiorly, the superior turbinate laterally, and the septum medially and always contains the ostium of the sphenoid sinus (Fig. 18.3a). The ostium can be well seen after decongesting the superior turbinate with local anesthesia and conservatively resecting its posterior-inferior third using cutting instruments.

Tips and Pearls

- The sphenoid ostium is always located medial to the turbinate, just posterior to its inferior edge in the sphenoethmoid recess.
- Jho [6] has described using the inferior edge of the middle turbinate as a landmark for orientation to the floor of the sella. This margin leads to the clival indentation, about 1 cm below the level of the sellar floor.

The posterior septal branch of the sphenopalatine artery crosses the inferior aspect of the sphenoethmoid recess on its way to supply the mucosa of the septum. Transection of this artery while performing the sphenoidotomy can lead to intraoperative bleeding but can usually be well controlled with bipolar cautery or topical decongestant packing. Vasoconstriction may be

further obtained by injection of lidocaine/epinephrine solution along the posterior septum, prior to any incision in the face of the sphenoid.

Tips and Pearls

- Once the sphenoid sinus ostium is identified, the sinus is entered and the ostium enlarged in an inferior and medial direction, away from critical structures along the lateral wall of the sinus

The ostium is enlarged to a point where the endoscope can be inserted into the sinus in order to visualize its lateral extent, while further enlargement is performed using a mushroom punch. The bone of the sphenoid rostrum is resected using a combination of Kerrison rongeurs and punches until the nasal septum is encountered; occasionally a high-speed drill is used for resection of this relatively thick bone. A partial posterior septectomy is then performed using backbiting forceps. This allows exposure of the contralateral face of the sphenoid. The intersinus septum is then resected, allowing bilateral exposure of the sella through the one nasal cavity. Great care is taken in resection of the intersinus septum, as it frequently attaches posteriorly over the carotid.

Medially, the sella is bordered by the tubercle rostrally, and the clivus caudally. As discussed earlier, the optic nerves are seen superior laterally, while the cavernous portions of the internal carotid arteries are located inferior to the optic nerves (Fig. 18.3b).

Tips and Pearls

- In approaching the sella via the endoscopic transsphenoidal approach, great caution must be exercised, especially around the carotid arteries and the optic nerves, as these can be dehiscent in approximately 20 and 10% of cases, respectively.

With adequate sellar exposure, the endoscope is attached to a fixed pneumatic holder with a custom-designed end piece, freeing up the surgeon's second hand (Fig. 18.6). Alternatively, an assistant can hold the scope for the operating surgeon.

The mucosa on the posterior wall of the sphenoid sinus is then coagulated with a bipolar cautery. The sella is then entered with a 4-mm chisel or high-speed drill, depending on the thickness of the sellar face and the opening enlarged with a Kerrison rongeur or mushroom punch (Figs. 18.3c, 18.7). Occasionally, bleeding can be encountered from anterior intercavernous connections; this can usually be readily controlled with microfibrillar collagen and temporary pressure. The dura is then cauterized and opened

Fig. 18.6. Specialized instruments utilized in endoscopic transsphenoidal hypophysectomy: **A** A 0° Hopkins rod with Endoscrub sheath; **B**, **C** 3-mm Kerrison rongeurs; **D**, **E** mushroom punch; *F*, I sickle knife; **G**, *J* rotating pituitary curette; **H**, *K* 90° rotating scissors

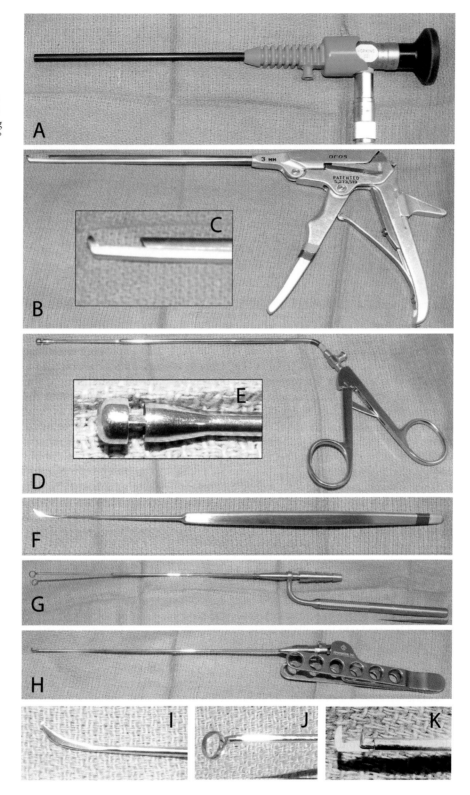

4. Couldwell WT (2004) Transsphenoidal and transcranial surgery for pituitary adenomas. J Neurooncol. Aug–Sep; 69(1–3):237–56.

5. Ezzat S, Asa SL, Couldwell WT, et al. (2004) The prevalence of pituitary adenomas. A systematic review. Cancer; 101(3): 613–619.

6. Jho HD (1999) Endoscopic pituitary surgery. Pituitary; 2:139–154.

7. Liu JK, Cohen-Gadol AA, Laws ER Jr. et al. (2005) Harvey Cushing and Oskar Hirsch: early forefathers of modern transsphenoidal surgery. J Neurosurg. Dec;103(6):1096–104.

8. Gray H (1918) The sphenoid bone. Gray's Anatomy.

9. Sonnenburg RE, White D, Ewend MG, Senior B (2003) Sellar reconstruction: is it necessary? Am J Rhinol; 17:343–346.

10. Parviz J, Montgomery WW, Joseph B. Nadol JB, Fabian RL, Galla R (2000) Surgical Anatomy of the Head and Neck. Publisher: Lippincott Williams & Wilkins.

11. Donald PJ (1998) Surgery of the Skull Base. Publisher: Lippincott Williams & Wilkins 1998.

12. White DR, Sonnenburg RE, Ewend MG, Senior BA (2004) Safety of minimally invasive pituitary surgery (MIPS) compared with a traditional approach. Laryngoscope; 114:1945–1948.

Chapter 19

Image-Guided Sinus Surgery

19

Martin J. Citardi, Pete S. Batra

Core Messages

- Computer-aided surgery (CAS) encompasses all semiconductor-based technologies for surgery.

- Image-guided surgery (IGS), a type of CAS, incorporates software-enabled imaging review and intraoperative surgical navigation.

- All IGS systems share similar hardware (computer workstation, display system, tracking system, surgical instrumentation) and software (data management, image review, surgical navigation) components.

- Registration is the process of establishing a one-to-one mapping relationship between corresponding points (termed "fiducial points") in the operative field volume and imaging data set volume.

- Registration protocols may be classified as paired-point, automatic and contour-based.

- Surgical navigation accuracy is best assessed through the index of target registration error (TRE), which is determined by the surgeon who visually estimates navigational error by localizing against known anatomic landmarks.

- TRE must be checked at different points in the operative field volume repeatedly throughout the case.

- Indications for IGS include revision sinus surgery, traumatic/congenital anomalies, sinonasal polyposis, disease involving frontal/posterior ethmoid/sphenoid sinuses, disease abutting the skull base, orbit, optic nerve and/or carotid artery, CSF rhinorrhea and encephaloceles, and benign and malignant neoplasms.

- IGS is performed with imaging obtained preoperatively and is not a substitute for surgical expertise.

- Both computed tomography (CT)–magnetic resonance (MR) image fusion and three-dimensional CT angiography (3 DCTA) may be utilized with selected IGS systems for advanced skull base lesions.

Contents

Disclosure: Martin Citardi was a consultant for CBYON (Mountain View, CA, USA) in 1999–2003. He has been a consultant for GE Healthcare Technologies (Waukesha, WI, USA) since 2003. Pete Batra is a consultant for Critical Therapeutics (since 2005).

Introduction

Since the late 1980s, rhinologic surgeons have increasingly incorporated image-guided surgery (IGS) technology into paranasal sinus surgery. By today's standards, early IGS systems were remarkably primitive; nonetheless, rhinologic surgeons quickly realized that IGS represented a significant technological advancement. Over the subsequent years, IGS technology has matured into a reliable, commonly utilized tool; in fact, it is difficult to conceive of advanced endoscopic sinus surgery without IGS.

This chapter presents a practical summary of contemporary IGS principles and practices. Because IGS is more fully developed for rhinology (compared with other subspecialties within otorhinolaryngology), the emphasis will be rhinologic applications. Of course, general IGS concepts may be applied to other disciplines within otorhinolaryngology and other surgical specialties.

Domain of Computer-Aided Surgery

The International Society for Computer Aided Surgery has proposed a broad definition of computer-aided surgery (CAS):

The scope of Computer-Aided Surgery encompasses all fields within surgery, as well as biomedical imaging and instrumentation, and digital technology employed as an adjunct to imaging in diagnosis, therapeutics, and surgery. Topics featured include frameless as well as conventional stereotaxic procedures, surgery guided by ultrasound, image-guided focal irradiation, robotic surgery, and other therapeutic interventions that are performed with the use of digital imaging technology [9].

CAS focuses upon semiconductor-based technologies in surgery. Surgical navigation, computer-aided image review, stereotactic surgery, robotic surgery, telemedicine and electronic medical records are all part of CAS.

Thus, IGS falls under the domain of CAS; specifically, IGS refers to intraoperative surgical navigation (Fig. 19.1) as well as preoperative, software-enabled image review and surgical planning. Within otorhinolaryngology, IGS is most commonly employed in rhinologic procedures, although interest in other applications (especially for otology and skull base surgery) is growing.

19

System Components

The underlying principles that permit the clinical application of IGS are similar for all IGS systems. The

Table 19.1.

IGS System Components
Hardware
– Computer workstation
– Display system
– Tracking system
– Surgical instrumentation
Software
– Data management
– Image review
– Surgical navigation

principles that govern IGS are uniform, and the individual components for all IGS systems are essentially identical [5, 6]. In practice, IGS systems from different vendors function in comparable ways.

Hardware

Each IGS system includes these individual components:

■ *Computer workstation.* The computer workstation serves to integrate the other hardware components and provides the central functionality of IGS. Standard input devices include a computer mouse and keyboard. Most workstations are also connected to a computer network.
■ *Display system.* A computer monitor obviously is necessary for the output of visual information. Today, high-resolution flat-panel monitors have supplanted older, cathode ray tube monitors.
■ *Tracking system.* The tracking system can monitor the position of devices (attached to instruments) in the surgical volume. The tracking system has also been termed a "digitizer" since it provides location information in digital format for processing by the computer software. The digitizer monitors specific devices, termed intraoperative localization devices (ILDs). Commercially available digitizers are either optical or electromagnetic. For optical tracking, the ILD is an array of light emitting diodes (LEDs) or highly reflective spheres (Fig. 19.2). During active optical tracking, the overhead camera tracks the LEDs; during passive optical tracking, an overhead infrared emitter bathes the reflective spheres with invisible light, which is then reflected back to the overhead camera. Obviously, line of sight must be maintained during optical tracking; minor adjustments in operating room setup and instrument design can minimize this potential problem. Electromagnetic tracking relies upon sensors that operate as ILDs. An electromagnetic field emitter

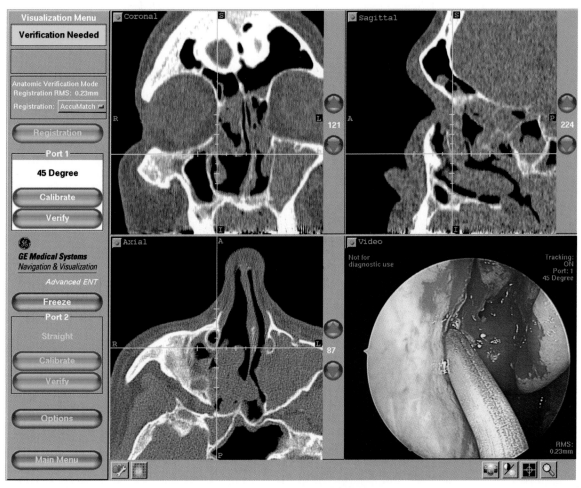

Fig. 19.1. This screen capture from the Instatrak 3500 Plus (GE Healthcare Navigation & Visualization, Lawrence, MA, USA) depicts the typical screen layout for intraoperative navigation. The position of the instrument tip, seen in the endoscopic picture-in-picture of the *lower-right quadrant* is depicted by the *crosshairs* seen on the axial, coronal and sagittal computed tomography (*CT*) images, which are shown in the *remaining three quadrants*. The controls for the software are present in the *far-left panel*. Because this system features a touch screen, the user can access the software by simply selecting the appropriate "soft" buttons. Both the sagittal and the coronal CT images were reconstructed from the axial CT image data set

generates an electromagnetic field that is sensed by the ILD; positional information is then sent to the computer software for processing (Fig. 19.3). The central limitation for electromagnetic tracking is perturbations of the electromagnetic field, although relatively simple maneuvers can prevent this from being a major clinical issue.

- *Surgical instrumentation.* Each IGS system has specific instrumentation for the operative field. In some instances, specific aspirators or forceps that incorporate an ILD must be used, while occasionally, the ILD may be designed so that it can be attached to almost any surgical instrument (including soft-tissue shavers).

Software

Software integrates the hardware components into a functional unit. Operationally, IGS system software performs a series of key tasks:

- *Data management.* The software must archive imaging data sets for retrieval for both image review and surgical navigation. Imaging data sets are large files, and in busy centers, there may be numerous data sets; thus, the software must be robust to avoid "choking" during this critical function.
- *Image review.* Image review at the computer workstation has emerged as a critical advantage offered by IGS. The software can process the axial image data to reconstruct both coronal and sagittal

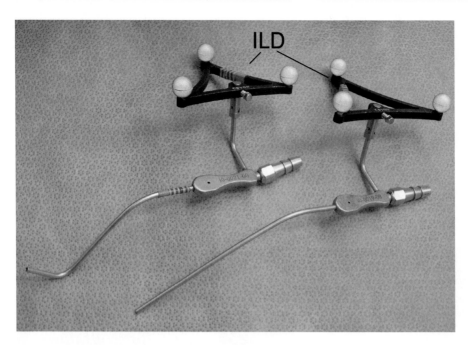

Fig. 19.2. An intra-operative localization device (*ILD*) simply permits the tracking of surgical instruments in the operative field. In this example, each ILD is an array of highly reflective spheres, whose position is monitored by the overhead camera system (also termed a "digitizer"). Since each array has a unique shape, it is possible to track each instrument separately

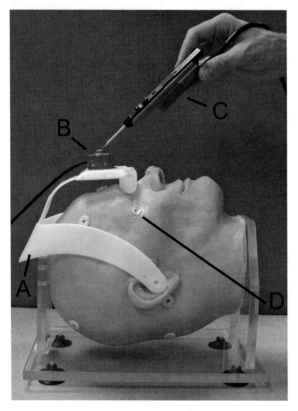

Fig. 19.3. The experimental model for image-guided surgery highlights the setup for surgical navigation for electromagnetic tracking, which is used by the InstaTrak 3500 Plus. This experimental model may be used for studies of registration in a dry laboratory setting. *A* headset, *B* electromagnetic field generator/emitter, *C* ILD, or electromagnetic sensor, incorporated into the handle of the surgical instrument, *D* external fiducial marker

images as well as three-dimensional models. By scrolling through these orthogonal views, the surgeon can better appreciate the three-dimensional relationships of the critical anatomy and formulate an effective surgical plan. In addition, the software typically includes other functions, including three-dimensional cut views, window width/level adjustments and trajectory views.

■ *Surgical navigation.* The software integrates registration (discussed in the next section), positional information (provided by the tracking system) and the preoperative imaging to present graphical representations of instrument tip position relative to the preoperative imaging.

Registration

Registration is the process of establishing a one-to-one mapping relationship between corresponding points (termed fiducial points) in the operative field volume and the imaging data set volume. Registration paradigms may be divided into paired-point registration, automatic registration and contour-based registration.

Although the terms "calibration" and "registration" are often use interchangeably, this usage is technically incorrect. Calibration is the process of defining (or confirming) the relationship between an instrument tip and an ILD.

19

Table 19.2.

Registration Paradigms
Paired-point registration
– Manually define fiducial points in the imaging data set
– Map corresponding anatomic points by sequentially localizing to each fiducial point.
– Computer calculates the registration
Automatic registration
– Headset contains fiducial markers.
– Headset positioning is reproducible.
– Computer calculates the registration after finding fiducial markers in the imaging data set.
Contour-based registration
– Computer builds 3D model to define surface in the imaging data set.
– Surgeon defines contour in operating field by localizing points along the external surface.
– Computer aligns corresponding points on each contour

Paired-Point Registration

Paired-point registration is a three-step process. In the first step, the fiducial points must be defined in the imaging data set. In the early era of CAS, fiducial points were typically bone-anchored screws. Later, taped-on fiducial markers were introduced. Obviously, such external markers had to be placed before imaging data set acquisition. More recently, anatomic points (such as the tragus, medial and lateral canthus) have been used as fiducial points. In the second step, the surgeon must manually map corresponding fiducial points by localizing to each fiducial point in the operating field volume with a tracked probe. Finally, the computer calculates the registration and thus aligns corresponding fiducial points.

Automatic Registration

The automatic registration headset, which incorporates a series of fiducial markers, is designed so that its exact positioning on each patient is reproducible; thus, the relationship between the fiducial markers and the patient is the same at the time of image acquisition and surgery. Of course, the patient must wear the headset for imaging and then the same or a functionally identical headset during surgery. The registration process is complete as soon as the computer software loads the imaging data set, recognizes the positions of the fiducial markers and calculates the registration. Intraoperative surgical navigation is based upon the assumption that the relationship between the patient and the headset fiducial markers is nearly identical during image acquisition and surgery.

Contour-Based Registration

Contour-based registration is a three-step process like paired-point registration. During the first step, the IGS software defines the surface contours by building a three-dimensional model from the axial imaging data. Next, the surgeon must define those contours in the operative field volume. This typically involves a quick paired-point registration with three anatomic fiducial points as an initial approximation. Subsequently, the user must define a large number (40 to 500) of points on relatively fixed contours by gently touching the surface in a nearly continuous fashion in a process that has been termed "painting." Alternatively, a handheld laser device may be used to define this contour. In the third step, the IGS software calculates the registration by aligning corresponding contours.

Assessment of Surgical Navigation Accuracy

Regardless of the registration process, errors in registration are inevitable. Importantly, even subtle errors of registration may have significant impact on the accuracy of surgical navigation. Discussion of the registration error theory [15] is beyond the scope of this chapter; nonetheless, the most critically relevant concepts will be discussed here.

Target registration error (TRE) is the error of surgical interest, since it alone is a measure of surgical navigation accuracy [11]. Clinically, TRE may only be assessed by a visual estimate of accuracy obtained by

Table 19.3.

Surgical Navigation Accuracy
– Target registration error (TRE) is the best index of surgical navigation accuracy.
– Clinically, TRE can only be estimated visually by assessing accuracy against known anatomic landmarks.
– TRE must be assessed at several points throughout the operating field volume.
– TRE must be re-assessed throughout the duration of surgery.
– TRE is best estimated by breaking TRE estimates into their vector components (x-direction, y-direction, z-direction).
– Published reports demonstrate TRE values of approximately 1.5–2.0 mm.

localizing to known anatomic structures. Root-mean-square values provided by some IGS systems are not reliable measures of TRE, and thus cannot reliably indicate surgical navigation accuracy.

Clinical determinations of TRE must be neither superficial nor casual. First, TRE may differ in different parts of the operating field volume. It has been a common clinical anecdote that surgical navigation accuracy deteriorates further posteriorly in the sinonasal space. Secondly, TRE may change during the same case for a variety of reasons, including headset slippage, bent instruments and tracking system errors. Finally, quick assessments of TRE are problematic since it is difficult to visually estimate TRE by inspection of a static endoscopic image, which is a two-dimensional representation with spherical distortion intrinsic to wide-angle optics.

In the clinical realm, TRE is best assessed by considering each of the directional components (i.e., x-axis, y-axis and z-axis) of error individually. For instance, localization against the posterior maxillary wall will provide a suitable landmark for assessing TRE along the z-axis (depth), while localization along the maxillary roof is helpful for determining TRE in the y-axis direction.

Table 19.4.

Surgical Navigation Accuracy
– TRE is the best index of surgical navigation accuracy. Clinically, TRE can only be estimated visually by assessing accuracy against known anatomic landmarks.
– TRE must be assessed at several points throughout the operating field volume.
– TRE must be reassessed throughout the duration of surgery.
– TRE is best estimated by breaking TRE estimates into their vector components (x-direction, y-direction, z-direction).
– Published reports demonstrate TRE values of approximately 1.5–2.0 mm.

Occasionally, some surgeons have proposed assessing TRE against external landmarks, but this practice should be discouraged. While such TRE estimates can provide a rough guide, they are quite far from the area of surgical interest, and thus there is considerable potential for significant differences between TRE at an external landmark and TRE at the operative site.

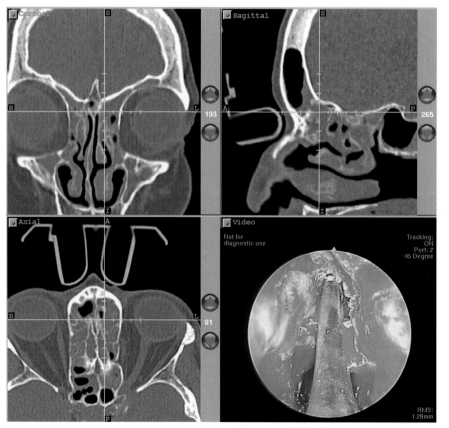

Fig. 19.4. This intraoperative screen capture, obtained with the InstaTrak 3500 Plus, shows the position of the curved aspirator in the posterior left frontal recess. The system was used for preoperative and intraoperative review of the preoperative CT images, and then during surgery, key anatomic boundaries, such as the skull base in the frontal recess, were confirmed through localization

19

Fig. 19.5. Surgical navigation is also critical for the recognition of the skull base in the posterior ethmoid, as seen in this intraoperative screen capture, obtained with the InstaTrak 3500 Plus

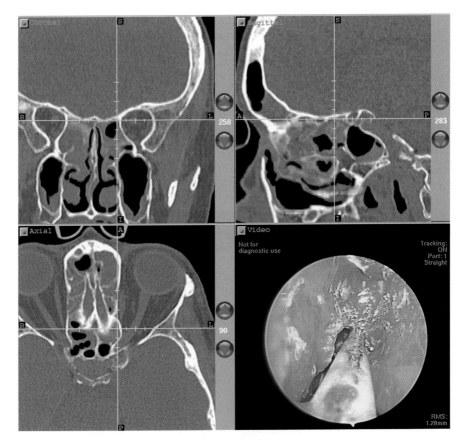

Fig. 19.6. This patient required debridement of clivus for skull base osteomyelitis after transsphenoidal hypophysectomy. This screen capture, obtained with the InstaTrak 3500 Plus, shows the relationship of the operative field to each internal carotid artery; thus, intraoperative surgical navigation facilitated the endoscopic clival "drill-out".

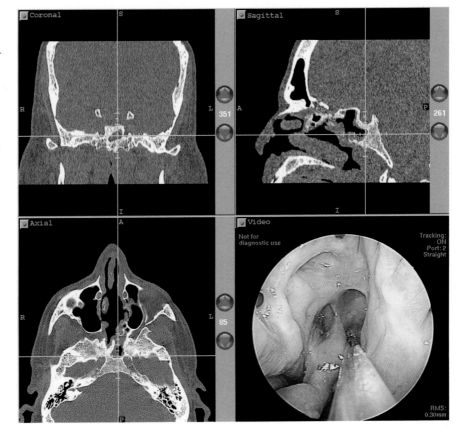

Literature reports of TRE for otorhinolaryngology inconsistently describe surgical navigation accuracy due to a lack of standardized methodology [12]. Early descriptions of surgical navigation using acrylic or plastic models reported an accuracy of approximately 2 mm [23–25]. More recent reports have highlighted an accuracy of approximately 1.5–2.4 mm [3, 8, 10, 17, 20, 22]. Today, real-world, intraoperative TRE at a level of 1.5–2.0 mm is achieved, although occasionally even lower levels of TRE may be observed.

Image-Guided Functional Endoscopic Sinus Surgery

The American Academy of Otolaryngology – Head and Neck Surgery policy statement on CAS provides a comprehensive summary of indications for IGS:

1. Revision sinus surgery
2. Distorted sinus anatomy of development, postoperative or traumatic origin
3. Extensive sinonasal polyposis
4. Pathology involving the frontal, posterior ethmoid and sphenoid sinuses

Table 19.5.

IGS Indications
– Revision sinus surgery
– Congenital and traumatic anomaly
– Extensive sinonasal polyposis
– Frontal sinus disease
– Posterior ethmoid disease
– Sphenoid disease
– Disease abutting skull base, orbit, optic nerve and/or carotid artery
– CSF rhinorrhea
– Benign and malignant neoplasia

5. Disease abutting the skull base, orbit, optic nerve or carotid artery
6. CSF rhinorrhea or conditions with a skull base defect
7. Benign and malignant sinonasal neoplasms [1]

The integration of IGS into functional endoscopic sinus surgery (FESS) creates the paradigm of image-guided FESS (IG-FESS) [19]. In this approach, the central concepts of FESS, including mucosal preservation, meticulous technique and restora-

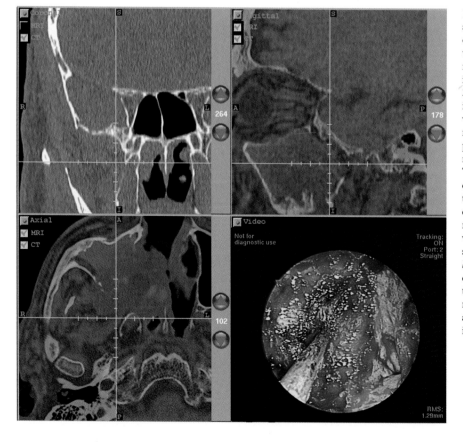

Fig. 19.7. Intraoperative screen capture, obtained during surgical navigation with CT–magnetic resonance (*MR*) fusion images with the InstaTrak 3500 Plus, demonstrates an immediate postresection view of the right pterygomaxillary fossa (*PMF*) in a patient with extensive sinonasal mucosal melanoma. The superb soft-tissue differentiation provided by the fused view facilitated endoscopic resection of the malignancy into the PMF with sparing of normal structures. The *upper-left image* is the standard coronal CT image, while the *lower-left* and upper-right images are the axial and sagittal CT–MR fusion images, respectively

19

tion of mucociliary clearance, are unchanged. IGS serves as an enabling technology by facilitating the comprehension of complex paranasal sinus anatomy. Thus, preoperative image review and surgical planning at the computer workstation are key parts of IG-FESS. During surgery, the rhinologic surgeon should use the IGS system interactively, rather than as a "point and hunt" device. For this reason, the IGS tower must be configured for simple ease of use, and the surgical instrumentation for IGS must be appropriately designed to facilitate its use during actual surgery. Clinical experiences have demonstrated that IG-FESS is most appropriate for revision sinus surgery, frontal sinus surgery, and posterior ethmoid and sphenoid surgery as well as for surgical procedures for allergic fungal rhinosinusitis and sinonasal polyposis (Figs. 19.4–19.6). Numerous reports attest to the utility of IGS in these applications [2, 7, 16–18, 21].

Limitations of Image-Guided Surgery

Although IGS is a remarkable technology, it is important to consider the limitations of IGS in the clinical realm:

- Robust surgical navigation relies upon robust registration. As a result, any problems with registration will severely compromise the reliability of the IGS system for surgical navigation. Rhinologic surgeons utilizing IGS should become familiar with registration concepts and troubleshooting.
- All intraoperative navigation is based on the preoperative imaging data set; thus, navigation cannot reflect changes from intraoperative manipulation in the operative field during surgery.
- IGS is an enabling technology, not a substitute for surgical expertise. This technology facilitates the completion of a specific procedure within the confines of accepted surgical principles.

Special Image-Guided Surgery Techniques

Most commonly, computed tomography (CT) images obtained without contrast are used for IGS in rhinology. These images provide little information about soft tissue differences and internal carotid artery (ICA) position. For most applications, this is satisfactory, but during extended endoscopic approaches to the skull base, more precise imaging is desirable. As a result, the incorporation of additional imaging modalities into IGS represents a significant technological advance.

Table 19.6.

IGS Limitations
– Satisfactory registration is critical for accuracy surgical navigation.
– Intraoperative surgical navigation uses preoperative imaging data.
– IGS is not a substute for surgical expertise

Computer software can now fuse corresponding CT and magnetic resonance (MR) images through a process of image-to-image registration. The principles that govern this process are remarkably similar to those that underlie image-to-patient registration employed for surgical navigation. Fused CT-MR images can be reviewed at the computer workstation; these hybrid images provide information that each imaging modality alone does not provide. Properly configured IGS systems can use fused CT-MR image data sets for surgical navigation (Fig. 19.7) [4, 13]. In these circumstances, the surgeon can navigate with both the bony information provided by CT and the soft-tissue information provided by MR. IGS with CT-MR fusion images may be most helpful during endoscopic skull base surgery, including tumor resection, as well as endoscopic marsupialization of loculated mucoceles.

Three-dimensional CT angiography (3D-CTA) is a technique for imaging the contrast-filled ICA with a rapid CT acquisition and a timed intravenous contrast bolus. Computer software can render three-dimensional images of the ICA and adjacent skull base, and intraoperative navigation with these 3D-CTA images is now feasible [14].

Conclusion

IGS, which combines both preoperative computer-aided image review and intraoperative surgical navigation, has become a mainstay of advanced endoscopic sinus surgery techniques. For surgical navigation, the critical initial step of registration defines a one-to-one, three-dimensional mapping relationship between the preoperative imaging data set and intraoperative surgical anatomy. Since even subtle errors of registration can have profound consequences on surgical navigation accuracy, rhinologic surgeons must consistently monitor surgical navigation accuracy. Numerous reports have confirmed that IGS technology has positively impacted contemporary surgical rhinology, and the current consensus, as

Table 20.1. Classification of some important issues leading to revision surgery

Environmental	General host	Local host
Cigarette smoke	Reactive airway	Iatrogenic
Chemical irritants	Immunodeficiency	Neosteogenesis
Inhalant allergy	Genetic factors:	Nasal polyps
Emotional stress	– Cystic fibrosis	
	– Kartagener's	
	Samter's triad	

Table 20.2. Iatrogenic factors

Lateralization of middle turbinate	Absence of middle turbinate
Mucus recirculation	Residual uncinate process
Scarring of bulla to middle turbinate	Residual ethmoid bony partitions
Scarring of frontal recess	Scarring of sphenoid sinus ostia

Preoperative Evaluation

History

The revision sinus surgery patient should undergo complete reassessment, especially in those cases where the prior surgery or surgeries were performed by another surgeon. It is important to secure the patient's initial complaints prior to the first surgery and the operative records. It is critical to understand whether the patient's complaints prior to the first surgery were truly of sinus origin, the evaluations and medical treatment performed prior to the surgery, the extent of the initial procedure, as well as whether any orbital or intracranial violation was present.

Some of the key areas to evaluate are potential genetic predisposition (cystic fibrosis, cilia dysmotility, immunodeficiency, autoimmune), allergy assessment if clinical suspicion exists and environmental exposure to dust, molds, chemicals and smoke. Certainly, it is inadvisable to perform elective sinus surgery and especially revision sinus surgery in a patient who has not yet stopped smoking.

Any patient who had their first operation for chronic sinusitis or polyposis before the age of 18 should be evaluated for a cystic fibrosis variant, if this has not been previously done. However, the possibility of cystic fibrosis should also be considered in patients who present even later in life, if they have had multiple disease recurrences.

Tips and Pearls

■ Samter's triad and asthma-associated nasal polyposis patients must understand that the nature of their disease process is chronic and will require ongoing medical care, and that in the absence of ongoing medical therapy and regular endoscopic follow up, further revision surgery is likely.

In any patient undergoing revision sinus surgery, evaluation of both active and passive immunocompetence is a consideration, in addition to allergy evaluation.

Physical Examination

A complete head and neck examination should be performed in the initial patient evaluation. The presence of lymphadenopathy may suggest sarcoidosis, chronic serous otitis media could be associated with Wegener's granulomatosis, or laryngeal findings of posterior glottic erythema and edema may reveal underlying gastroesophageal reflux.

Diagnostic nasal endoscopy is an essential component of the preoperative physical examination and typically, particularly in the previously operated on patient, provides more information regarding the anatomy and the disease present than is provided by imaging. Reactive nasal mucosa, when identified on endoscopy, should be controlled prior to surgical intervention with topical and oral steroids. Typically a course of 20–30 mg of prednisone daily for 3–7 days before surgery is sufficient. The steroids will also help stabilize lower-airway reactivity as well as reduce bleeding intraoperatively. In addition, any purulence within the sinonasal cavity should be cultured and treated with the appropriate antibiotic. The cavity is assessed for evidence of iatrogenic factors (Table 20.2).

Radiographic Evaluation

The radiologic assessment should include review of films taken prior to the first surgical procedure whenever possible and these should be compared with the present imaging. Stereotactic computer-assisted navigation systems are commonly used for revision sinus surgery cases. The key areas for review in the preoperative computed tomography (CT) evaluation are shown in Table 20.3.

20

Table 20.3. Preoperative computed tomography evaluation

Site	Evaluation
Skull base	Slope, height, erosions, asymmetry, neosteogenesis
Medial orbital wall	Integrity, residual uncinate position, erosion
Ethmoid vessels	Anterior/posterior ethmoid vessels relative to skull base
Posterior ethmoid	Vertical height, presence of Onodi cell, neosteogenesis
Maxillary sinus	Infraorbital ethmoid cells, accessory ostia
Sphenoid sinus	Position of intersinus septum, location and appreciation of a bony dehiscence of the carotid artery and optic nerve
Frontal recess/sinus	Presence of agger nasi and supraorbital pneumatization, frontal sinus drainage, anterior-posterior diameter of frontal sinus

Endoscopic Revision Sinus Surgery

General Concepts

It is important to appreciate that normal anatomic relationships have been altered in a revision sinus surgery case; thus, the identification of constant landmarks at the outset of the surgery is vital. The key landmarks to identify are the maxillary sinus roof, the medial orbital wall and the skull base within either the posterior ethmoid or the sphenoid sinus. The roof of the maxillary sinus serves as a landmark for two things: the level of the sphenoid ostium and a safe height for posterior dissection through the ethmoids to the sphenoid sinus. Once we are in the sphenoid, the lowest height of the skull base is identified. Dissection can now proceed in a posterior to anterior direction forwards along the skull base. As the dissection is brought anteriorly it is performed laterally, skeletonizing the medial orbital wall so as to avoid the area of attachment of the middle turbinate where the skull base both slopes inferiorly and is significantly thinner. Indeed the bone may even be absent in the region of the anterior ethmoid artery where it enters the skull base medially. Dissection is therefore only performed in this area after the anatomy of the skull base has clearly become evident.

Tips and Pearls

- Key anatomic areas to identify during surgery are the maxillary sinus roof, the medial orbital wall and then the skull base.
- Avoid relying on the middle turbinate as a major landmark in revision surgery.
- Identify the skull base in the posterior ethmoid sinus or sphenoid sinus.
- Superior dissection should be performed from posterior to anterior following skull base identification.

Instrumentation

The revision sinus surgery case will require both manual and powered instrumentation and the manual instrument set should be extensive. Through-cutting instruments are essential for the removal of bony partitions without stripping mucosa. Non-through-cutting instruments such as the Blakesley forceps are helpful in fracturing thickened osteitic bone along the skull base or medial orbital wall. When thickened bone is fractured with non-through-cutting forceps, it is not typically removed in the jaws of these forceps because of the possibility of stripping mucosa. Rather, it is teased out from the mucosa and then removed.

Powered instrumentation includes angled microdebriders and diamond burr drills. Microdebriders allow the expeditious removal of bony partitions and loose mucosa without stripping mucoperiosteum. In addition, use of angled debriders of 60° and 90° is an efficient way of removing polyps from the frontal recess and from the maxillary sinus. Powered drills play a role in the removal of osteitic bone that is not amenable to manual instrumentation. The 15° and 70° diamond burr drills are used in areas where the osteitic bone is too thick or cannot be fractured with forceps. However, when the diamond burrs are used, it is with the understanding that mucosal sacrifice is inevitable and adjacent mucosa will need to resurface the area; thus, they should be used very selectively.

Maxillary Sinus

The most common problems related to the maxillary sinus are a segment of residual uncinate process, resulting in either blunting or scarring at the anterior aspect of the antrostomy or failure to communicate the true and iatrogenic ostia with resultant mucus recirculation. Residual infraorbital ethmoid (Haller) cells are also identified relatively frequently and may result in persistent inflammation. In addition, if the maxillary sinus extends medially into the nasal cavity, entrapment of airflow occurs with mucosal drying and secondary impairment of mucociliary clearance.

The following are typical problems, the instruments used and the technique employed:

- *Residual uncinate process.* The instruments used are a Backbiter, a ball-tip seeker and a Stammberger downbiter. Most commonly the residual uncinate process is anterior to the antrostomy and a 45° endoscope will be required to obtain a better view of the area in question. A ball-tip seeker is then used to medialize this segment of uncinate and the curved 60° microdebrider is used for tissue removal. Another option is to use the backbiter for both dissection and removal of residual uncinate in this area (Fig. 20.1).
- *Failure to communicate the true ostium and the accessory or iatrogenic ostium.* The instruments used are a 45° endoscope, a backbiter and a curved 60° microdebrider. The backbiter is placed within the more posteriorly located accessory ostium and gently biting anteriorly until the dissection connects with true ostium (Fig. 20.2). An angled 60° microdebrider can be used to do obtain the same result.
- *Presence of infraorbital ethmoid (Haller) cell.* The instruments used are a J curette, a right-angled curette, 45° or 90° Blakesley, side-to-side giraffe forceps and a curved microdebrider. Fracture or entry into the cell can be done with a curette. Once the cell is exposed, 45° or 90° Blakesley forceps depending on the angle needed can be used to remove the cell walls or the bone can be fractured with giraffe forceps and then teased out. Another option is to use the curved 60° or 90° microdebrider to remove the bony partitions of the cell.
- *Medial projection of maxillary sinus.* The instruments used are straight through-cutting and Blakesley forceps. The medial wall of the maxillary sinus is removed so that it is flush with the posterior wall of the sinus. Care must be taken to avoid extending the dissection too far posteriorly and risking injury to the sphenopalatine artery.

Tips and Pearls

- A 45° or 70° endoscope is frequently necessary to identify residual uncinate and the natural ostium of the maxillary sinus.
- The backbiter can be used for both dissection and resection of residual uncinate process.

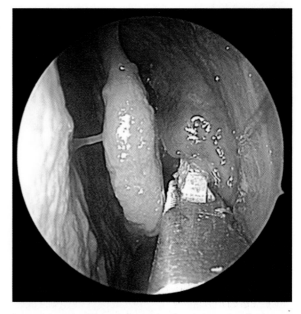

Fig. 20.1. A backbiter is being used to remove residual uncinate process

Ethmoid Sinus

The ethmoid region is a common area for residual bony partitions along the skull base and medial orbital wall. These areas may be sources of persistent inflammation and cellular obstruction with secondary neo-osteogenesis. In addition, if prior surgery has removed or perforated the middle turbinate, clearing the skull base of bony partitions or polyps becomes dangerous as the site of attachment of the middle turbinate and the dural invagination which occurs at this site may be difficult to identify, with subsequent increased risk of CSF leak The use of stereotactic navigation can be helpful in these cases. The location of the anterior ethmoid artery should be evaluated on a preoperative CT scan since at times the artery may be traveling through an area of neo-osteogenic bone, or may be hanging freely from the ethmoid roof.

A typical problem is residual bony partitions and/or neo-osteogenesis along skull base or medial orbital wall. The instruments used are 45° through-cutting forceps, a microdebrider, a 15° and 70° diamond burr self-irrigating drill, frontal sinus and J curettes, and in select cases 45° Blakesley forceps. The medial orbital wall should be identified initially in order to establish the lateral extent of the dissection. This is best achieved by using through-cutting forceps to remove these bony partitions while preserving mucosa. The medial wall of the maxillary sinus can be used as a reference point for the plane of the lamina papyracea. Angled Blakesley forceps can be used to palpate

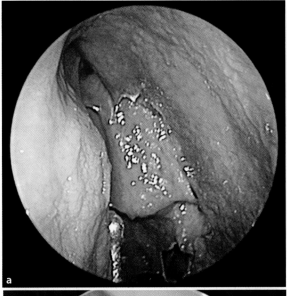

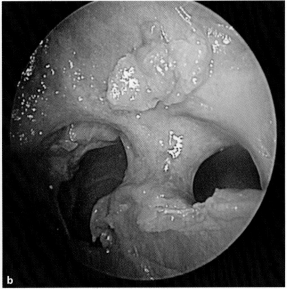

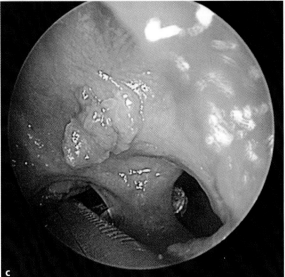

Fig. 20.2. **a** View with a0° endoscope revealing residual unci-nate process superiorly and inferiorly. The iatrogenic ostium is visualized. **b** View with a 45° endoscope revealing the failure of communication of the iatrogenic and natural ostium. **c** A backbiter is used to bring both ostia into continuity

the medial orbital wall for residual bony partitions. Once the medial orbital wall is cleared, the skull base can be identified in the sphenoid sinus or posterior ethmoid region. In all surgical procedures, a 0° tele-scope should be utilized until the medial orbital wall and skull base have been identified. If the skull base is not readily identified in the posterior ethmoid sinus, it is important to identify the sphenoid sinus ostium and widen the ostium to determine the location of the skull base roof within the sphenoid sinus. This is the lowest point of the skull base; thus, moving from pos-terior to anterior, staying adjacent to the medial or-bital wall, is the safest way to avoid intracranial en-try. The key to safely clearing the skull base is palpat-ing behind each bony partition before removal (Fig. 20.3). If space can be felt behind a bony partition, it is safe for removal. In addition, the instrument should be angled laterally to decrease the risk of intracrani-al penetration medially. If the bone is too thick to re-move with through-cutting forceps, it may be gently fractured with Blakesley forceps, teased away from the surrounding mucosa with a curette or ball-tip seeker and then removed. In certain circumstances, a wide area of bony neoosteogenesis may be present and a curved drill will be necessary. Mucosal sacrifice is inevitable in this situation, and reliance on adjacent mucosa and postoperative debridement and antibiot-ic coverage will be necessary until the area is resur-faced. In the posterior ethmoid region, a 15° drill is adequate; however, as the dissection progresses an-teriorly, transition to an angled endoscope and a 70° drill will be necessary.

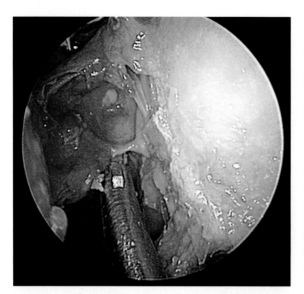

Fig. 20.3. Palpation behind bony partitions along the ethmoid skull base. Note the lateral orientation of the instrument away from a medial low-lying skull base

Tips and Pearls

- The 0° endoscope is used until the skull base is identified in order to avoid disorientation created by angled endoscopes.
- Palpate behind bony partitions along the skull base before removal.
- Angle instruments laterally along the skull base to avoid inadvertent intracranial entry.
- Review CT scans carefully to determine the location of the anterior ethmoid artery.

Sphenoid Sinus

The sphenoid sinus serves as a critical structure to be identified in the revision sinus surgery case. It anatomically defines the lowest point of the skull base, marks the posterior extent of the dissection and serves as a posterior landmark for the medial orbital wall. The most common iatrogenic sequela of the sphenoid sinus is scarring of the ostium. At times the ostium may be densely osteitic, requiring a drill for entry. In these cases, stereotactic navigation is very helpful.

A typical problem is scarring of sphenoid ostia. The instruments used are a J curette, thin Frazier suction tubing, a Stammberger mushroom punch, a Hajek rotating sphenoid punch, 45° small through-cutting forceps and a 15° diamond drill. There are two main approaches to the sphenoid sinus: the transethmoid and endoscopic transnasal. The transethmoid approach is used if the ethmoid sinus has already been dissect-

ed or if a concurrent ethmoidectomy is required. The transnasal approach is usually used if an isolated sphenoidotomy is required. In the transethmoid approach, the last posterior ethmoid cell typically has a pyramidal shape with the apex pointing superolaterally towards the anterior clinoid process. Once this has been identified, attention is directed medially and the superior meatus is identified by palpation. The posterior boundary of the superior meatus is the superior turbinate and the inferior portion of the superior turbinate is then resected with through-cutting forceps. This leads the surgeon directly back to the natural ostium, which lies medial to the superior turbinate, and the ostium can then be palpated and widened. Once entry has been established, widening of the ostium can be accomplished using either a mushroom punch or a rotating sphenoid punch (Fig. 20.4). At times the superior wall can be removed more easily with small 45° through-cutting forceps rather than the mushroom punch. Palpation is performed behind the superior wall to confirm the presence of space and then the wall is resected until it is flush with the skull base. Occasionally, a drill may be required when the bone is very thick. We prefer a wide sphenoidotomy, with the superior and lateral walls flush with the skull base and the medial orbital wall, respectively, to reduce the chances of postoperative restenosis. In addition, any Onodi cells should be brought into continuity with the sphenoid sinus.

Tips and Pearls

- Identify the superior meatus medially within the ethmoid sinus
- Resect the inferior portion of the superior turbinate
- Identify the ostium medial to the superior turbinate
- Widen the ostium to the level of the medial orbital wall and the skull base

Frontal Sinus

Revision endoscopic frontal sinus surgery has been an area of significant recent advancement. With the appropriate anatomy, frontal sinus inflammatory disease can be treated endoscopically (Video 20.1), with only a select few cases requiring open approaches such as trephination or an osteoplastic flap. The main iatrogenic sequelae causing frontal sinus obstruction are residual uncinate process, bulla ethmoidalis or agger nasi cells obstructing the frontal recess region. In addition, mucosal stripping in the region of the frontal recess can result in secondary neoosteogenesis. The key concepts to remember are to remove all bony par-

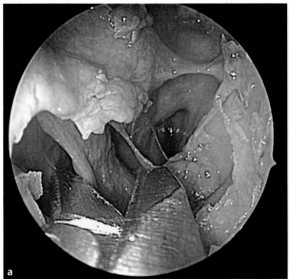
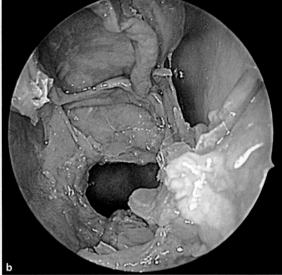
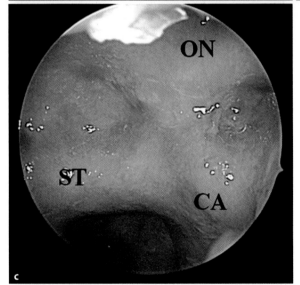

Fig. 20.4. **a** Resection of the inferior superior turbinate is performed. **b** Note the appearance of the sphenoid ostium after superior turbinate removal. **c** Endoscopic view within the sphenoid. *ON* optic nerve, *CA*, carotid artery, *ST* sella turcica

titions within the frontal recess while leaving a fully mucosalized ostium of at least 4–5-mm diameter. This can be a challenging task in the setting of neoosteogenesis.

Table 20.4. Classification of Draf frontal sinusotomy

Type	Description
Draf I	Anterior ethmoidectomy, frontal recess drainage pathway confirmed
Draf IIa	Create an opening between lamina papyracea and middle turbinate insertion
Draf IIb	Removal of frontal sinus floor between lamina papyracea and nasal septum
Draf III	Bilateral IIb with removal of upper nasal septum and lower frontal sinus septum

Endoscopic management of the frontal sinus requires angled endoscopes (45° or 70°) and the proper instrumentation. Draf [7] has described three classifications of frontal sinus dissection (Table 20.4). In the revision sinus surgery case, the minimum of a Draf IIa procedure is usually recommended. In cases where a prior Draf II procedure failed, a transseptal frontal sinusotomy (Draf III) can be performed if the anatomy is amenable.

Draf IIa

This procedure has also been described by Stammberger [2] as "uncapping the egg" and involves expanding the frontal sinus ostia from the lamina papyracea to the middle turbinate by removing residual

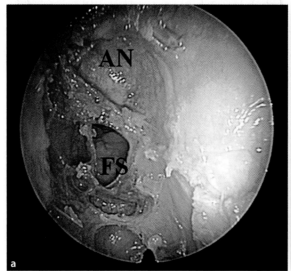

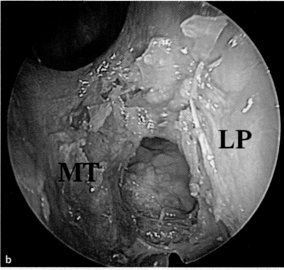

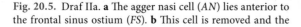

Fig. 20.5. Draf IIa. **a** The agger nasi cell (*AN*) lies anterior to the frontal sinus ostium (*FS*). **b** This cell is removed and the frontal recess is enlarged from the lamina papyracea (*LP*) to the middle turbinate (*MT*)

bony partitions. The indications are persistent frontal sinus or frontal recess disease on the CT scan with bony partitions amenable to removal. The instruments used are a 60° microdebrider, cobra forceps, side-to-side and forward–backward angled through-cutting and giraffe forceps (55° and 90°), a curved mushroom punch and a frontal sinus curette. On the preoperative CT scan determine the location of the anterior ethmoid, and the presence of supraorbital ethmoid cells, residual uncinate process, bulla ethmoidalis, and agger nasi cells. Use triplanar reconstructions or interactive imaging to identify the frontal sinus drainage pathway and conceptualize the anatomy as it will be seen endoscopically. The technique is the following. The first step is confirmation of the frontal sinus drainage pathway. This can be done very gently with a malleable probe. The ostium often lies between the uncinate process and the middle turbinate in a medial location. The ostium is identified using a probe. This area can then be expanded using additional instrumentation. Anterior expansion with a frontal sinus curette will fracture any residual agger nasi cell. This should be done in an anterolateral direction. Once fracture of the bony partitions is complete, a curved microdebrider may be used to remove bony fragments and mucosal tags. Alternatively, larger bony fragments can be teased out with a curved probe and removed with giraffe forceps. This anterior exposure facilitates working in the frontal recess and is termed "uncapping the egg"[4, 5]. Lateral extension of the ostium is performed with a curved mushroom punch to the medial orbital wall. An alternative is to downfracture fragments with a curved hook. Medial dissection is

expanded to the middle turbinate insertion and posterior dissection is conducted to the posterior table of the frontal sinus. In most cases, there is a supraorbital ethmoid air cell posteriorly of variable size. When this is identified, the bony partition between the supraorbital ethmoid cell and the frontal sinus should be removed. Once this has been completed, a wide fully mucosalized frontal sinus ostium will be present (Fig. 20.5).

Tips and Pearls

- Conceptualize the anatomy and frontal sinus drainage pathway preoperatively
- Identify the drainage pathway with a probe intraoperatively
- Fracture residual bony partitions anteriorly and laterally
- Tease out all bony fragments
- Remove mucosal tags with a curved microdebrider
- Preserve mucosa covering residual bone

Draf IIb

This involves expansion of the frontal sinus from the lamina papyracea to the nasal septum. The anterior third of the middle turbinate is resected up to the skull base. A drill or through-cutting punch is used to expand the sinus ostia medially. Although this may result in loss of mucosa in this area, the remaining walls of the ostia are mucosalized. The indica-

20

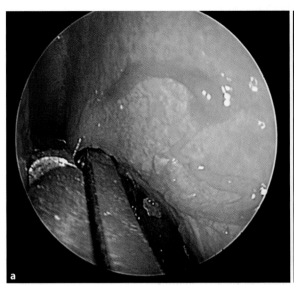

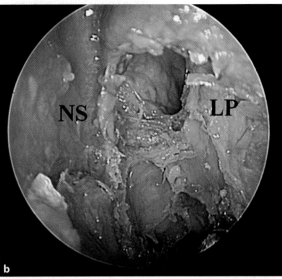

Fig. 20.6. **a** After completing a Draf IIa procedure, the anterior third of the middle turbinate is resected at the skull base using a 30° scope and a straight through-cutting instrument.

b Once this has been done, the frontal sinus ostium is enlarged from the lamina papyracea (*LP*) to the nasal septum (*NS*)

tions are failure of a prior Draf I or Draf IIa procedure, especially when due to an osteitic middle turbinate and scarring to the medial orbital wall. The instruments used are the same as those used for the Draf IIa procedure, with the addition of a 70° diamond burr drill and 1-mm Acufex through-cutting forceps. The technique consists of the same steps for the Draf IIa procedure. The anterior third of the middle turbinate can be resected using the Acufex forceps (Fig. 20.6a). In the revision case, a prior partial middle turbinate resection may have been performed. If this is the case, the anterior resection should be carried superiorly to the level of the skull base, taking care more posteriorly not to resect the region where the dura invaginates into the turbinate attachment. Side-to-side through-cutting or giraffe forceps are an ideal instrument for the delicate superior part of the resection. Before expanding the ostium medially, care must be taken to expand the ostium as far anteriorly as possible; this may be done with through-cutting "cobra" forceps or with a 70° diamond drill. In essence, the floor of the sinus is removed from the lamina papyracea to the nasal septum (Fig. 20.6b).

Tips and Pearls

■ Resect the anterior middle turbinate completely
■ Widen the ostium anteriorly before extending it medially
■ Be conservative posteriorly where the dura invaginates into the middle turbinate attachment

Draf III (Transseptal Frontal Sinusotomy)

This procedure is essentially the performance of bilateral Draf IIb procedures with resection of both the intervening segment of the nasal septum and the adjacent intersinus septum. There is up to a 10% risk of CSF leak, and all patients do not have suitable anatomy for this procedure. An anteroposterior diameter of at least 5 mm is required. Evaluation of the preoperative CT scan is required with careful attention to the anteroposterior diameter of the frontal sinus, the width of the ethmoid cavity and the thickness of the nasofrontal beak. A thick nasofrontal beak translates into additional denuded bone, increased drilling time and an increased incidence of postoperative scarring. The instruments used are the same as those used for the Draf IIb procedure, with the addition of instruments needed to resect the superior nasal septum: an angled beaver blade or a sickle knife and a suction Freer elevator. The procedure is typically begun by identifying the more open frontal sinus; however, when both sinuses are involved, it may be initiated with the septal resection and creation of the septal window (transseptal frontal sinusotomy). The skull base is then identified posteriorly, and the frontal sinuses are opened from within the septal space. More commonly, bilateral Draf IIb procedures are first performed. Once the ostia have been enlarged to the nasal septum, the superior septum is resected after injecting it with 1% lidocaine with 1:100,000 epinephrine solution. A sickle knife or beaver blade is used to make a superiorly based U-shaped flap on the nasal septum. This mucosa is removed with a 60° micro-debrider. The frontal sinus is reidentified and the segment of bony septum at the floor of the frontal sinus is removed. The nasofrontal "beak" is then removed with a 70° diamond drill under direct visualization, taking care to preserve the mucosa posteriorly. After this has been done, the intersinus septum of the frontal sinus comes into view and this can be removed in one of two ways. Side-to-side through-cutting SSI forceps can be used if the bone is not too thick; however, when bone density is a factor, a 70° diamond burr drill can be used to resect the septum.

Tips and Pearls

- Carefully evaluate the triplanar CT scans for anatomic suitability for this procedure.
- Start on the side of the most easily identified frontal sinus and open this side. If both frontal sinuses are closed, consider a transseptal approach initially.
- Remember the two frontal sinuses cannot be connected with a straight line; the opening must be brought anteriorly in an inverted-U shape to avoid the midline skull base.
- Use the drill anteriorly to create a wide antero-posterior diameter opening.
- Preserve the mucosa posteriorly.

Complications of Endoscopic Sinus Surgery

The major complications of endoscopic sinus surgery can be narrowed to two main categories: intracranial and intraorbital injuries [(Table 20.5). In most series, these potential complications appear to occur in approximately one in 200 cases, but are essential in the preoperative discussion of informed consent and the incidence may be higher in revision procedures. The risk of CSF leak should be adjusted accordingly in those patients having multiple revision procedures, those with dense osteitic bone or neo-osteogenesis

Table 20.5. Complications of endoscopic sinus surgery

Major	Minor
Orbital	Scarring
Hemorrhage	Bleeding
Muscle injury	Infection
Optic nerve injury	Epiphora
Internal carotid injury	
Central nervous system	
CSF leak	
Encephalocele	
Brain abscess	

along the skull base and those undergoing transseptal frontal sinusotomy.

Although the major complications are rare, more minor complications such as scarring, disease persistence, synechiae formation and mucoceles are much more common.

Postoperative Care and Debridement

The long-term success of revision sinus surgery is dependent on diligent postoperative medical management and office debridement. The office setting should have a complete set of instruments available for removal of residual bony partitions and lysis of synechiae. Endoscopically directed cultures should be performed as needed. The mucosal appearance is the critical sign of whether a postoperative cavity has healed completely and is likely to remain stable. Residual areas of edema along the skull base or medial orbital wall are suggestive of residual bony partitions. Palpation and removal of these areas with curettes or through-cutting instruments can be performed after topical anesthesia. In addition, in select cases intralesional steroids can be administered, especially in the frontal recess.

Medical management involves the use of antibiotics, nasal steroids, nasal saline irrigations and antibiotic irrigations. The duration of oral steroids and other medical management is dependent on the endoscopic appearance of the postoperative cavity. Aggressive irrigations are not initiated until 2 weeks after surgery in order to alleviate the risk of introducing infection. Nasal saline preparations are easily available over the counter to keep the cavity moist between debridements. Patients are seen in the office for 4–6 weeks of weekly debridement. Topical nasal steroids are usually continued long term, especially in the revision patient who may need indefinite treatment.

Open Revision Sinus Surgery

Caldwell–Luc

The use of the Caldwell–Luc approach to the maxillary sinus is essentially of little utility in the management of inflammatory sinus disease. In patients with neoplastic processes, including inverted papilloma, the Caldwell–Luc approach is an ideal adjunct to the endoscopic approach, especially in those tumors with anterior or lateral attachment. For this reason a brief description of the procedure is presented since it has already been well described [1, 3]. An incision is made in the upper gingivobuccal sulcus leaving a cuff of mucosa for reapproximation on the dental side of the incision. Unipolar cautery can be used to take the dissection to the face of the maxilla. An incision is made through the periosteum, and a periosteal elevator is used to elevate superiorly. Medial elevation to the piriform aperture and lateral extension to the lateral wall of the maxilla is performed. As the periosteum is elevated superiorly, the infraorbital nerve bundle is identified. Entry into the maxillary sinus is performed with a 2-mm osteotome and mallet in the canine fossa. A small square is created to accommodate a Kerrison rongeur. Closure of the incision is performed with a 3-0 chromic suture in a running horizontal mattress fashion. We feel the horizontal mattress everts the mucosal edges well and prevents retraction of mucosa and food trapping in the wound.

Frontal Sinus Trephination

The indications are as follows: frontal sinus cells inaccessible via an endoscopic approach; evaluation of the posterior table frontal sinus or examination of the integrity of the frontal sinus ostia; aid in resection of frontal sinus neoplasm. The technique involves an infrabrow incision made down to the bone. Whereas for frontal sinus irrigation the opening is typically made in the sinus floor, when the primary purpose of the trephine is for endoscopic examination and manipulation, the bony entry is usually made in the anterior wall. Transillumination or image guidance can be used to confirm the location of the frontal sinus. A 5-mm cutting burr is used to enter the frontal sinus. Care is taken to avoid the area of the supraorbital nerve. Once entry has been gained into the sinus, expansion of the entry site can be done with a drill or rongeur if necessary. Once widening has been done, dissection can be performed via the trephination site under endoscopic visualization or using a combined above-and-below approach, using endoscopic visualization both intranasally and through the trephine.

Tips and Pearls
- Carefully evaluate the sinus imaging before performing the trephine
- Feel for the supraorbital notch
- Use a round burr to remove the bone and then carefully open the mucosa

Osteoplastic Flap

The indications are intractable frontal sinus inflammatory disease not amenable to a transseptal frontal sinusotomy, failure of Draf III frontal sinusotomy, and for resection of selected frontal sinus tumors. The technique is a standard coronal incision typically extending from each helical crus. A subgaleal plane is identified and elevated to 2 cm above the supraorbital rims. At this point blunt dissection is used to further elevate the flap and identify the supraorbital neurovascular bundles. A safe dissection area is the midline. A radiographic template is cut to the dimensions of the frontal sinus or, preferably, computer-assisted imaging is used to identify the outline of the frontal sinus. The periosteum is incised a few millimeters outside the template and elevated 2 mm on either side. Low-profile miniplates are drilled and then removed. An oscillating saw is used to make a 2-mm vertical trough and then the saw is beveled towards the sinus until entry into the frontal sinus itself. The vertical cuts at the supraorbital rim can be completed with an osteotome if desired and a horizontal saw cut can be made in the midline above the root of the nose to make it easier to fracture the sinus in this region. If obliteration is planned, all mucosa is removed by both Freer elevation and drilling the entire bony surface under magnification with the operating microscope in order to ensure complete mucosal removal. In cases of tumor or fungal disease, obliteration is avoided and a wide opening is made into the nasal cavity. This combined above-and-below approach involves combining a classic Lothrop procedure from above with a bilateral endoscopic anterior ethmoidectomy transseptal frontal sinusotomy from below. Typically, the transnasal endoscopic procedure is performed initially and, if it is clear that all the disease cannot be removed, the external approach is performed. For reconstruction at the end of the procedure, the bone flap is then replaced and miniplates are reapplied. The wound is closed with the use of 2-0 Vicryl sutures in an interrupted fashion. This layer must incorporate the galea aponeurosis. The skin is closed with staples. Suction drains are placed for 24 h. Staple removal is done at 10 days.

Tips and Pearls
- Reserve the osteoplastic approach for when other procedures fail.
- Use computer-assisted imaging to outline the frontal sinus whenever possible, but have a 6-ft posteroanterior Caldwell view for backup use as a template.
- Bevel the saw during the osteotomy.

- Use the 0° and 30° scopes interchangeably during the procedure.
- Avoid trauma to the middle turbinate; this will decrease the incidence of adhesions considerably.
- If the frontal sinus is not diseased, stay away form the frontal recess area to prevent scarring in that area. If frontal recess surgery is needed, it should be minimal.

- Extreme caution is needed while doing the uncinectomy in children to avoid orbital fat herniation.
- The anterograde approach to the maxillary sinus ostium will decrease the chances of stripping the mucosa of the maxillary sinus and injury of the nasolacrimal duct because there will be no need to use the side biter anteriorly.

Complications

Complications are very rare in children. They can be intraoperative or postoperative:

1. Intraoperative complications
   (a) *Cerebrospinal fluid leak.* This needs to be recognized during the procedure and repaired immediately.
   (b) *Orbital entry with fat herniation.* In most instances the procedure can be completed and no intervention is needed.
   (c) *Orbital hemorrhage with increased pressure.* An immediate lateral canthotomy with removal of all the packing in the ethmoid on that side. An ophthalmology consult should be obtained.
   (d) *Stripping of the maxillary sinus mucosa.* This needs to be recognized otherwise, even though the bony ostium is open, the mucosa inside the sinus will be collapsed with no ventilation of the inside of the sinus.
   (e) *Inadvertent injury to the middle turbinate.* All attempts should be made to preserve it in place.
   (f) *Bleeding.* If bleeding is impairing vision considerably, the procedure should be aborted. There is no need to put the patient at risk for blood transfusion. If the bleeding is excessive with respect to the blood volume of the child, then the procedure should also be aborted.
2. Postoperative complications
   (a) *Bleeding.* In most instances it is self-contained. Rarely packing or examination in the operating room is needed.

(b) *Adhesions.* These can be very common depending on the age of the child. If they are not causing any symptoms, then they can be left alone. If symptomatic and severe, a second-look to deal with them would be appropriate.
(c) *Orbital swelling and ecchymosis.* If eye pressure is high, then proceed as for intraoperative increased pressure. If the pressure is normal and the child is cooperative enough, remove the packing and observe.
(d) *Cerebrospinal fluid leak.* Place the patient on complete bed rest, with head elevation, and give stool softeners for 1 week. There is no support in the literature for a lumbar drain. If the cerebrospinal fluid leak persists, then consider endoscopic repair.

Conclusion

The endoscopic technique provides superb visualization and can be used safely for sinus surgery in children once medical therapy fails. It is important though to recognize that the majority of children with sinus disease respond to medical treatment.

References

1. Andrews TM. (2003) Current concepts in antibiotic resistance. Curr Opin Otolaryngol Head Neck Surg 11(6):409–415.
2. Bhattacharyya N, Jones DT, Hill M, Shapiro NL. (2004) The diagnostic accuracy of computed tomography in pediatric chronic rhinosinusitis. Arch Otolaryngol Head Neck Surg 130(9): 1029–1032.
3. Garbutt JM, Goldstein M, Gellman E, et al. (2001) A randomized, placebo-controlled trial of antimicrobial treatment for children with clinically diagnosed acute sinusitis. Pediatrics 107:619–625.
4. Kennedy DW, Zeinreich SJ. (1989) Functional Endoscopic Surgery: Advances in Otolaryngology Head and Neck Surgery. Chicago: Year Book, 1–26.
5. Lusk RP, Muntz HR. (1990) Endoscopic sinus surgery in children with chronic sinusitis. Laryngoscope 100:654–658
6. Manning S. (2001) Surgical intervention for sinusitis in children. Curr Allergy Asthma Rep 1:289–296.
7. Norante JD. (1984) Surgical management of sinusitis. Ear Nose Throat J 63:155–162.
8. Parsons DS, Phillips SE. (1993) Functional endoscopic surgery in children: a retrospective analysis of results. Laryngoscope 103(8):899–903.
9. Phipps CD, Wood WE, Gibson WS, et al. (2000) Gastroesophageal reflux contributing to chronic sinus disease in

21

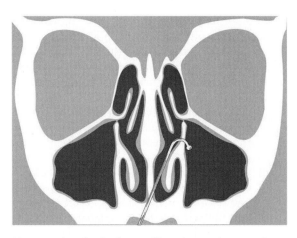

Fig. 21.4. A seeker in the maxillary sinus ostium anterior to the uncinate process

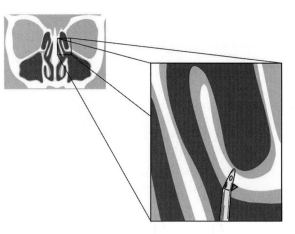

Fig. 21.7. Straight Blakesley forceps

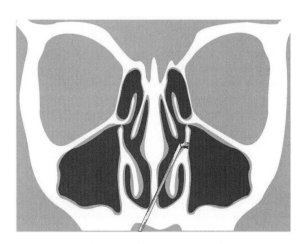

Fig. 21.5. Straight cutting forceps removing the uncinate process

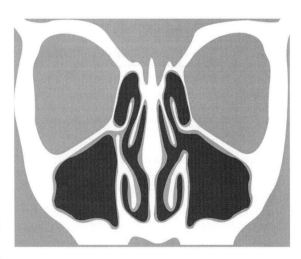

Fig. 21.6. The ostium open after the uncinate has been removed

nus is diseased, then opening of the frontal recess and ostium is needed.

In most instances, once the uncinectomy is performed, a small residual piece superiorly can be identified. The seeker is used to palpate just posterior to that piece (if not present, palpation in that area is done) to enter into the frontal sinus opening. A curved suction cannula is then introduced into the sinus for inspection. In most instances, the surgeon will alternate between right and left nasal cavities using pledgets impregnated with 0.5% oxymetazoline solution for control of hemostasis while performing part of the procedure on the other side.

Once the procedure is complete, the cavities are packed with hyaluronic acid pledgets rolled up in thirds and placed in the ethmoid cavity next to the middle turbinate. A nasal drip pad is placed on the nose. The eyes are then inspected for any swelling, edema, increased pressure or ecchymosis.

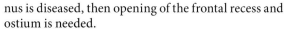

Postoperative Care

All patients are given oral antibiotics for 10–14 days. It is recommended that they sleep with the head elevated for 7 days. We discourage blowing of the nose or use of nasal sprays for 1–2 weeks. A second-look procedure is not needed on most patients. Packing will be absorbed by around 2–3 weeks and debridement in children is not necessary.

Tips and Pearls

- Use a 4-mm scope for better visualization whenever possible. In most children a 4-mm scope can be used instead of a 2.7-mm scope.

Contraindications for surgery are:

- Children with chronic rhinitis without evidence of rhinosinusitis
- Children with a normal CT scan of the sinuses

Anesthesia

- ESS is done under general anesthesia in children.
- Pledgets impregnated with 0.5% oxymetazoline solution are used for topical vasoconstriction.
- Injection of the middle turbinates, uncinate processes, bulla ethmoidalis and septum adjacent to the middle turbinates with 1% lidocaine solution with 1:100,000 epinephrine.

Preparation for Surgery

The child is placed supine with the head of table slightly elevated. The results of a CT scan should always be in the operating suite to be used as a road map. The surgeon should be facing the patient with the monitor facing the surgeon. The surgeon can operate looking through the scope using a beam-splitter camera, or, if so trained, can operate by looking at the monitor. If the surgeon is skilled in the procedure, the eyes do not need to stay uncovered. A small tape can be used to cover them. At this point the anesthesiologist is directed to make sure that the patient received a 0.15 mg/kg decadron intravenous bolus.

Instruments Used in Surgery

The following instruments are used in surgery:

- Rigid scopes (0°, 30° and 70°)preferably 4 mm in size
- Straight and upturned Blakesley forceps of different sizes.
- Straight and upturned through-cutting forceps.
- A double-blind ostium seeker
- Short and long curved antrum cannulas.
- Right side and left side backward punch cutting forceps
- Frazier suction tubes (3, 5 and 7 French)
- A Cottle elevator
- If possible, a powered microdebrider with aggressive 2.9- and 4-mm blades

- Additional instruments as deemed appropriate by the surgeon for frontal sinus and sphenoid surgery

Surgical Procedure

The 0° 4-mm scope is introduced into the nasal cavity after the pledgets have been removed (see "Anesthesia"). If more injection is needed it can be performed at this stage. With use of the cottle elevator, the middle turbinate is medialized until the uncinate process and bulla are visualized. With use of the seeker, the area of the maxillary sinus ostium is found and the ostium palpated. This can be performed in a retrograde or an anterograde manner. I prefer the antegrade technique because it prevents the posterior maxillary mucosa from stripping (Fig. 21.4).The ostium can then be widened posteriorly by removing the inferior edge of the uncinate process with straight cutting forceps (Figs. 21.5, 21.6). For retrograde technique, the right-sided backbiter can be used to remove the uncinate process anteriorly. Care should be taken not to injure the nasolacrimal duct with this technique.

A curved angled cannula is then introduced into the maxillary sinus for suction. Polyps, cysts or other debris can be suctioned and removed. All attempts should be made not to strip the mucous membrane of the sinus. The remainder of the uncinate process is then removed using up-biting and backbiting forceps. The ethmoid bulla should be now fully visualized. A straight biter is used to enter the bulla inferiorly and medially. These cells are then removed using straight and up-biting forceps (Fig. 21.7). The lamina papyracea and skull base should be visualized during this procedure to avoid any injuries.

If a posterior ethmoidectomy is needed, the ground lamella of the middle turbinate should be identified. Penetration through the lamella with a 5-mm Frazier suction tube can be performed. Any pathologic contents inside can be suctioned or removed. The anterior table of the posterior ethmoid can be widened. Removal of the mucous membrane of the sinus is not encouraged.

A posterior to anterior dissection is then performed along the skull base, which is easily identified in the posterior ethmoid air cells. This can be facilitated by using a 30° 4-mm endoscope. Exenteration of these cells along skull base can be performed using the J curette. These cells can be removed under visualization using up-biting forceps.

If a posterior ethmoidectomy is not needed, then identification of the skull base can be done anterior to the basal lamella and a similar posterior to anterior dissection is then done. At this point if the frontal si-

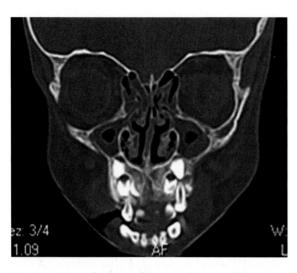

Fig. 21.3. Coronal computed tomography scan of the sinuses of a child with chronic rhinosinusitis through the ostiomeatal complex area. It shows disease in the anterior ethmoid, maxillary sinuses and maxillary sinus ostium

Medical Treatment

Oral antibiotics are the mainstay of treatment of rhinosinusitis in children according to the 2005 practice guidelines [15]. High-dose amoxicillin or amoxicillin–clavulanic acid is recommended as first line of treatment. Cephalosporins or macrolides can be used as a second line of treatment or for those with penicillin allergy. There is no consensus on the duration of treatment, but most agree that it should be at least 3–4 weeks. Antibiotics can be repeated, depending on the response of the child. Adjunct treatment consists of topical nasal steroids and oral antihistamines for those with allergic rhinitis. Topical or systemic decongestants can be used, although studies have not shown them to be effective [3].

The role of intravenous antibiotics for the treatment of children with persistent or recurrent symptoms despite oral antibiotic management is still controversial. Parenteral antibiotics did not seem to contribute to a lasting resolution of children with chronic rhinosinusitis [16]. Gastroesophageal reflux disease has been noted to have a role in the pathophysiology of chronic rhinosinusitis in children. The role of reflux treatment in these children, however, is still not universally accepted [9]. Antibiotic prophylaxis to prevent infection in children who have recurrent episodes is also controversial. Little support is expressed for this approach based on the otitis media model, because of concerns of increasing prevalence of antibiotic-resistant organisms. Antibiotic prophylaxis may be used in patients with cystic fibrosis, immunodeficiency and immotile cilia disorders [1].

Surgical Treatment

There is no consensus and there are no guidelines on surgical treatment for chronic rhinosinusitis in children. Several surgical techniques were used in the past for the treatment of children with sinusitis, including Caldwell–Luc, intranasal ethmoidectomy, maxillary antrostomy and other external procedures. Endoscopic sinus surgery (ESS) has been the surgical treatment of choice for the last 15 years. The success with the procedure has been very rewarding [5–8,].

Absolute Indications

Most otolaryngologists agree that the absolute indications for surgery are:

- Orbital complications, most commonly subperiosteal abscess
- Central nervous system complications
- Severe nasal polyposis
- Suspected benign lesions, tumor or fungal infection

Relative Indications

This category includes children who have signs and symptoms of chronic rhinosinusitis or children who have recurrent acute rhinosinusitis despite adequate medical treatment. Controversy prevails about when to operate and what procedure to perform [10]. Some physicians are of the opinion that an adenoidectomy should be performed on all children prior to ESS [18]. Agreements exist that surgery should be a last resort for children with CT evidence of disease who fail maximal medical treatment [11, 12].

Relative indications for surgery are:

- Chronic rhinosinusitis with anatomical abnormalities
- Children with cystic fibrosis who have complicated pulmonary disease
- Children with symptoms of asthma secondary to refractory chronic rhinosinusitis who are not responding to systemic steroids
- Children with immotile cilia or immune deficiency who are not responding to medical treatment of culture and irrigation.

Classification

Rhinosinusitis is classified into four categories:
1. *Acute rhinosinusitis*: symptoms last up to 2 weeks but not more than 4 weeks.
2. *Subacute rhinosinusitis*: symptoms last 2–4 weeks but not more than 3 months.
3. *Chronic rhinosinusitis*: symptoms last more than 3 months.
4. *Recurrent acute rhinosinusitis*: four or more episodes per year of acute rhinosinusitis.

Clinical Presentation

The diagnosis of rhinosinusitis in children can be difficult. Symptoms can be similar to those of a viral illness or may mimic allergic symptoms. Also symptoms can be similar to those of adenoiditis or sometimes reflux symptoms. Since children average six to eight colds a year, the physician should have a high index of suspicion for rhinosinusitis. Generally, most agree that if symptoms of a cold are not improving by 10–14 days, rhinosinusitis should be considered [21].

History

Symptoms of rhinosinusitis in children may vary by age. Younger children present with colored nasal discharge and cough, while older ones will complain of nasal stuffiness/obstruction and headache. The most common symptoms of chronic rhinosinusitis include nasal discharge (75%), cough (73%), nasal congestion (72%) and headache (72%) (Fig. 21.1) [10, 13, 21].

Physical Examination

Physical examination in children is usually difficult and findings are rarely helpful. Nasal endoscopy can be performed in an older cooperative child. Findings such as a concha bullosa, nasal polyps, purulent discharge or enlarged adenoids can be helpful findings (Fig. 21.2) [21].

Laboratory Studies

Diagnostic workup of children with chronic rhinosinusitis should include an allergy evaluation, immune deficiency testing, cilia biopsy and reflux evaluation.

On the basis of the findings, appropriate management should be considered.

Imaging Studies

Coronal computed tomography (CT) of the sinuses is the imaging study of choice for the evaluation of children with chronic rhinosinusitis. Plain films in these patients have a poor sensitivity and specificity. Plain films can be helpful in cases of acute rhinosinusitis.

For the CT scan to help in the management of children with chronic rhinosinusitis, it should be performed at the end of maximal medical management. A CT scan is also the preferred imaging modality in evaluating children with complicated rhinosinusitis [2, 14] (Fig. 21.3).

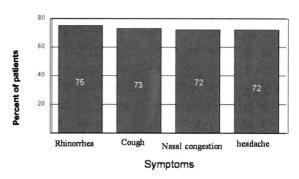

Fig. 21.1. The most common presenting symptoms of chronic rhinosinusitis in that children

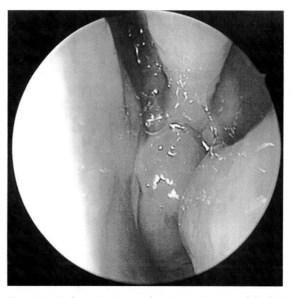

Fig. 21.2. Endoscopic view with a 4-mm 0° scope of the left nasal cavity of a child showing complete blockage of the choana by adenoid tissue

21

Pediatric Sinus Surgery

Hassan H. Ramadan

Core Messages

- Chronic rhinosinusitis is a very common condition in children.

- Diagnosis can be confused with a viral infection, adenoiditis or allergy symptoms.

- The majority of children respond to medical treatment.

- Coronal computed tomography scan is the imaging modality of choice in children with chronic rhinosinusitis.

- Pathophysiology in these children is blockage of the ostiomeatal complex area.

- Surgery is recommended for children who fail medical treatment.

- Endoscopic sinus surgery is the surgical modality of choice.

Contents

Development of the Sinuses

The ethmoid and maxillary sinuses are present at birth. They can be detected radiographically at 5–6 months of age. The ethmoid sinuses grow rapidly in the first few years of life. Their growth slows significantly by 7 years of age. They reach full size by 12–14 years of age. The maxillary sinuses also grow rapidly in the first few years of life, mainly during the third and fourth years of life. After 7 years of age, growth accelerates inferiorly after the permanent teeth have erupted. They reach full growth by 15 years of age. The frontal and sphenoid sinuses start aerating by 4 years of age. Their development starts accelerating by 8 years of age and full development is reached by 18 years of age. Because of this development, the main sinuses involved in children with chronic rhinosinusitis are the ethmoid and maxillary sinuses [17].

Pathogenesis

The majority of cases of rhinosinusitis are secondary to obstruction of the ostiomeatal unit, which is an area located in the middle meatus. This obstruction will lead to poor ventilation and stasis of secretions, resulting in inflammation or infection. Obstruction can be due to several causes, the most common being anatomical anomalies, viral infections and allergic rhinitis. Certain conditions that can affect mucociliary clearance of the sinuses can also cause rhinosinusitis. Such conditions include cystic fibrosis, ciliary dyskinesia and immotile cilia. Several other conditions can affect the development of rhinosinusitis. Other than allergic rhinitis, immune deficiencies and reflux disease are conditions that may impact the response to treatment of rhinosinusitis [4, 19, 20].

- Remove all the mucosa (including the supraorbital ethmoid cells) if obliteration is to be performed.
- Consider beginning with a Draf III procedure or transseptal frontal sinusotomy in cases of tumor. It may be possible to remove all tumor and drill the sites of attachment from below using a 70° diamond drill.

Conclusion

Revision sinus surgery for the treatment of inflammatory disease has been revolutionized with the advent of endoscopic sinus surgery. In only select cases is open surgery required. The keys to successful revision surgery are adjunctive medical management, aggressive postoperative debridement, mucosal preservation and removal of osteitic bone.

References

1. Bailey BJ, Calhoun KH, Friedman NR, Newlands SD, Vrabec JT (2001). Atlas of Head and Neck Surgery-Otolaryngology. Philadelphia, Lippincott, Williams and Wilkins.
2. Stammberger H (2004). "Uncapping the Egg" – The Endoscopic Approach to Frontal Recess and Sinuses." Tuttlingen, Endo, pp 15–17.
3. Kennedy DW (2001). Diseases of the Sinuses Diagnosis and Management. Hamilton, Ontario, BC Decker.
4. Kuhn FA, Bolger WE, Tisdahl RG (1991). "The agger nasi cell in frontal recess obstruction: an anatomic, radiologic and clinical correlation." Operative Techniques in Otolaryngology-Head and Neck Surgery 2:226–231.
5. Palmer JN, Kennedy D W (2005). Revision Endoscopic Sinus Surgery. Philadelphia, Elsevier Mosby.
6. Senior BA, Kennedy DW, Tanabodee J, et al (1998). "Long-term results of functional endoscopic sinus surgery." Laryngoscope 108:151–157.
7. Weber R, Draf W, Kratzsch B, Hosemann W, Schaefer SD (2001). "Modern concepts of frontal sinus surgery." Laryngoscope 111:137–146.

20

ing a cuff of mucosa for reapproximation on the dental side of the incision. Unipolar cautery can be used to take the dissection to the face of the maxilla. An incision is made through the periosteum, and a periosteal elevator is used to elevate superiorly. Medial elevation to the piriform aperture and lateral extension to the lateral wall of the maxilla is performed. As the periosteum is elevated superiorly, the infraorbital nerve bundle is identified. Entry into the maxillary sinus is performed with a 2-mm osteotome and mallet in the canine fossa. A small square is created to accommodate a Kerrison rongeur. Closure of the incision is performed with a 3-0 chromic suture in a running horizontal mattress fashion. We feel the horizontal mattress everts the mucosal edges well and prevents retraction of mucosa and food trapping in the wound.

Frontal Sinus Trephination

The indications are as follows: frontal sinus cells inaccessible via an endoscopic approach; evaluation of the posterior table frontal sinus or examination of the integrity of the frontal sinus ostia; aid in resection of frontal sinus neoplasm. The technique involves an infrabrow incision made down to the bone. Whereas for frontal sinus irrigation the opening is typically made in the sinus floor, when the primary purpose of the trephine is for endoscopic examination and manipulation, the bony entry is usually made in the anterior wall. Transillumination or image guidance can be used to confirm the location of the frontal sinus. A 5-mm cutting burr is used to enter the frontal sinus. Care is taken to avoid the area of the supraorbital nerve. Once entry has been gained into the sinus, expansion of the entry site can be done with a drill or rongeur if necessary. Once widening has been done, dissection can be performed via the trephination site under endoscopic visualization or using a combined above-and-below approach, using endoscopic visualization both intranasally and through the trephine.

Tips and Pearls

- Carefully evaluate the sinus imaging before performing the trephine
- Feel for the supraorbital notch
- Use a round burr to remove the bone and then carefully open the mucosa

Osteoplastic Flap

The indications are intractable frontal sinus inflammatory disease not amenable to a transseptal frontal sinusotomy, failure of Draf III frontal sinusotomy, and for resection of selected frontal sinus tumors. The technique is a standard coronal incision typically extending from each helical crus. A subgaleal plane is identified and elevated to 2 cm above the supraorbital rims. At this point blunt dissection is used to further elevate the flap and identify the supraorbital neurovascular bundles. A safe dissection area is the midline. A radiographic template is cut to the dimensions of the frontal sinus or, preferably, computer-assisted imaging is used to identify the outline of the frontal sinus. The periosteum is incised a few millimeters outside the template and elevated 2 mm on either side. Low-profile miniplates are drilled and then removed. An oscillating saw is used to make a 2-mm vertical trough and then the saw is beveled towards the sinus until entry into the frontal sinus itself. The vertical cuts at the supraorbital rim can be completed with an osteotome if desired and a horizontal saw cut can be made in the midline above the root of the nose to make it easier to fracture the sinus in this region. If obliteration is planned, all mucosa is removed by both Freer elevation and drilling the entire bony surface under magnification with the operating microscope in order to ensure complete mucosal removal. In cases of tumor or fungal disease, obliteration is avoided and a wide opening is made into the nasal cavity. This combined above-and-below approach involves combining a classic Lothrop procedure from above with a bilateral endoscopic anterior ethmoidectomy transseptal frontal sinusotomy from below. Typically, the transnasal endoscopic procedure is performed initially and, if it is clear that all the disease cannot be removed, the external approach is performed. For reconstruction at the end of the procedure, the bone flap is then replaced and miniplates are reapplied. The wound is closed with the use of 2-0 Vicryl sutures in an interrupted fashion. This layer must incorporate the galea aponeurosis. The skin is closed with staples. Suction drains are placed for 24 h. Staple removal is done at 10 days.

Tips and Pearls

- Reserve the osteoplastic approach for when other procedures fail.
- Use computer-assisted imaging to outline the frontal sinus whenever possible, but have a 6-ft posteroanterior Caldwell view for backup use as a template.
- Bevel the saw during the osteotomy.

children: a prospective analysis. Arch Otolaryngol Head Neck Surg 126(7):831–836.

10. Ramadan HH. (2004) Surgical management of chronic sinusitis in children. Laryngoscope 114(12):2103–2109.

11. Ramadan HR. (1999) Adenoidectomy vs. endoscopic sinus surgery for the treatment of pediatric sinusitis. Arch Otolaryngol Head Neck Surg 25:1208–1211.

12. Rosenfeld RM. (1995) Pilot study of outcomes in pediatric rhinosinusitis. Arch Otolaryngol Head Neck Surg 121:729–736.

13. Siegel JD. (1987) Diagnosis and management of acute sinusitis in children. Pediatr Infect Dis J 6:95–99.

14. Sobol SE, Smadi DS, Kazahaya K, Tom LW. (2005) Trends in the management of pediatric chronic sinusitis: survey of the American Society of Pediatric Otolaryngology. Laryngoscope 115(1):78–80.

15. Subcommittee on Management of Sinusitis and Committee on Quality Improvement. (2001) Clinical Practice Guideline: Management of Sinusitis. Pediatrics 108:798–808.

16. Tanner SB, Fowler KC. (2004) Intravenous antibiotics for chronic rhinosinusitis: are they effective? Curr Opin Otolaryngol Head Neck Surg 12(1):3–8.

17. Van Alyea OE. (1951) Nasal sinuses. In: Anatomic and Clinical Considerations. 2nd ed. Baltimore: Williams and Wilkins.

18. Vanderberg SJ, Heatley DG. (1997) Efficacy of adenoidectomy in relieving symptoms of chronic sinusitis in children. Arch Otolaryngol Head Neck Surg 123:675–678.

19. Wald ER. (1988) Diagnosis and management of acute sinusitis. Pediatr Ann17:629–638.

20. Wald ER. (1985) Epidemiology, pathophysiology and etiology of sinusitis. Pediatr Infect Dis J 4(Suppl 6):551–554.

21. Wald ER. (1988) Management of sinusitis in infants and children. Pediatr Infect Dis J 7:449–452.

Chapter 22

External Approaches to the Paranasal Sinuses

22

Mark C. Weissler

Core Messages

- During the Caldwell–Luc procedure, since there is no longer any active transport of mucous within the sinus, drainage must be created inferiorly through the inferior meatus.

- Since the floor of the maxillary sinus is lower than the floor of the nose, gravity does not serve entirely to drain the sinus. Hence, after a Caldwell–Luc procedure, plain films (Caldwell views) of the maxillary sinus will forever be abnormal with some degree of opacification.

- The external ethmoidectomy approach is a classic approach that has been used to address a large variety of conditions of the sinuses, orbit and skull base.

- Frontal sinus trephination is indicated to drain the acutely infected frontal sinus with impending orbital or intracranial complications and as an adjunct to endoscopic exploration of the nasofrontal drainage system.

- The Lynch procedure was used in the treatment of chronic frontal sinusitis in an attempt to reconstruct a large nasofrontal drainage pathway via an external approach.

- For the osteoplastic frontal sinus procedure, a coronal flap is elevated in a plane *superficial* to the periosteum.

- The lateral rhinotomy is an approach used for lesions of the anterior nasal cavity including the nasal floor, septum and vestibule. When combined with a medial maxillectomy, lesions of the posterior nasal cavity, nasal sidewall, maxillary sinus cavity and pterygomaxillary space can be approached.

- The Weber–Ferguson approach combines the lateral rhinotomy with an upper lip splitting incision and a lateral horizontal incision below the orbit at the level of the inferior orbital rim.

- The midfacial degloving approach provides exposure to the bilateral nasal cavities and maxillae.

- The craniofacial resection approach is used for sinonasal neoplasia involving the skull base.

- The subcranial approach is an alternative to formal craniofacial resection for tumors of the superior nasal cavity and anterior cranial base.

Contents

Introduction

The external approaches to the paranasal sinuses form a group of procedures which build on one another and can be combined in various ways to gain access and exposure to the anatomic regions of the paranasal sinuses, orbit, face, anterior and middle skull base. These procedures are germane not only to surgery for acute and chronic disease of the paranasal sinuses, but also to neoplasia that involve these areas and trauma. An endoscope, an operating microscope and/or brilliant illumination with a headlight and operating loupes, all of which are really just means of improving visualization, can certainly be used with these "greater" surgical access procedures or with more minimally invasive or transnasal approaches. Instrumentation is by no means tied to access procedures, and the wise surgeon will use those instruments and those access procedures which best allow him/her to adequately visualize the relevant anatomy and abnormality in such a way as to do his/her patient the maximal good with the least amount of harm. Some of these open procedures are essentially of historical interest in the treatment of chronic rhinosinusitis, but remain worthy of some attention for the treatment of complicated acute infections, neoplasia, some inflammatory orbital conditions and trauma.

Approaches to the Maxillary Sinus and Nasal Sidewall

The Caldwell–Luc Procedure and Antrostomy (Nasoantral Window)

Indications are:

- Chronic polypoid maxillary sinusitis unresponsive to conservative intranasal procedures
- Acute complicated maxillary sinusitis
- In the treatment of oroantral fistulae
- As a route to biopsy
- Infraorbital nerve
- Maxillary sinus mass
- As an approach to the orbital floor
- To treat fracture
- For orbital decompression of Grave's ophthalmopathy

The Caldwell–Luc procedure is a sublabial approach to the maxillary sinus through the anterior wall under the upper lip. Traditionally it was used to treat chronic maxillary sinusitis with irreversible changes of the maxillary sinus respiratory epithelium. During the procedure all the lining mucosa of the maxillary sinus is removed and will be replaced by a rind of scar tissue covered by cuboidal nonciliated epithelium as the sinus heals. Because there is no longer any active transport of mucous within the sinus, drainage must be created inferiorly through the inferior meatus. Since the floor of the maxillary sinus is lower than the floor of the nose, gravity does not serve entirely to drain the sinus. After a Caldwell–Luc procedure, plain films (Caldwell views) of the maxillary sinus will forever be abnormal with some degree of opacification. In recent times, it has been felt that creating aeration of the maxillary sinus via the natural ostium will allow for healing of the damaged mucosa of chronic sinusitis and reestablishment of the natural drainage system. Theoretically, respiratory epithelium within the sinus will regenerate. There may still, however, be a role for this operation in cases in which maximal medical and "functional" surgery of the sinus has failed to restore healthy mucosa to a sinus. Attempts have been made at obliterating the maxillary sinus with fat and other substances, but these have never been successful. After a well-performed Caldwell–Luc operation, the sinus is to some extent "obliterated" by the natural course of healing. Other indications for a Caldwell–Luc approach include the treatment of oroantral fistulae, the treatment of malignant exophthalmos, as an approach to biopsy the infraorbital nerve in cases of suspected perineural invasion by cancer, as an approach to the orbital floor in the treatment of trauma, as an approach to the pterygomaxillary space for ligation of the internal maxillary artery in the treatment of resistant epistaxis, and as part of a larger operation to treat benign and malignant neoplasms of the lateral nasal wall, pterygomaxillary space and nasopharynx.

The operation is performed by retracting the upper lip superiorly, most effectively with a Johnson-type retractor. The soft tissues overlying the canine fossa are infiltrated with local anesthetic and epinephrine. An incision is made centered on the canine fossa, slightly convex inferiorly and extending from just short of the midline back to the second or third maxillary molar. The incision is kept at least 5 mm above the gingival edge to allow enough tissue for closure. The incision in carried down to bone and then elevated in a subperiosteal plane superiorly to expose the infraorbital foramen and nerve. This elevation is done most expeditiously by beginning with a McKenty or other small periosteal elevator and then pushing on a gauze sponge for further elevation. A 2-mm osteotome is used to create a small opening into the maxillary sinus above the level of the maxillary tooth roots and this is then enlarged with a Kerrison-type rongeur. Most of the enlargement occurs superiorly up

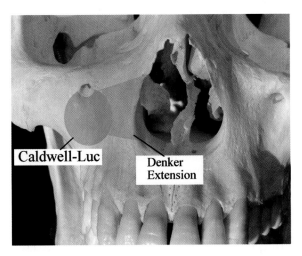

Fig. 22.1. Bone incisions used for the Caldwell–Luc and Denker procedures

to and even around the infraorbital nerve (Fig. 22.1). The offending maxillary sinus mucosa is then completely stripped from the sinus. The roof is saved for last, realizing that the infraorbital nerve is frequently dehiscent within the sinus. Great care is taken to avoid damage to the infraorbital nerve. A variety of small curettes and pituitary-type forceps are used to remove all of the mucosa. Slow, steady traction is better than rapid tearing to remove large portions of the lining mucosa in a single piece.

Since the respiratory mucosa has been removed, the sinus will no longer drain via the natural ostium. A nasoantral window is therefore created via the inferior meatus. A mosquito-type clamp is inserted approximately 1 cm back into the inferior meatus to avoid the opening of the nasolacrimal duct. The clamp is directed toward the lateral canthus and bluntly inserted through the lateral wall of the inferior meatus and spread. A rat-tail rasp, Kerrison forceps or large Blakesley forceps are then used to enlarge the new ostium anteriorly and posteriorly to about 1.5–2.0 cm in diameter. If there is no significant bleeding, no packing is necessary. If bleeding persists, the sinus is packed with 0.5-in. gauze impregnated with antibiotic ointment, brought out via the nasoantral window. The gauze can be used as a file, much like dental floss, to smooth the opening of the new antrostomy by sliding it back and forth through the antrostomy. Finally the sublabial incision is closed with interrupted simple absorbable sutures. If packing is used, it is left for 1 or 2 days and then removed through the nose.

The Denker Procedure

Indications are:

- To gain exposure for removal of lesions of the nasal sidewall or posterior nasal cavity and pterygomaxillary space
- Inverting papilloma
- Juvenile nasopharyngeal angiofibroma

The Denker procedure is just a modification of the Caldwell–Luc operation in which the inferior portion of the ascending portion of the maxilla is removed along the lateral aspect of the pyriform aperture, essentially connecting the inferior meatal nasoantral window with the opening via the canine fossa (Fig. 22.1). In recent times such an approach has been termed a partial facial degloving approach and may be useful as an approach to benign tumors such as juvenile nasopharyngeal angiofibromas or inverting papillomas.

Approach to the Pterygomaxillary Space

Indications are:

- Control branches of the internal maxillary artery in the treatment of refractory epistaxis
- Biopsy lesions of the pterygomaxillary space
- Approach to the foramen rotundum or pterygoid canal
- Vidian neurectomy

A transantral approach to the pterygomaxillary space can be carried out via a Caldwell–Luc approach without stripping of the sinus mucosa. After opening the canine fossa, an operating microscope is used to visualize the posterior wall of the maxillary sinus. A mucosal flap is raised and a small chisel used to crack the posterior wall bone. The bone is picked away with a curette and then the opening enlarged with Kerrison forceps. The posterior periosteum is opened with a cruciate cautery cut and the pterygomaxillary space then explored with a nerve hook or long alligator forceps. Generally, this procedure is used for ligation of the sphenopalatine artery. It can also be used as an approach to the vidian nerve.

Approaches to the Ethmoid and Sphenoid Sinuses

For external ethmoidectomy/sphenoidotomy indications are:

- Chronic ethmoid sinusitis unresponsive to conservative intranasal procedures.
- As an approach to the orbital apex for optic nerve decompression.
- As an approach to the anterior skull base or sphenoid sinus in the treatment of CSF rhinorrhea or other abnormality, such as encephalocele.
- As an approach to the lacrimal sac for dacryocystorhinostomy.
- As an approach to the anterior and posterior ethmoid arteries in the treatment of refractory epistaxis.
- No true ethmoidectomy is necessary, just the exploration of the medial orbital wall.
- For the treatment of acute complicated ethmoid sinusitis.
- Orbital abscess or subperiosteal abscess.

The external ethmoidectomy approach is a classic approach that has been used to address a large variety of conditions, including acute and chronic infection of the ethmoid and sphenoid sinus; as an approach to infections of the orbit; as an approach to the cribriform and fovea ethmoidalis in the treatment of CSF fistulae and defects of the anterior skull base; as an approach to the anterior and posterior ethmoid arteries in the treatment of recalcitrant epistaxis; and as a portion of several larger operations, such as approaches to the nasofrontal drainage system, maxillectomy and craniofacial resection.

Prior to beginning an external ethmoidectomy, the nasal cavity is packed with cottonoid pledgets that have been impregnated with vasoconstrictor. The external ethmoidectomy is performed via a gullwing incision centered midway between the medial canthus and the midline dorsum of the nose (Fig. 22.2). The incision is carried down through skin and orbicularis muscle. The angular vessels are ligated and the periosteum is elevated medially and laterally and retracted with stay sutures that are weighted with small hemostats and laid over gauze sponges covering the eyes. Sequentially, the anterior lacrimal crest, lacrimal fossa and posterior lacrimal crest are identifiers. The medial canthal tendon is released by dissecting the periosteum from the medial orbital wall and retracting the orbital contents laterally with a Sewell retractor. The lacrimal sac is elevated out of the fossa and reflected medially. The lacrimal duct is preserved. If the lacrimal duct is to be sacrificed as for maxillectomy, it is cannulated at the end of the procedure with a double-ended silastic lacrimal stent, one end inserted through each lacrimal punctum.

With use of a Sewell retractor to retract the orbital contents laterally, the dissection extends from superficial to deep along the medial orbital wall and the lamina papyracea. The anterior and posterior ethmoidal arteries are identified and ligated. These serve as a landmark to the level of the floor of the anterior cranial fossa. The pressure head to these arteries is from the ophthalmic artery on the orbital side of the wound. They must not be allowed to retract back into the orbit unligated. A hemaclip is applied to the orbital side, a bipolar cautery used to cauterize the nasal side, and then the vessel is transected medial to the hemaclip. Care is taken to avoid opening the periorbita, which leads to the herniation of orbital fat. The ethmoid sinus is then entered via the lacrimal fossa and this opening is enlarged toward the nasal dorsum with a Kerrison rongeur. The anterior ethmoid cells (agger nasi) are entered with a mastoid curette and the mucosa forming the lateral nasal wall anterior to the middle turbinate is exposed. An incision is made in this mucosa and the nasal pledgets previously placed in the nose are identified and removed. The middle turbinate and nasal septum can now be visualized. Using the lamina papyracea, middle turbinate and ethmoid foraminae as landmarks, one removes the ethmoid cells from anterior to posterior with Blakesley or Takahashi forceps. Approximately the anterior half of the lamina papyracea is resected to allow visualization. Remember that the plane of the fovea ethmoidalis falls inferiorly as one proceeds from anterior to posterior. The orbital contents, cribriform plate and nasal

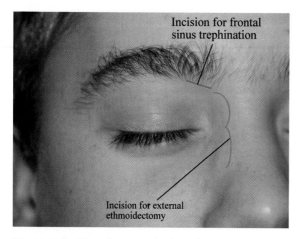

Fig. 22.2. Incisions for external ethmoidectomy and frontal sinus trephination

septum are avoided by direct visualization. If necessary, the sphenoid sinus is entered medially and inferiorly and its front wall removed with Kerrison-type forceps. The middle turbinate is resected at its attachment to the skull base with turbinate scissors and removed. The maxillary sinus can easily be entered and any Haller cells removed. The frontal sinus drainage system is immediately accessible. Onodi cells can be directly visualized along the posterior orbital wall. If an orbital abscess is suspected, the periorbita can be incised and the medial orbital contents explored (Fig. 22.3).

At the conclusion of the procedure, the medial orbital periosteum with its attached medial canthal tendon is reattached to the nasal periosteum.

Approaches to the Frontal Sinus

Trephination

Indications are:

- Acute frontal sinusitis with impending or present complications
- As an adjunct to the endoscopic exploration of the nasofrontal drainage system

Frontal sinus trephination is indicated to drain the acutely infected frontal sinus with impending orbit-

Fig. 22.3. Acute ethmoiditis complicated by orbital abscess treated by external ethmoidectomy

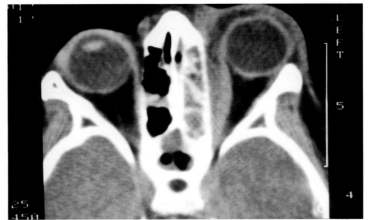

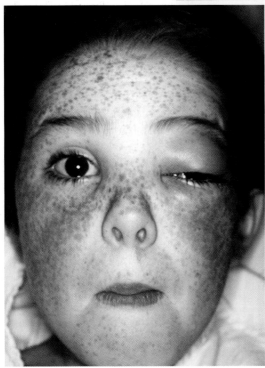

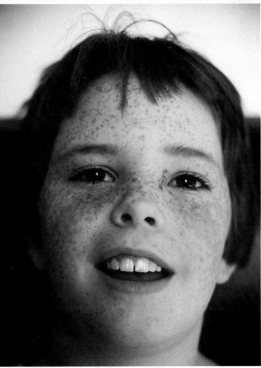

al or intracranial complications and as an adjunct to endoscopic exploration of the nasofrontal drainage system. In the former case, it can be thought of essentially as draining an abscess. In the treatment of acute frontal sinusitis, an incision is made in the superomedial orbit below the medial brow and carried down to the bone of the floor of the frontal sinus in a stabbing manner. The incision need only be about 1 cm in length (Fig. 22.3). Traditionally the trephination is carried out through the horizontal cancellous bone of the roof of the orbit rather than through the vertical diploic bone of the anterior frontal sinus wall to avoid spreading infection to the diploic space. A 2- or 3-mm cutting burr is used to create the trephine and the frontal sinus is then irrigated with saline via an angiocatheter until this flows freely out the nose. An angiocatheter is left in the trephine and irrigated 3 or 4 times a day with saline and/or a dilute vasoconstrictor such as oxymetazoline. The patient is treated with intravenous antibiotics and the catheter is left in place for 3 days. There should be free flow of the irrigant out the nose (Fig. 22.4).

When the trephination is used as an adjunct to endoscopic surgery in the frontal recess, the catheter is irrigated with dilute methylene blue that can be visualized in the nose and used as a guide to the frontal sinus drainage pathway. In this case, the catheter is removed at the end of the operation.

The Lynch Procedure

Indications are:

- Chronic frontal sinusitis unresponsive to conservative intranasal procedures where hope still exists of reconstructing the nasofrontal drainage system

- Acute, complicated frontal sinusitis

The Lynch procedure was used in the treatment of chronic frontal sinusitis in an attempt to reconstruct a large nasofrontal drainage pathway via an external approach. The operation began with an external ethmoidectomy as described in "Approaches to the Ethmoid and Sphenoid Sinuses," but with the upper limb of the incision extending further laterally beneath the brow. There are so many permutations of the "Lynch procedure" that no single method is universally accepted. The original operation involved removal of the entire bony floor of the frontal sinus and stripping of all mucosa along with a complete ethmoidectomy and removal of the middle turbinate. Removal of the frontal sinus mucosa was difficult because of the limited exposure high and lateral. Eventually, many surgeons stopped trying to remove the mucosa and simply attempted to reconstruct the drainage system. The lateral nasal wall mucosal flap was fashioned with a superior base and turned up at the conclusion of the operation to reline the nasofrontal drainage system medially. The reconstructed frontal drainage was stented for about 3 months with an endless variety of materials. The most popular were rolled silastic sheeting and cut portions of endotracheal tubes that were sewn to the nasal septum. The major complication of this procedure was restenosis of the nasofrontal drainage duct and subsequent mucocele formation or recurrent frontal sinus obstruction and infection.

The Lothrop Procedure

Indications are chronic frontal sinusitis unresponsive to conservative intranasal procedures where hope still exists of reconstructing the nasofrontal drainage system.

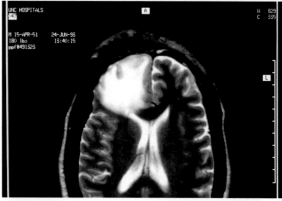
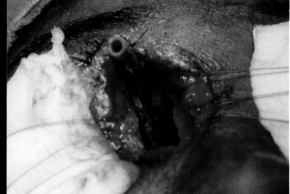

Fig. 22.4. A frontal sinus trephination and lynch procedure for acute frontal and ethmoid sinusitis complicated by cerebritis and brain abscess

The Lothrop procedure is performed via a unilateral or bilateral anterior ethmoidectomy and middle turbinectomy. The frontal intersinus septum is resected along with the most anterosuperior portion of the nasal septum, creating a large drainage pathway. In cases of unilateral disease, the opposite nasofrontal drainage system could theoretically serve as a pathway for egress of frontal sinus secretions. Like its endoscopic counterpart, it works best in frontal sinuses with wide anteroposterior dimensions.

Osteoplastic Frontal Sinus Obliteration

Indications are:

- Chronic frontal sinusitis unresponsive to conservative intranasal procedures.
- As a portion of a craniofacial resection.
- As treatment for fractures of the frontal sinus involving the posterior table or with significant damage to the nasoethmoid drainage system.

Contraindications are acute frontal sinusitis. This may lead to infection of the bone flap.

The osteoplastic frontal sinus obliteration procedure remains an important part of the sinus surgeon's armamentarium. Although it can be carried out unilaterally, it is generally performed bilaterally (Fig. 22.5). The keys to success are *complete* removal of *all* frontal sinus mucosa and burring of the inner table of bone of the sinus cavity. Generally the sinus is

obliterated with abdominal fat harvested from the left lower quadrant of the abdomen so as not to be confused in the future with an appendectomy incision. Montgomery [1] has shown in cats, and personal experience corroborates, that fat can survive long term within the sinus cavity.

Preoperatively, the patient has a Caldwell-view X-ray taken from 6-ft away and the frontal sinus is cut out of the film to be used as a template during surgery. Alternatively, one can use intraoperative CT guidance or transillumination to delineate the borders of the frontal sinus. A coronal flap is elevated in a plane *superficial* to the periosteum, down to the supraorbital rim. The supratrochlear and supraorbital nerves are spared and may be released from foramina as needed. With utilization of the template, or other method, the sinus is outlined and an oscillating or sagittal saw used to cut the frontal bone slightly inside the limits shown by the template. There is no need to follow the exact lateral contours of the sinus. The saw blade should be greatly beveled in toward the central sinus. At the supraorbital rims, the very thick bone must be completely transected; a horizontal bone incision is made at the nasal root. A fine osteotome is inserted through the superior bony kerf and used to divide the interfrontal sinus septum. The osteoplastic flap with vascularized periosteum adherent to its anterior wall is then fractured inferiorly through the roofs of the orbits. Next, all mucosa is painstakingly removed from the frontal sinus, and the lining cortical bone is drilled with a cutting burr. Small 1–2-mm burrs can be helpful in removing mucosa from small extensions of the sinus. The intersinus septum is completely drilled away. This dissection extends down into the nasofrontal drainage system.

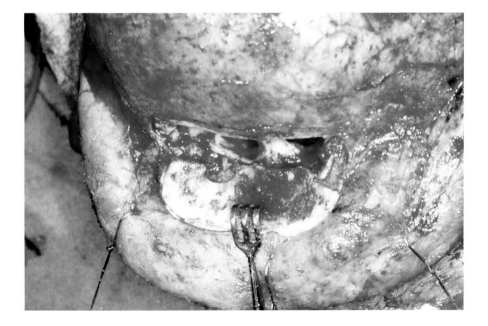

Fig. 22.5. Osteoplastic frontal sinus operation

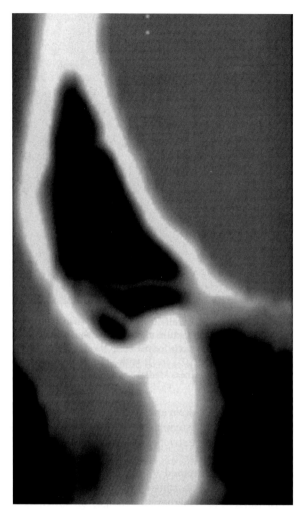

Fig. 24.5. Sagittal CT scan demonstrating narrow anterior–posterior dimensions of the frontal sinus. (Reprinted from [8], with permission from Elsevier)

Operative Technique

All surgical procedures are performed under general anesthesia. The patient is positioned, prepped, and draped as for routine endoscopic sinus surgery. Although this technique was first utilized without computer-aided technique, it is now typically performed using image guidance. This helps confirm critical anatomic landmarks throughout a technically demanding procedure. At the outset of the procedure, oxymetazoline on pledgets is instilled in each nasal cavity to achieve maximal vasoconstriction. Injections with 1% lidocaine with 1:200,000 epinephrine are performed bilaterally on the septum, lateral nasal wall (agger nasi region), and middle turbinate remnant. A bilateral greater palatine foramen block is also performed with the same agent. Adjacent paranasal sinus disease, if present, is addressed prior to performing the TSFS, as superiorly created bleeding with TSFS

can result in significant difficulty in performing the remaining procedures.

The septum may be endoscopically mobilized to one side for surgical access; this facilitates improved visualization and instrumentation in cases of a narrow nasal vault. The technique for endoscopic septoplasty has been previously described [6]. A hemitransfixion incision is created with an ophthalmic crescent knife (Alcon Labs, Ft. Worth, TX, USA) at the mucocutaneous junction on the appropriate side of the septum. After adequate subperichondral dissection, the quadrilateral cartilage is separated at the bony-cartilaginous junction and the anterior septum is mobilized from the maxillary crest. Resection of any deviated portions of septal cartilage and bone further improves surgical exposure. A high septal perforation is then created.

Regardless of whether or not septal mobilization is required, a 1.5–2-cm endoscopic partial septectomy including bone and mucosa is performed. This leads to a permanent superior septal perforation that is created just across from the leading edge of the middle turbinate/agger nasi region below the skull base. This permits further exposure, ventilation, future endoscopic inspection, and sinus debridement through the nasal cavity postoperatively. The incisions for the perforation are created utilizing an ophthalmic crescent knife. Through-cutting endoscopic forceps or a soft-tissue shaver help complete the perforation.

The floor of the frontal sinus is identified intraoperatively by surgical navigation or, alternatively, by using anatomic landmarks that are helpful in gauging the position of the frontal sinus relative to the cribriform plate.

Tips and Pearls

■ The midline position of floor of the frontal sinus is typically located posterior–superior to the most anterior–superior aspects of the septal bony-cartilaginous junction.

This location is approximated adjacent to the most anterior remnant or root of the middle turbinate and the agger nasi region. This is considerably more anterior than the position of the naturally occurring frontal recess area. In patients with a Y-shaped septum at the floor of the frontal sinus, the midline floor of the frontal sinus has an appearance similar to that of the anterior wall of the sphenoid sinus that has been described during transsphenoidal surgery. It appears as the "prow of a ship," albeit in a much narrower region.

After careful inspection of the roof of the nasal vault, the frontal sinus is entered. The evolution of surgical instrumentation has permitted the use of angled drills with concurrent suction/irrigation to minimize heat-related damage to bone and surrounding soft tissues. Straight drills may also be used without concurrent suction irrigation; in these cases, irrigation can be applied through a 5-Fr ureteral catheter positioned into the operative field through the contralateral nares. Alternatively, depending upon the thickness of the floor of the sinus, curetting may be sufficient to enter the frontal sinus and resection of the floor may be performed using through-cutting punches [3].

After successful entry into the frontal sinus lumen, the opening can be enlarged further by drilling anteriorly and laterally, if clinically indicated. Depending on the extent of the disease, dissection can be carried laterally to include the frontal recess.

Tips and Pearls

■ Note that the frontal recess is located posteriorly relative to the midline frontal sinus floor and, thus, drilling directly across from one frontal recess to the other should be avoided.

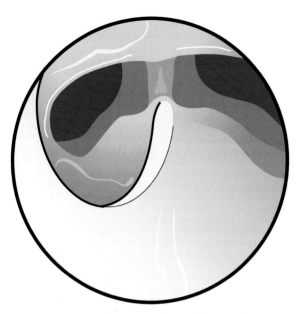

Fig. 24.6. C-shaped "neoostium" surgically created via TSFS. (Reprinted from Fig. 27.4b in [1] with kind permission from Springer Science+Business Media)

This straight path of drilling will traverse the olfactory fossa and anterior cranial vault and place the patient at risk for iatrogenic CSF leak or even intracranial injury. Meticulous preservation of the mucosa within the frontal sinus/recess is imperative throughout the procedure. The reduction of mucosal injury minimizes bone exposure and reduces risk of delayed frontal stenosis. The inferior aspect of the intersinus septum may be resected to create a "neoostium" and to provide a common outlet for both right and left frontal sinuses at the midline (Fig. 24.6).

If septal dislocation is required at the beginning of the procedure, this is now corrected. The hemitransfixion incision is closed with interrupted 4-0 chromic sutures. The septal flaps are reapproximated with a running transseptal mattress type closure with 4-0 plain gut suture on a Keith needle. Packing is not typically required in these cases.

Postoperative Care

All extended frontal sinus approaches require commitment to postoperative care. Meticulous debridement of fibrin and clots is initiated 1 week after surgery and continues on a weekly to biweekly basis until all healing is complete. Culture-directed antibiotics and systemic steroids, if clinically indicated, and aggressive saline irrigations are continued during the healing process. Figure 24.7 demonstrates the healed endoscopic appearance of the "neoostium" at 1 year after TSFS.

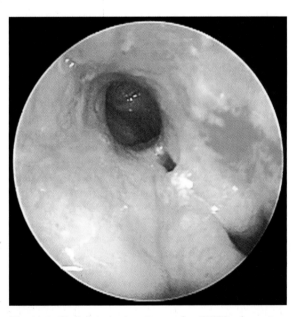

Fig. 24.7. Healed neoostium 1 year after TSFS in the patient with frontal sinus mucocele presented in Figs. 24.1 and 24.2

Advantages and Disadvantages

Advantages are:

■ Functional approach with restoration of frontal sinus drainage
■ Permits mucosal preservation of the frontal recess

24

- Uses inherent anatomic landmarks to facilitate surgery
- Allows for endoscopic and radiographic surveillance postoperatively
- Improved cosmesis through avoidance of facial incisions
- Decreased morbidity compared to open frontal sinus approaches
- May resort to open approaches if required

Disadvantages are:

- Requirement of endoscopic expertise and specialized surgical instrumentation
- Risk of inadvertent CSF leak and skull base injury greater than with routine frontal sinus surgery
- Possible bone loss at radix
- Drill-related heat injury to sinonasal tissues
- Controlled septal perforation with potential for chronic crusting

Clinical Outcomes

The initial results on TSFS were reported by McLaughlin et al. [9]. Twenty patients were presented with endoscopic examination and a telephone questionnaire with a mean follow-up of 12 and 16 months, respectively. The primary indication of surgery was frontal recess stenosis after previously failed endoscopic frontal sinusotomy. Endoscopic patency was reported in all 20 patients, with a diameter of 3-mm confirmed by passage of a curved suction in 19 of 20 (95%) patients. Of the patients evaluated by the telephone questionnaire, 17 of 19 patients (89.5%) reported symptom improvement and 12 of 18 patients (67%) reported reduction in medication requirements [9].

In an updated series Lanza et al. [8] reported on 29 patients undergoing TSFS between 1995 and 1999. The main indication for TSFS was chronic frontal sinusitis in the setting of previously failed endoscopic surgery; other indications included mucocele formation and nasofacial trauma. Twenty-four patients (83%) were available for telephone interview postoperatively with a mean follow-up period of 45 months (range 9–69 months). In this subset of patients, 18 of 24 (75%) reported at least 50% improvement of symptoms, while 14 of 24 (58%) reported 80% or greater improvement of their symptoms. Four (16.6%) patients underwent further frontal sinus surgery, with three having frontal sinus obliteration [8]. Complications included CSF leaks (two cases), unplanned anterior inferior septal perforation (one case), and chronic crusting at the planned perforation (one case). One

leak was attributable to surgical trauma with a drill in a patient with narrow anterior–posterior dimensions, and the second occurred during debridement of scarred mucosa within the frontal sinus in a patient with history of severe maxillofacial trauma. Both CSF leaks were identified and repaired intraoperatively without further sequelae. Both patients with septal difficulties had undergone prior septoplasty.

Conclusions

TSFS represents an additional endoscopic advance in the surgical paradigm for management of chronic frontal sinus disease, especially in the setting of osteoneogenesis. The technique utilizes the unique relationship of the frontal sinus floor to the nasal septum. It permits entry into the thin medial frontal sinus floor, which is clearly advantageous in cases with extensive osteoneogenesis that preclude identification and cannulation of the frontal recess. TSFS is a functional approach that offers several potential advantages over frontal sinus obliteration, including decreased morbidity, improved cosmesis, and ease of radiographic and endoscopic surveillance of the frontal sinus postoperatively.

References

1. Batra PS, Lanza DC (2005) Endoscopic trans-septal frontal sinusotomy. In: Kountakis S, et al (eds) The Frontal Sinus. Springer, New York
2. Draf W (1991) Endonasal micro-endoscopic frontal sinus surgery: the Fulda concept. Op Tech Otolaryngol Head Neck Surg 2:234–40.
3. Dubin MG, Kuhn FA (2005) Endoscopic modified Lothrop (Draf III) with frontal sinus punches. Laryngoscope 115:1702–3.
4. Gross W, Gross C, Becker D, et al (1995) Modified transnasal endoscopic Lothrop procedure as alternative to frontal sinus obliteration. Otolaryngol Head Neck Surg 113:427–34.
5. Hardy JM, Montgomery WM (1976) Osteoplastic frontal sinusitis: an analysis of 250 operations. Ann Otol Rhinol Laryngol 85:523–32.
6. Hwang PH, McLaughlin RB, Lanza DC, et al (1999) Endoscopic septoplasty: indications, technique, and complications. Otolaryngol Head Neck Surg 120:678–82.
7. Kennedy DW (1985) Functional endoscopic sinus surgery: technique. Arch Otolaryngol 111:643–9.
8. Lanza DC, McLaughlin RB, Hwang PH (2001) The five year experience with endoscopic trans-septal frontal sinusotomy. Otolaryngol Clin North Am 34:139–52.

9. McLaughlin RB, Hwang PH, Lanza DC (1999) Endoscopic trans-septal frontal sinusotomy: The rationale and results of an alternative technique. Am J Rhinol 13:279–87.

10. Stammberger H (1986) Endoscopic endonasal surgery – concepts in treatment of recurring rhinosinusitis. Part II. Surgical technique. Otolaryngol Head Neck Surg 94:147–56.

11. Swanson PB, Lanza DC, Vining EM, et al (1995) The effect of middle turbinate resection upon the frontal sinus. Am J Rhinol 9:191–7.

12. Weber R, Draf W, Keerl R, et al (2000) Osteoplastic frontal sinus surgery with fat obliteration: technique and long-term results using magnetic resonance imaging in 82 operations. Laryngoscope 110:1037–44.

27

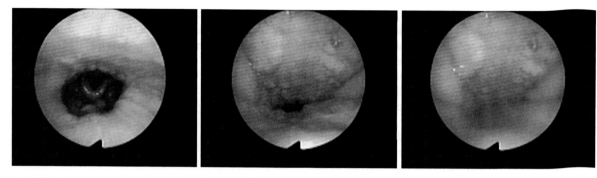

Fig. 27.3. Progressive collapse at the velopharyngeal level during a Müller maneuver

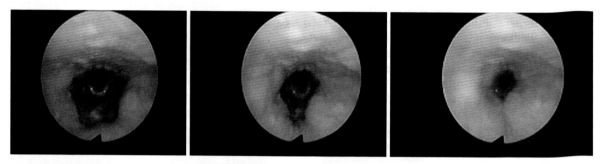

Fig. 27.4. Progressive collapse at the oropharyngeal level during a Müller maneuver

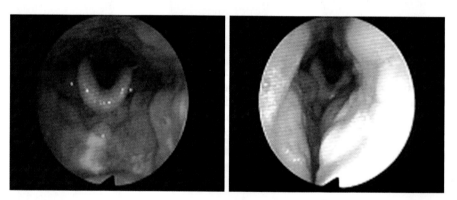

Fig. 27.5. Progressive collapse at the retroglossal level during a Müller maneuver

In addition to inspection, flexible fiberoptic nasopharyngoscopy can be performed. A thorough examination of the nose, nasopharynx, oropharynx, hypopharynx and larynx can reveal different causes of airway obstruction. This technique provides the possibility to assess the oropharynx in a more physiological state, i.e., without active opening of the mouth. In addition to this, fiberoptic evaluation can provide dynamic information. The observer can evaluate which soft tissues are involved in snoring when the patient produces snoring sounds. An idea about the collapsibility of the pharyngeal structures and the site of collapse can be offered by a Müller maneuver (Figs. 27.3–27.5). While the physician is inspecting the pharynx, the patient is asked to make an inspiratory effort against a closed nose and mouth. The degree of collapse is noted at the velopharyngeal and retroglossal levels (as a percentage from the baseline). Several considerations have to be taken into account concerning this technique:

- The degree of collapse is only a subjective estimation of the examiner.
- The negative pressure generated is variable and is highly dependent on the effort generated by the patient.
- Since the maneuver is performed during wakefulness, the changes in pressure and shape do not necessarily mimic the physiological changes that occur while breathing during sleep.

Nevertheless, the degree of collapse of the velopharynx during a Müller maneuver is highly correlated with the severity of OSA, whereas the collapse of the lateral walls during a Müller maneuver is only moderately correlated [38]. In addition to this, the Müller maneuver has a predictive value in determining the outcome of velopharyngeal surgery. Collapse in the retroglossal regions is correlated with a low success rate of velopharyngeal surgery [2,19]. After multilevel pharyngeal surgery, the change in velopharyngeal collapse during a Müller maneuver was significantly correlated with the change in AHI [38].

Considering the static and the dynamic data, it is important to realize that no single finding alone is pathognomonic for snoring and OSA. On the other hand, even when the velopharynx appears normal, the diagnosis cannot be excluded.

Cephalometric Evaluation

Cephalometry is based on a standardized lateral radiograph of the head and neck on which several landmarks are identified. The distance between these landmarks and the angles between the lines connecting the landmarks are measured (Figs. 27.6, 27.7).

Originally, this technique was used to assess bony abnormalities in the craniofacial skeletal structure and to a lesser extent to evaluate upper-airway soft-tissue anatomy. In 1983, Riley et al. [26] described specific landmarks, which included soft-tissue contours, for the use of cephalometry in evaluation of OSA patients.

Concerning the velopharynx, a lot of attention has been given to the length of the soft palate, i.e., the length of the line constructed from the posterior nasal spine to the tip of the soft palate contour. A mean of 37 mm in a group of normal subjects was calculated by Riley et al. [26]. Several studies described a longer soft palate in OSA patients (AHI>10) [3, 4, 20, 22, 26, 37] and in snorers (AHI≤10) [22] compared with controls. When OSA patients and snorers are compared, the soft palate is longer in OSA patients [22, 39]. The soft palate is also thicker and has an increased area in OSA patients than in controls [20, 37]. Battagel and L'Estrange [5] had slightly different results: in this study the soft palate was not longer but did have an increased area in OSA patients versus controls. Battagel and L'Estrange also calculated a four-variable model, including soft palate area and the width of the pharynx where the soft palate was at its thickest. This model, with two velopharyngeal parameters, provided a 100% discrimination between OSA and control groups [5]. The cephalopmetric evaluation of the velopharynx is not only limited to the description of the soft palate. Several studies documented a re-

duced airway space at the level of the velopharynx [5, 20, 35, 37].

A disadvantage of this technique is the fact that one is limited to the assessment of static measure-

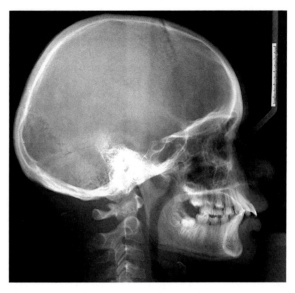

Fig. 27.6. An example of a cephalogram

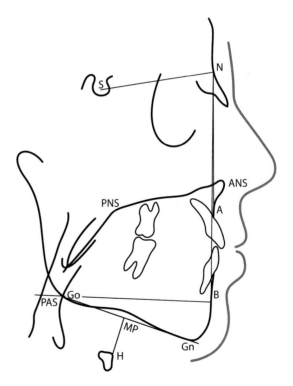

Fig. 27.7. Cephalogram with indication of different landmarks according to Riley et al. [26]. *S* sella, *N* nasion, *ANS* anterior nasal spine, *PNS* posterior nasal spine, *A* subspinale, *Pg* pogonion, *B* supramentale, *Gn* gnathion, *Go* gonion, *MP* mandibular plane, *H* hyoid, *PAS* posterior airway space. (From [26] with permission)

ments, so dynamic information, which may be of clinical significance, cannot be obtained. Another disadvantage of this technique is that subjects have to be dentated.

CT and MRI

Another way to investigate the upper airway is CT and MRI. Compared with CT, MRI has an improved soft-tissue contrast and the ability to create multiplanar imaging. In addition to this, on magnetic resonance images there are no dental amalgam artifacts and beam-hardening artifacts from the dense mandible as is the case with CT images. Specific metals do produce artifacts on magnetic resonance images; however, this image distortion is limited to the immediate area of the offending material and does not produce the global image disruption that occurs on CT scans.

Several CT and MRI studies have detected a smaller upper airway in OSA patients [6, 12, 14, 30–32]. In addition to this, the upper airway of the OSA patient has a different geometric configuration as opposed to that of controls. This finding was first described by Rodenstein et al. [27]. In normal subjects, the cross-sectional airway has an elliptic shape with the major axis in the laterolateral dimension. However, in OSA patients and snorers the cross section of the upper airway is circular or elliptic, with the major axis in the anteroposterior dimension. This difference in shape is due to a reduction of the laterolateral diameter [27] (lateral narrowing) (Figs. 27.8, 27.9). Schwab et al. [31] confirmed these findings and found the lateral narrowing to be the result of thickening of the lateral walls.

When interpreting these MRI data, one must take into account the relatively long scanning time. As a consequence, magnetic resonance images are means of multiple respiratory cycles. These mean values might not be representative of the actual situation since OSA and snoring are dynamic processes. Recently ultrafast MRI has become available to give some information of the dynamic aspects. Using this technique, Ciscar et al. [7] found the velopharyngeal airway to be smaller in OSA patients than in controls only during part of the respiratory cycle! In this study, measurements were not only obtained during wakefulness, but also during sleep. During sleep the differences between OSA patients and controls in velopharyngeal airway area intensified. Dynamic measurements showed that in OSA patients the variations of the velopharyngeal airway during the respiratory cycle are larger than in controls. These variations were also accentuated during sleep [7].

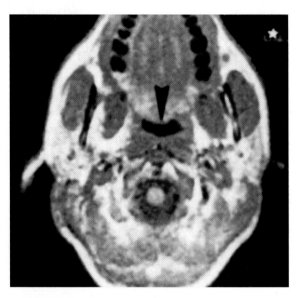

Fig. 27.8. Magnetic resonance image of the pharynx in a normal subject. (From [27] with permission)

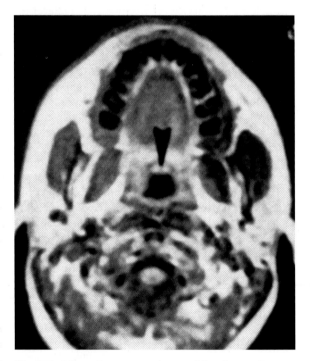

Fig. 27.9. Magnetic resonance image of the pharynx in a patient with simple snoring. (From [27] with permission)

Discussion

The most relevant abnormalities of the velopharynx in the snorer and the OSA patient are a long soft palate and uvula, and narrowing of the cross-sectional area.

The importance of the velopharyngeal structures in the pathogenesis of snoring and OSA has already been established; hence the assessment of these velopharyngeal structures in the patient with snoring (and possibly OSA) plays a pivotal role in determining possible surgical treatment modalities. This is illustrated by the significantly higher success rate of velopharyngeal surgery, such as uvulopalatopharyngoplasty, as a treatment for OSA in patients with type I narrowing or collapse (only at the velopharyngeal level) [34]. Unfortunately there is no standard way to describe the clinical features associated with snoring and OSA. Moreover, there are no clear descriptions of the normal velopharyngeal anatomy to our knowledge. Consequently the clinical examination should be performed by a physician with experience in the assessment of patients with sleep-disordered breathing. Even so, clinical evaluation remains based on subjective measurements of the observer, so one has to take into account the interobserver variability. Concerning the Mallampati technique (in predicting difficult intubation) for example, a poor interobserver reliability has been documented [18]. Nevertheless, clinical evaluation remains a vital keystone in the overall assessment.

Cephalometry and CT and MRI are also very helpful in screening for velopharyngeal abnormalities and the site of pharyngeal collapse. According to Sher et al. [34], the methods most clinically useful in determining the site of collapse are fiberoptic endoscopy (with or without a Müller maneuver) and cephalometry.

Several considerations have to be made concerning the everyday assessment of the patient with snoring and OSA. One must realize that the findings obtained during wakefulness might not be applicable during sleep! The site of collapse cannot always be predicted using awake measurements [16], partly because the additional effect of muscle relaxation during sleep [24, 28] can result in an increased collapsibility. Variations in airway narrowing are greater in the sleeping versus the awake patient [7]. For this reason, sleep nasendoscopy can be performed in order to decide if a certain patient is a candidate for velopharyngeal surgery. Before, this technique was only used in research settings, but now it is becoming more and more a routine examination in the assessment of the snoring patient.

One must also not forget the effect of posture and head position on pharyngeal narrowing. Cross-sectional area decreases when lying down [17, 23], and hyperextension of the neck increases the pharyngeal dimension [31].

Finally, the physiological function of the velopharynx in deglutition and speech may not be underestimated and must be respected when surgical alterations are made for treating snoring and OSA.

References

1. Practice parameters for the treatment of obstructive sleep apnea in adults: the efficacy of surgical modifications of the upper airway. Report of the American Sleep Disorders Association. Sleep 1996;19:152–155.
2. Aboussouan LS, Golish JA, Wood BG, Mehta AC, Wood DE, Dinner DS: Dynamic pharyngoscopy in predicting outcome of uvulopalatopharyngoplasty for moderate and severe obstructive sleep apnea. Chest 1995;107:946–951.
3. Bacon W, Berreur C, Krieger J, Hildwein M, Stierle JL: Pharyngeal obstruction and the functional adaptation of the natural posture of the head and the hyoid bone in sleep apnea syndrome. Orthod Fr 1992;63 Pt 2:595–602.
4. Bacon WH, Turlot JC, Krieger J, Stierle JL: Cephalometric evaluation of pharyngeal obstructive factors in patients with sleep apnea syndrome. Angle Orthod 1990;60:115–122.
5. Battagel JM, L'Estrange PR: The cephalometric morphology of patients with obstructive sleep apnoea (OSA). Eur J Orthod 1996;18:557–569.
6. Bohlman ME, Haponik EF, Smith PL, Allen RP, Bleecker ER, Goldman SM: CT demonstration of pharyngeal narrowing in adult obstructive sleep apnea. AJR Am J Roentgenol 1983;140:543–548.
7. Ciscar MA, Juan G, Martinez V, Ramon M, Lloret T, Minguez J, Armengot M, Marin J, Basterra J: Magnetic resonance imaging of the pharynx in OSA patients and healthy subjects. Eur Respir J 2001;17:79–86.
8. Croft CB, Brockbank MJ, Wright A, Swanston AR: Obstructive sleep apnoea in children undergoing routine tonsillectomy and adenoidectomy. Clin Otolaryngol Allied Sci 1990;15:307–314.
9. Croft CB, Pringle M: Sleep nasendoscopy: a technique of assessment in snoring and obstructive sleep apnoea. Clin Otolaryngol 1991;16:504–509.
10. Friedman M, Tanyeri H, La Rosa M, Landsberg R, Vaidyanathan K, Pieri S, Caldarelli D: Clinical predictors of obstructive sleep apnea. Laryngoscope 1999;109:1901–1907.
11. Goldberg AN, Schwab RJ: Identifying the patient with sleep apnea: upper airway assessment and physical examination. Otolaryngol Clin North Am 1998;31:919–930.
12. Haponik EF, Smith PL, Bohlman ME, Allen RP, Goldman SM, Bleecker ER: Computerized tomography in obstructive sleep apnea. Correlation of airway size with physiology during sleep and wakefulness. Am Rev Respir Dis 1983;127:221–226.
13. Hiremath AS, Hillman DR, James AL, Noffsinger WJ, Platt PR, Singer SL: Relationship between difficult tracheal intubation and obstructive sleep apnoea. Br J Anaesth 1998;80:606–611.
14. Horner RL, Shea SA, McIvor J, Guz A: Pharyngeal size and shape during wakefulness and sleep in patients with obstructive sleep apnoea. Q J Med 1989;72:719–735.
15. Houghton DJ, Camilleri AE, Stone P: Adult obstructive sleep apnoea syndrome and tonsillectomy. J Laryngol Otol 1997;111:829–832.
16. Hudgel DW: Variable site of airway narrowing among obstructive sleep apnea patients. J Appl Physiol 1986;61:1403–1409.
17. Jan MA, Marshall I, Douglas NJ: Effect of posture on upper airway dimensions in normal human. Am J Respir Crit Care Med 1994;149:145–148.

27

18. Karkouti K, Rose DK, Ferris LE, Wigglesworth DF, Meisami-Fard T, Lee H: Inter-observer reliability of ten tests used for predicting difficult tracheal intubation. Can J Anaesth 1996;43:554–559.

19. Katsantonis GP, Maas CS, Walsh JK: The predictive efficacy of the Muller maneuver in uvulopalatopharyngoplasty. Laryngoscope 1989;99:677–680.

20. Lyberg T, Krogstad O, Djupesland G: Cephalometric analysis in patients with obstructive sleep apnoea syndrome: II. Soft tissue morphology. J Laryngol Otol 1989;103:293–297.

21. Mallampati SR, Gatt SP, Gugino LD, Desai SP, Waraksa B, Freiberger D, Liu PL: A clinical sign to predict difficult tracheal intubation: a prospective study. Can Anaesth Soc J 1985;32:429–434.

22. Maltais F, Carrier G, Cormier Y, Series F: Cephalometric measurements in snorers, non-snorers, and patients with sleep apnoea. Thorax 1991;46:419–423.

23. Martin SE, Mathur R, Marshall I, Douglas NJ: The effect of age, sex, obesity and posture on upper airway size. Eur Respir J 1997;10:2087–2090.

24. Orem J, Lydic R: Upper airway function during sleep and wakefulness: experimental studies on normal and anesthetized cats. Sleep 1978;1:49–68.

25. Potsic WP, Wetmore RF: Sleep disorders and airway obstruction in children. Otolaryngol Clin North Am 1990;23:651–663.

26. Riley R, Guilleminault C, Herran J, Powell N: Cephalometric analyses and flow-volume loops in obstructive sleep apnea patients. Sleep 1983;6:303–311.

27. Rodenstein DO, Dooms G, Thomas Y, Liistro G, Stanescu DC, Culee C, Aubert-Tulkens G: Pharyngeal shape and dimensions in healthy subjects, snorers, and patients with obstructive sleep apnoea. Thorax 1990;45:722–727.

28. Sauerland EK, Harper RM: The human tongue during sleep: electromyographic activity of the genioglossus muscle. Exp Neurol 1976;51:160–170.

29. Schellenberg JB, Maislin G, Schwab RJ: Physical findings and the risk for obstructive sleep apnea. The importance of oropharyngeal structures. Am J Respir Crit Care Med 2000;162:740–748.

30. Schwab RJ, Gefter WB, Hoffman EA, Gupta KB, Pack AI: Dynamic upper airway imaging during awake respiration in normal subjects and patients with sleep disordered breathing. Am Rev Respir Dis 1993;148:1385–1400.

31. Schwab RJ, Gupta KB, Gefter WB, Metzger LJ, Hoffman EA, Pack AI: Upper airway and soft tissue anatomy in normal subjects and patients with sleep-disordered breathing. Significance of the lateral pharyngeal walls. Am J Respir Crit Care Med 1995;152:1673–1689.

32. Shellock FG, Schatz CJ, Julien P, Steinberg F, Foo TK, Hopp ML, Westbrook PR: Occlusion and narrowing of the pharyngeal airway in obstructive sleep apnea: evaluation by ultrafast spoiled GRASS MR imaging. AJR Am J Roentgenol 1992;158:1019–1024.

33. Shepard JW, Jr., Gefter WB, Guilleminault C, Hoffman EA, Hoffstein V, Hudgel DW, Suratt PM, White DP: Evaluation of the upper airway in patients with obstructive sleep apnea. Sleep 1991;14:361–371.

34. Sher AE, Schechtman KB, Piccirillo JF: The efficacy of surgical modifications of the upper airway in adults with obstructive sleep apnea syndrome. Sleep 1996;19:156–177.

35. Solow B, Skov S, Ovesen J, Norup PW, Wildschiodtz G: Airway dimensions and head posture in obstructive sleep apnea. Eur J Orthod 1996;18:571–579.

36. Stauffer JL, Buick MK, Bixler EO, Sharkey FE, Abt AB, Manders EK, Kales A, Cadieux RJ, Barry JD, Zwillich CW: Morphology of the uvula in obstructive sleep apnea. Am Rev Respir Dis 1989;140:724–728.

37. Tangugsorn V, Skatvedt O, Krogstad O, Lyberg T: Obstructive sleep apnoea: a cephalometric study. Part II. Uvuloglossopharyngeal morphology. Eur J Orthod 1995;17:57–67.

38. Yao M, Utley DS, Terris DJ: Cephalometric parameters after multilevel pharyngeal surgery for patients with obstructive sleep apnea. Laryngoscope 1998;108:789–795.

39. Zucconi M, Ferini-Strambi L, Palazzi S, Orena C, Zonta S, Smirne S: Habitual snoring with and without obstructive sleep apnoea: the importance of cephalometric variables. Thorax 1992;47:157–161.

40. Zucconi M, Strambi LF, Pestalozza G, Tessitore E, Smirne S: Habitual snoring and obstructive sleep apnea syndrome in children: effects of early tonsil surgery. Int J Pediatr Otorhinolaryngol 1993;26:235–243.

Chapter 28

Risks of General Anesthesia in People with Obstructive Sleep Apnea

28

Cindy den Herder, Joachim Schmeck, Nico de Vries

Core Messages

- Obstructive sleep apnea (OSA) is a significant health problem. The cardinal symptoms of OSA are heavy habitual snoring, witnessed intermittent apneas, and excessive daytime sleepiness.

- Patients with OSA are at high risk of developing postoperative complications when undergoing surgery under general anesthesia. This holds true for surgery to cure OSA and for any other surgery.

- Surgeons of all specialties, and especially anesthetists, should be aware that undiagnosed OSA is common. They should be alert to patients who are at risk of having OSA and be aware of the potential preoperative and postoperative complications in such patients.

- Surgeons and anesthetists should cooperate in developing a protocol whereby patients in whom the possibility of OSA is suspected on clinical grounds are evaluated long enough before the day of surgery to allow preparation of a perioperative management plan.

- Management options include alternative methods of pain relief, use of nasal continuous airway pressure before and after surgery, and postoperative airway surveillance, especially after nasal and upper-airway surgery.

- An algorithm for management of difficult airways should be established preoperatively

Contents

Tips and Pearls

1. Consider the possibility of OSA in patients with the following signs and symptoms:
   (a) Snoring and witnessed apneas
   (b) Excessive daytime sleepiness
   (c) Hypertension
   (d) A large neck circumference (more than 43 cm)
   (e) Maxillary hypoplasia
   (f) Retrognathia (receding chin)
   (g) Body mass index above 30
2. If you suspect a patient has OSA, you should refer him/her to a specialist in the management of this disorder (this may be a respiratory physician, an ENT surgeon, or a sleep physician, depending on local expertise). You should postpone any elective general anesthesia until the patient has seen a specialist. Consider local anesthesia if this is feasible.
3. Avoid giving sedative premedication to patients with OSA. You should also avoid using opioids and benzodiazepines perioperatively in these patients.

4. Tell patients using continuous positive airway pressure at home to bring the apparatus to the hospital with them and to use it frequently preoperatively. The system must be available for immediate use postoperatively.
5. High-dependency nursing is advisable for patients with severe OSA or for patients in whom the disease was suspected perioperatively.

28

Sleep and the Upper Airway

Sleep is an integral part of human existence and is now, more than ever, the subject of clinical and research interest. Why do we spend approximately one third of our lives asleep? Sleep probably has a recovery function, especially for the brain. Theories of nonrapid eye movement sleep suggest a role in energy conservation and in nervous system recuperation. Rapid eye movement sleep may have a role in localized recuperative processes and emotional regulation. Especially during this state the body is at its most relaxed state, owing to loss of skeletal muscle tone, and the upper airway may collapse in a three-dimensional way when preexistent slackening and narrowing of the upper airway is present owing to excess fatty tissue [12, 32]. Two important consequences will arise when airflow accelerates through the narrowed upper airway: vibration due to turbulent flow patterns and a tendency to collapse completely (apnea: complete cessation of oronasal airflow in a minimum of 10 s) or partially (hypopneas: 50% reduction in oronasal airflow accompanied by a decrease of more than 4% in ongoing PaO_2) as a result of the Bernoulli effect [34]. This in turn causes repetitive arousal from sleep to restore airway patency. The prevalence of obstructive sleep apnea (OSA) in middle age is 2% for women and 4% for men [39]. In practice, OSA seems to be underreported; OSA is undiagnosed in an estimated 80% of patients [38]. Patients with OSA are particularly vulnerable during anesthesia and sedation [7, 21]. This is not only the case for operations or other invasive interventions aiming at alleviation of OSA through reduction of the obstructive upper airway; even after surgery not related to OSA, such as hip and knee operations, patients with OSA are at risk of developing respiratory and cardiopulmonary complications postoperatively. Serious complications include reintubations and cardiac events [13]. Anesthetic management must focus on and address the likelihood of morphological alterations of the upper airway leading to an increased rate of difficulties in securing and maintaining a patent airway [8].

Preoperative Aspects

Anesthetists are the key figures in the early recognition of undiagnosed OSA, because of their role in preoperative screening. Heavy and persistent snoring, sudden awakenings accompanied by choking, apneas as observed by the bed partner [8], and excessive sleepiness during daytime [30] are characteristic symptoms of OSA. OSA can also be associated with a wide variety of other symptoms (Table 28.1) and signs (Table 28.2), which unfortunately are not very specific. The Epworth sleepiness scale can be used to screen for OSA, but its specificity and sensitivity are also low. Ideally, full-night polysomnography is used to determine if OSA is present. Obesity (body mass index above 30) and especially a large neck circumference (more than 43 cm) have a positive correlation with severe OSA, because these conditions involve extensive soft-tissue enlargements of the upper airway [24]. Other predisposing factors include increasing age, [39] male sex [39], and use of alcohol [33].

The risk of developing perioperative complications is increased not only by the presence of OSA but also, not surprisingly, by comorbidity associated with OSA. There is evidence that patients with OSA have an increased risk of developing hypertension, arrhythmias, heart attacks, right heart failure, pulmonary hypertension, and strokes [15, 19, 20, 26, 27]. Polycythaemia, initiated by a hypoxia-driven production of erythropoietin by the kidneys, is common [4]. The American Society of Anesthesiologists' Task Force has constructed practice guidelines for the perioperative management of patients with OSA [1]. They propose a scoring system which may be used to estimate whether a patient is at increased perioperative risk of complications from OSA. It must be emphasized that this scoring system is not yet validated and is meant only as a guide, and clinical judgment should be used to assess the risk of an individual patient (Tables 28.3, 28.4).

Assessment of Risk that Tracheal Intubation May Be Difficult

OSA is, by definition, a problem of the upper airway. Its presence indicates an increased likelihood of difficult intubation and airway maintenance under anesthesia. Three different groups of patients undergoing general anesthesia can be defined that require three different strategies for managing the upper airway: patients who have been diagnosed with OSA, patients with symptoms suggestive for OSA and patients who lack signs of the syndrome or in whom such features are missed preoperatively.

Table 28.1. Symptoms associated with obstructive sleep apnea (OSA)

Adults	Children
Heavy persistent snoring	Snoring
Excessive daytime sleepiness	Restless sleep
	Sleepiness
Apneas as observed by bed partner	Hyperactivity
Choking sensations while waking up	Aggression and behavioral disturbance
Gastroesophageal reflux	Frequent colds or coughing
Reduced ability to concentrate	Odd sleeping positions
Memory loss	
Personality changes	
Mood swings	
Night sweating	
Nocturia	
Dry mouth in the morning	
Restless sleep	
Morning headache	
Impotence	

Table 28.2. Physical characteristics associated with OSA

Nasal obstruction (deviation of the septum or hypertrophic conchae inferiors)
Edematous or long soft palate or uvula
Hypertrophic tongue tonsils
Narrow oropharynx
  (large tonsils, redundant pharyngeal arches)
Adiposity or large neck circumference
Retrognathia
Maxillary hypoplasia

Tips and Pearls

- No staging system can prevent unexpected difficulties in tracheal intubation, so any patient diagnosed as having OSA or in whom problematic intubation is anticipated on the basis of clinical signs (obesity, limited mouth opening, or a large tongue) should be treated as having a difficult airway until this has been proved otherwise.

A difficult airway is defined as the clinical situation in which a conventionally trained anesthetist experiences difficulty with face mask ventilation of the upper airway, difficulty with tracheal intubation, or both. The purpose of the American Society of Anesthesiologists' guidelines is to reduce the likelihood of adverse outcomes by providing basic recommendations [2].

Orotracheal intubation, especially in severely obese patients with OSA, may be extremely difficult and postoperative airway obstruction due to swelling or bleeding should be anticipated. Alterations in craniofacial morphology contributing to OSA – such as macroglossia, retrognathia, a narrow hypopharynx because of fat deposition in the lateral walls of the pharynx, or an anteriorly displaced larynx – also have an impact on anesthetic management [11, 22, 36].

Although no strong relation between cephalometric variables and the incidence of OSA has been found, two anatomical landmarks were shown to be important in patients with OSA:

1. Inferiorly positioned hyoid (distance between chin and hyoid bone) [3, 14]
2. Increased length of the soft palate [3, 14]

Mallampati et al. [22] constructed a staging system to predict difficult tracheal intubation. In general, oral intubation is hindered when patients are categorized as Mallampati stage 3 or 4, [22, 36] although Siyam and Benhamou [31] failed to find a correlation of this preoperative staging system with more difficult intubation.

Whenever possible, an airway history, physical examination, and review of medical records may improve the detection of difficult airway in patients with OSA, thereby enabling the anesthetist to prepare the patient and the anesthesia team for the occurrence of airway difficulties. In some patients, additional evaluation may be indicated to further judge the likelihood of the anticipated airway difficulty.

Perioperative Aspects

Premedication

Preoperative sedation with benzodiazepines before the induction of general anesthesia has muscle-relaxing effects on the upper-airway musculature, causing an appreciable reduction of the pharyngeal space. Consequently, a higher risk of preoperative phases of apnea and/or hypopnea and consecutive hypoxia and hypercapnia arises after administration, and oxygen saturation needs to be monitored adequately [9, 28]. If needed, oxygen can be given by an insufflation mask preoperatively, and application of nasal continuous positive airway pressure (with oxygen) might be nec-

28

Table 28.3. Identification and assessment of OSA: Example

A. Clinical signs and symptoms suggesting the possibility of OSA [1]
   1. Predisposing physical characteristics:
      a. BMI 35 kg/m2 [95th percentile for age and gender]*
      b. Neck circumference 17 in. (men) or 16 in. (women)
      c. Craniofacial abnormalities affecting the airway
      d. Anatomical nasal obstruction
      e. Tonsils nearly touching or touching in the midline

   2. History of apparent airway obstruction during sleep (two or more of the following are present; if patient lives alone or sleep is not observed by another person, then only one of the following needs to be present):
      a. Snoring (loud enough to be heard through closed door)
      b. Frequent snoring
      c. Observed pauses in breathing during sleep
      d. Awakens from sleep with choking sensation
      e. Frequent arousals from sleep
      f. [Intermittent vocalization during sleep]*
      g. [Parental report of restless sleep, difficulty breathing, or struggling respiratory efforts during sleep]*

   3. Somnolence (one or more of the following is present):
      a. Frequent somnolence or fatigue despite adequate "sleep"
      b. Falls asleep easily in a nonstimulating environment (e.g., watching TV, reading, riding in or driving a car) despite adequate "sleep"
      c. [Parent or teacher comments that child appears sleepy during the day, is easily distracted, is overly aggressive, or has difficulty concentrating]*
      d. [Child often difficult to arouse at awakening time]*

   If a patient has signs or symptoms in two or more of the above categories, there is a significant probability that he or she has OSA. The severity of OSA may be determined by sleep study. If a sleep study is not available, such patients should be treated as though they have moderate sleep apnea unless one or more of the signs or symptoms above is severely abnormal (e.g., markedly increased BMI or neck circumference, respiratory pauses that are frightening to the observer, patient regularly falls asleep within minutes after being left unstimulated), in which case they should be treated as though they have severe sleep apnea.
   usual awakening time]*

B. If a sleep study has been done, the results should be used to determine the perioperative anesthetic management of a patient. However, because sleep laboratories differ in their criteria for detecting episodes of apnea and hypopnea, the Task Force believes that the sleep laboratory's assessment (none, mild, moderate, or severe) should take precedence over the actual AHI (the number of episodes of sleep-disordered breathing per hour). If the overall severity is not indicated, it may be determined by using the table below:

BMI body mass index, *AHI* apnea-hypopnea index

essary postoperatively, especially when severe OSA is present [7].

Intubation Technique

The main goal in all patients is to avoid inadequate ventilation and oxygenation resulting in hypoxemia or hypercapnia and any associated hemodynamic changes (such as tachycardia, arrhythmia, and hypertension) leading to increased morbidity and mor-tality. Death, brain injury, cardiopulmonary arrest, airway trauma, and damage to teeth are among the adverse events associated with difficult airway management.

One important strategy in patients with a known or suspected difficult airway may be the avoidance of the necessity for invasive airway management. Whenever feasible, local anesthesia infiltration or regional blockades should be preferred in these patients.

Components of the preoperative physical examination of the airway are shown in Table 28.5. It is widely accepted that preparatory effects will help minimize

Table 28.4. OSA scoring system: example [1]

A. Severity of sleep apnea based on sleep study (or clinical indicators if sleep study not available). Point score _____ (0–3)		C. Requirement for postoperative opioids. Point score _____ (0–3)	
Severity of OSA**		None	0
None	0	Low-dose oral opioids	1
Mild	1	High-dose oral opioids, parenteral or neuraxial opioids	3
Moderate	2		
Severe	3		

D. Estimation of perioperative risk. Overall score
The score for A plus the greater of the score for either B or C.
Point score _____ (0–6)

B. Invasiveness of surgery and anesthesia.
Point score _____ (0–3)

a.	Superficial surgery under local or peripheral nerve block anesthesia without sedation	0
b.	Superficial surgery with moderate sedation or general anesthesia	1
c.	Peripheral surgery with spinal or epidural anesthesia (with no more than moderate sedation)	1
d.	Peripheral surgery with general anesthesia	2
e.	Airway surgery with moderate sedation	2
f.	Major surgery, general anesthesia	3
g.	Airway surgery, general anesthesia	3

A scoring system similar to this table may be used to estimate whether a patient is at increased perioperative risk of complications from OSA. This example, which has not been clinically validated, is meant only as a guide, and clinical judgment should be used to assess the risk of an individual patient.

*One point may be subtracted if a patient has been on CPAP or NIPPV before surgery and will be using his or her appliance consistently during the postoperative period

†One point should be added if a patient with mild or moderate OSA also has a resting arterial carbon dioxide tension (PaCO2) greater than 50 mmHg
‡Patients with a score of 4 may be at increased perioperative risk from OSA: patients with a score of 5 or 6 may be at significantly increased perioperative risk from OSA

Severity of OSA	**Adult AHI**	**Pediatric AHI**
None	0–5	0	
Mild OSA	6–20	1–5
Moderate OSA	21–40	6–10
Severe OSA	40	10

CPAP continuous positive airway pressure, NIPPV noninvasive positive pressure ventilation

the risk in patients presenting with a difficult airway. In these cases, the patient should be informed of particular risks and management protocols of the difficult airway. Equipment for management of a difficult airway should be in place before induction of general anesthesia and it is recommended to have another experienced anesthetist on standby. Before intubation, preoxygenation for 3 min or more is a must.

When general anesthesia is induced in patients with a known or suspected difficult airway, tracheal intubation will still be successful in a number of patients without problems, especially when performed by an experienced anesthetist. If the initial intubation attempt fails, an additional anesthetist should be called if not already present, and the option of wakening the patient and returning to spontaneous ventilation should be considered depending on the urgency of the surgical procedure. The possibility of face mask ventilation is the key issue for all further proceedings: when face mask ventilation and oxygenation of the patient are possible, repeated attempts at tracheal intubation can be attempted, with modified techniques where necessary. Alternative approaches may be the use of a fiberoptic bronchoscope, the use of special laryngoscope blades such as the McCoy blade with the option of additional leverage of the epiglottis (Fig.

28.1), or the use of an intubation stylet. The McCoy blade allows a major problem in many OSA patients to be overcome: the enlarged tongue. In many patients, correct positioning of the head will further aid in achieving the goal of tracheal intubation. Pressure on the cricoid cartilage by an assistant, ideally backward, upward, and toward the right (BURP – backward, upward, rightward pressure) may also facilitate identification of the glottis. Any "blind" intubation attempts without visualization of the glottis should be avoided for they may lead to trauma and swelling interfering with further management of the airway.

Whenever face mask ventilation is difficult or impossible in a patient after induction of general anesthesia and a failed intubation attempt, supraglottic airway devices such as a laryngeal mask airway or a laryngeal tube (Figs. 28.2, 28.3) should be inserted to ensure oxygenation of the patient while reconsidering intubation strategies. One approach can be to attempt fiberoptic intubation via the supraglottic airway device, directly or with a tube-exchange catheter, after preoxygenation of the patient. Using the intubating laryngeal mask airway, which provides a curved steel shaft guiding the fiberscope towards the glottis, will facilitate fiberoptic intubation (Fig. 28.4). Reconsidering the necessity of tracheal intubation versus the pos-

28

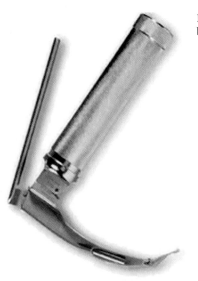

Fig. 28.1. McCoy blade

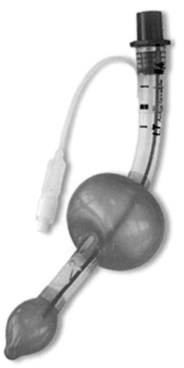

Fig. 28.3. Laryngeal tube

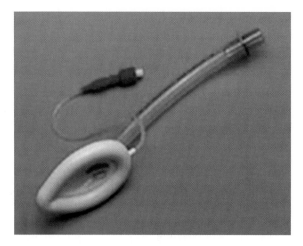

Fig. 28.2. Laryngeal mask airway

Table 28.5. Components of preoperative physical examination of airway that may indicate difficult intubation [2]

Airway investigation element	Disturbing findings
Length of neck	Short
Thickness of neck	Thick
Range of motion of head and neck	Patient cannot touch tip of chin to chest or cannot extend neck
Visibility of uvula	Not visible when tongue is protruded with patient in sitting position
Shape of palate	
Thyromental distance[a]	
Compliance of mandibular space	Highly arched or very narrow
Length of upper incisors	Less than three ordinary finger breadths
Normal jaw closure	
Interincisor distances	Stiff, indurated, occupied by mass, or nonelastic
	Prominent "overbite"
	Less than 3 cm

[a] Measured along a straight line from the thyroid notch to the lower border of the mandibular mentum with the head fully extended

sibility of maintaining the airway with a supraglottic airway device for the surgical procedure planned may be another option. Innovative substitutes to tracheal intubation and face mask ventilation such as laryngeal tube suction (Fig. 28.5) or the ProSeal laryngeal mask airway (Fig. 28.6) provide an additional lumen allowing positioning of a gastric tube and suctioning and should be favored over the ordinary devices in obese patients since a better airway seal is achieved.

Life-Threatening Conditions

The presence of a preformulated strategy to ensure oxygenation and achieve tracheal intubation is absolutely mandatory in any situation requiring urgent airway maintenance. The emergency airway should be basically the same as described already, but the choice of the options and strategies should be narrowed down to the techniques the anesthetist is most familiar with.

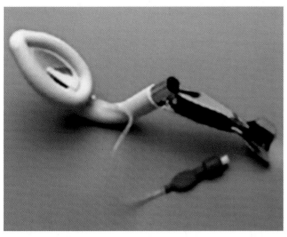

Fig 28.4. Laryngeal mask airway with a curved steel shaft guiding the fiberscope towards the glottis

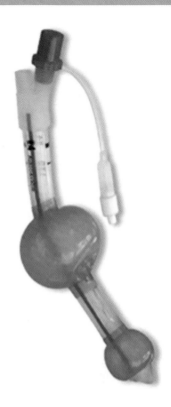

Fig 28.5. Laryngeal tube suction with an additional lumen allowing placement of a gastric tube and suctioning

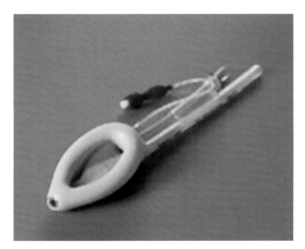

Fig 28.6. ProSeal laryngeal mask airway

Tips and Pearls

■ Patients with extreme anatomical anomalies should be intubated in alert condition with optimal local anesthesia [10].

Once the glottis has been successfully identified, the tracheal tube can be advanced and general anesthesia can be inducted. If the procedure fails owing to lack of patient cooperation, difficulties in identifying the glottic aperture caused by anatomical aberrations, or massive secretion, the case may be canceled.

In any patient requiring urgent oxygenation, supraglottic airway devices should be inserted early even when face mask ventilation is possible since the airway seal with these devices is superior and the rate of gastric insufflation is therefore lower. Fiberoptic intubation via these devices or the use of a newer supra-

glottic alternative providing access to the alimentary tract for suctioning should be considered. In the case of a ventilation emergency, surgical tracheostomy or needle cricothyroidotomy should be considered early, especially if the problem is caused by airway obstruction on the glottic level [29]. The latter might be considered as the first choice in some patients with the options of surgical or percutaneous tracheostomy and surgical or needle cricothyroidotomy with the option of jet ventilation. ENT surgeons and anesthetists should cooperate closely in these critical incidents, and also in the preoperative and perioperative management of all patients with OSA undergoing surgery.

Postoperative Aspects

Extubating the Difficult Airway

The surgical procedure and the condition of the patient, as well as any known or suspected trauma to the upper airway due to manipulations during the process of securing the airway, will influence the anesthetist's strategy for extubating the patient with a difficult airway. Despite the fact that removal of the tracheal tube will not be a problem, reinsertion, if required, will certainly not be easier than during the first effort.

28

Tracheal extubation should be carried out only when the patient is conscious, communicative, and breathing spontaneously with an adequate tidal volume and oxygenation. Full reversal of neuromuscular block should be verified and extubation is preferred in lateral, semiupright, or nonsupine position [9]. After adequate suctioning of secretions in the pharynx, the cuff should be deflated with closure of the tube to check breathing sounds around the tube. Complete airway obstruction is possible if breathing sounds are negative and the patient should be taken to an intensive care unit for extended weaning. Most patients do not need continuous monitoring in the postoperative phase, but the decision to discharge these patients from the recovery room to a regular ward, an intermediate care unit, or an intensive care unit should be based on the type of procedure, the overall condition of the patient, the severity of OSA, and the infrastructure of the hospital.

Respiratory Depression (Arrest)

Respiratory depression and repetitive apneas often occur directly after extubation in patients with OSA [7]. Use of opioids increases this risk, and intravenous administration may cause delayed (4–12 h after administration) respiratory depression [6, 16, 25]. We believe that opioids should only be used when nonsteroid anti-inflammatory drugs or regional anesthesia cannot be administered or is insufficient. In some cases it may be wise to titrate short-acting opioid variants until pain sensation is sufficiently diminished. When patient-controlled systemic opioids are used, continuous infusions should be used with extreme caution or avoided entirely [1].

Ostermeier et al. [25] state that patients with OSA are at increased risk of developing respiratory problems postoperatively in the absence of pain. Pain would prevent the rebound of rapid eye movement sleep and diminish stage 3 and stage 4 sleep, which also predisposes to collapse of the upper airway, around the third day postoperatively [18]. It is postulated that the number of possible breathing depressions would thus decline [25]. Use of nasal continuous positive airway pressure preoperatively and immediately postoperatively could reduce the risk of developing respiratory depression and is strongly advised in severe OSA [7]. Corrective airway surgery does not alleviate OSA immediately and patients undergoing these procedures should be assumed to remain at risk for OSA complications unless a normal sleep study has been obtained and symptoms have not recurred [1].

Obstruction of the Upper Airway

Surgery of the upper airway – especially uvulopalatopharyngoplasty and (adeno) tonsillectomy – causes tissue damage and produces edema and occasionally (considerable) hematomas. These changes can instigate or increase narrowing of the upper airway and even lead temporarily to severe OSA, particularly when opioids and sedating drugs are administered as well [5, 23]. Mortality after reconstruction of the soft palate (palatoschisis, uvulopalatopharyngoplasty – 30-day mortality rate 0.2%), due to obstruction of the upper airway, has been reported [17, 35]. Patients with severe OSA will need prolonged tracheal intubation or tracheotomy. Supplemental oxygen should be administered with caution, because the ventilation process may be dependent on its "hypoxic" drive and may increase the duration of apneic episodes and may hinder detection of atelectasis, transient apnea, and hypoventilation by pulse oximetry [1].

Nasal obstruction also has a role in the natural history of OSA, but its impact as a contributing factor remains unclear. Nasal surgery alone seems to cure only 16% of patients with OSA and nasal obstruction [37]. A decreased nasal passage may not be the major contributor to OSA, but nasal or sinus surgery with use of packs does constitute an extra risk. Observation in a medium or high care unit as long as the packs are in place is advisable, and in the case of severe OSA full-face continuous positive airway pressure is needed to prevent dangerous apneas. The effectiveness of a therapeutic alternative – a ventilation channel inside the nasal pack – is often very disappointing. Use of mattress sutures alone, without packing, could be of great value. Gupta et al. [13] found a twofold increased risk of developing complications in patients with OSA who had knee or hip surgery compared with patients without OSA after the same operation. Use of nasal continuous airway pressure preoperatively and postoperatively may reduce this complication risk [8].

Conclusion

▼

Extreme caution should be exercised when providing perioperative anesthesia to patients with OSA. Careful airway history, physical examination, and review of medical records may improve the detection of a difficult airway in patients with OSA, and allow the anesthetist to prepare the patient and the anesthesia team for the occurrence of airway difficulties.

References

1. American Society of Anesthesiologists Task Force. (2006) Practice guidelines for the perioperative management of patients with obstructive sleep apnea. *Anesthesiology*;104:1081–1093.
2. American Society of Anesthesiologists Task Force on Management of the Difficult Airway. (2003) Practice guidelines for management of the difficult airway. *Anesthesiology*;98:1269–77.
3. Baik UB, Suzuki M, Ikeda K, Sugawara J, Mitani H. (2002) Relationship between cephalometric characteristics and obstructive sites in OSA syndrome. *Angle Orthod*;72:124–34.
4. Boushra NN. (1996) Anesthetic management of patients with sleep apnea syndrome. *Can J Anaesth*; 43:599–616.
5. Burgess LP, Derderian SS, Morin GV, Gonzalez C, Zajtchuk JT. (1992) Postoperative risk following uvulopalatopharyngeoplasty for OSA. *Otolaryngol Head Neck Surg*;106:81–6.
6. Chauvin M, Samii K, Schermann JM, Sandouk P, Bourdon R, Viars P. (1982) Plasma pharmacokinetics of morphine after i.m., extradural and intrathecal administration. *Br J Anaesth*;54:843–7.
7. Chung F, Crago RR. (1982) Sleep apnea syndrome and anesthesia. *Can Anaesth Soc J*;29:439–45.
8. Chung F, Imarengiaye C. (2002) Management of sleep apnea in adults. *Can J Anaesth*;49:R1–6.
9. Connolly LA. (1991) Anesthetic management of OSA patients. *J Clin Anesth*;3:461–9.
10. Craddock M, Lees DE. (1989) Anesthesia for OSA patients: risks, precautions, and management. In: Fairbanks DNF, ed. *General anesthesia*, 5th ed. London/Boston: Butterworths;346–57.
11. Do KL, Ferreyra H, Healy JF, Davidson TM. (2000) Does tongue size differ between patients with and without sleep-disordered breathing? *Laryngoscope*;110:1552–5.
12. Gleadhill IC, Schwartz AR, Schubert N, Wise RA, Permutt S, Smith PL. (1991) Upper airway collapsibility in snorers and in patients with obstructive hypopnea and apnea. *Am Rev Respir Dis* 1991;143:1300–3.
13. Gupta RM, Par vizi J, Hanssen AD, Gay PC. (2001) Postoperative complications in patients with OSA syndrome undergoing hip or knee replacement: a case-control study. *Mayo Clin Proc*;76:897–905.
14. Hoekema A, Hovinga B, Stegenga B, De Bont LG. (2003) Craniofacial morphology and OSA: a cephalometric analysis. J Oral Rehabil;30:690–6.
15. Hung J, Whitford EG, Parsons RW, Hillary DR. (1990) Association of sleep apnea with myocardial infarction in men. Lancet;336:261–4.
16. Kafer ER, Brown JT, Scott D, Findlay JW, Butz RF, Teeple E, et al. (1983) Biphasic depression of ventilatory responses to CO2 following epidural morphine. Anesthesiology;58:418–27.
17. Kezirian EJ, Weaver EM, Yueh B, Deyo RA, Khuri SF, Daley J, Henderson W. (2004) Incidence of serious complications after vulopalatopharyngoplasty. Laryngoscope; 114(3):450–3.
18. Knill RL, Moote CA, Skinner MI, Rose EA. (1990) Anesthesia with abdominal surgery lead to intense REM sleep during the first postoperative week. Anesthesiology;73:52–61.
19. Lavie P, Herer P, Hoffstein V. (2000) OSA syndrome as a risk factor for hypertension population study. BMJ;320:479–82.
20. Lavie P, Herer P, Peled R, Berger I, Yoffe N, Zomer J, Rubin AH. (1995) Mortality in sleep apnea patients: a multivariate analysis of risk factors. Sleep;18:149–57.
21. Loadsman JA, Hillman DR. (2001) Anesthesia and sleep apnea. Br J Anaesth;86:254–66.
22. Mallampati SR, Gatt SP, Gugino LD, Desai SP, Waraksa B, Freiberger D, et al. (1985) A clinical sign to predict difficult tracheal intubation: a prospective study. Can Anaesth Soc J;32:429–34.
23. McColley SA, April MM, Carroll JL, Naclerio RM, Loughlin GM. (1992) Respiratory compromise after adenotonsillectomy in children with OSA. Arch Otolaryngol Head Neck Surg;118:940–3.
24. Mortimore IL, Marshal I, Wraith PK, Sellar RJ, Douglas NJ. (1998) Neck and total body fat deposition in non-obese and obese patients with sleep apnea compared with that in control studies. Am J Respir Crit Care Med;157:280–3.
25. Ostermeier AM, Roizen MF, Hautkappe M, Klock PA, Klafta JM. et al. (1997) Three sudden postoperative respirator y arrests associated with epidural opioids in patients with sleep apnea. Anesth Analg;85:452–60.
26. Partinen M, Jamieson A, Guilleminault C. (1988) Long-term outcome for OSA syndrome patients. Mortality. Chest;94(6):1200–1204.
27. Peppard PE, Young TB, Palta M, Skatrud J. (2000) Prospective study of the association between sleep-disordered breathing and hypertension. N Engl J Med;342:1378–84.
28. Pharmaceutic Therapeutic Compass 2003. Chapter 1: Central nervous system (psychic diseases):51–66.
29. Rafferty TD, Ruskins A, Sasaki C, Gee JB. (1980) Perioperative considerations in the management of tracheotomy for the OSA patient: three illustrative case reports. Br J Anaesth;52:619–22.
30. Reimer MA, Flemons WW. (2003) Quality of life in sleep disorders. Sleep Med Rev;7:335–49.
31. Siyam MA, Benhamou D. (2002) Difficult endotracheal intubation in patients with sleep apnea syndrome. Anesth Analg;95:1098–102.
32. Strohl KP, Cherniack NS, Gothe B. (1986) Physiologic basis of therapy for sleep apnea. Am Rev Respir Dis;134:791–802.
33. Taasan VC, Block AJ, Boysen PG, Wynne JW. (1981) Alcohol increases sleep apnea and oxygen desaturations in asymptomatic men. Am J Med;71:240–5.
34. American Academy of Sleep Medicine Task Force. (1999) Sleep-related breathing disorders in adults: recommen-

of 2 or above is considered as pathological. Newborns should not have any obstructive apneas [19]. Concerning adults, no generally accepted consensus exists. He et al. [10] were able to demonstrate in an examination of 385 men with SDB that the mortality risk rises significantly above an apnea index of 20.

In our sleep laboratories in Mannheim and Hamburg we therefore use the following distinction:

- Mild OSA $10 \leq AHI < 20$
- Moderate OSA $20 \leq AHI < 40$
- Severe OSA $40 \leq AHI$

Below an AHI of 10 it is necessary to make a differential diagnosis between harmless primary snoring and a potentially health-impairing UARS. One should consider that the above values are applicable to 30-year-olds. In the case of a 70-year-old, an AHI up to 15 may not necessarily need treatment if the patient does not have any daytime symptoms.

Apart from the AHI, the symptoms of the patient play a role. That is, a patient with a UARS and an AHI significantly below 10, but suffering from intense daytime sleepiness, may be in need of treatment, whereas an older patient with an AHI of 15 may not require treatment. The concomitant diagnoses also need to be considered. Since SDB constitutes risk factors for myocardial infarction, arterial hypertension and strokes, patients with a corresponding history need to be sufficiently treated early on. One should also take special note of traffic accidents in the history-taking, as these are frequently a result of sleepiness behind the wheel, which again suggests the existence of a SDB.

In the meantime, a multitude of treatment options for SDB exist. They can be classified into conservative, apparative and surgical methods. This chapter focuses on the surgical treatment options for OSA. However, the surgeon has always to keep in mind, that respiratory treatment with continuous positive airway pressure (CPAP) with its various modifications remains the gold standard procedure. The CPAP ventilation therapy according to Sullivan et al. [22], which is for the most part nasally applied, splints the upper airway pneumatically from the nares to the larynx (Fig. 29.1), whereas surgical procedures often only address a limited segment of the upper airway.

Concerning the implementation of CPAP therapy, and its diverse modifications, please refer to the specialized literature [4–6]. With a primary success rate of 98%, CPAP therapy is alongside tracheotomy the most successful therapy modality available. Only these two treatment modalities achieve sufficient cure rates in cases of extreme obesity and severe OSA; therefore, nasal CPAP therapy is considered to be the gold standard in the treatment of OSA. All other therapies for OSA must be measured against this method. Unfortunately, the long-term acceptance rate of CPAP therapy lies below 70% [14]. The acceptance rate of CPAP therapy especially decreases the younger the patient is, and the less his/her subjective symptoms improve with CPAP therapy [12]. As a consequence, many patients with moderate and severe OSA in need of treatment have to be secondarily guided into another therapy. Often surgery may help in these cases [21].

The most widespread and scientifically evaluated surgical procedures are listed in Table 29.1. On one

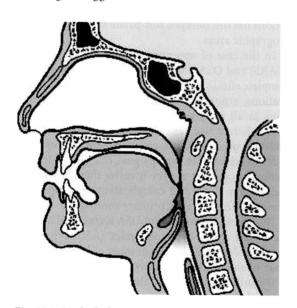 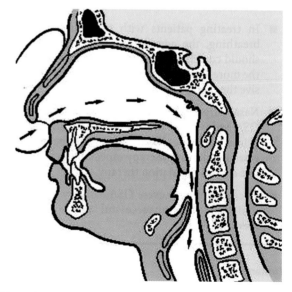

Fig. 29.1. Method of pneumatic stenting of the upper airway with continuous positive airway pressure. *Left*: Airway collapse. *Right*: Stabilization with continuous positive airway pressure

Table 29.1. Surgical treatment modalities for obstructive sleep apnea

Anatomic area	Minimally invasive	Invasive
Nose	Laser-assisted surgery of the turbinates	Septoplasty
	Electrosurgery of the turbinates	Septorhinoplasty
	Radiofrequency surgery of the turbinates	Inferior turbinoplasty
Soft palate/tonsils	Radiofrequency surgery of the soft palate	Laser-assisted uvulopalatoplasty
	Palatal implants	Uvulopalatopharyngoplasty
	Cautery-assisted palatal stiffening operation	Uvulopalatal flap
	Injection snoreplasty	Transpalatal advancement pharyngoplasty
	Radiofrequency surgery of the tonsils	Tonsillectomy/tonsillotomy
		Genioglossus advancement
Base of tongue/ hypopharynx	Radiofrequency surgery of the base of the tongue	Hyoid suspension (thyreohyoidopexy)
		Tongue-base reduction
		Repose® tongue suspension
Larynx/trachea		Laryngeal laser surgery
		Tracheotomy
Maxillofacial surgeries		Maxillomandibular advancement
		Distraction ostegenesis

hand, they can be grouped according to the anatomic area addressed and, on the other hand, they can be divided into minimally invasive and in invasive techniques. Procedures are regarded as minimally invasive if they (1) can be performed on an outpatient basis, (2) require only local anesthesia and (3) produce little intraoperative and postoperative morbidity and complications.

Within the first years after the implementation of uvulopalatopharyngoplasty (UPPP) as treatment for OSA in 1981 [7], most authors focused on the proper selection of candidates for UPPP by identifying the site(s) of obstruction [26]. However, ENT surgeons only assumed two sites of obstruction. Fujita [8], for example, classified OSA patients into those with an obstruction solely behind the soft palate (type I), those with an obstruction solely behind the tongue (type II) and those with an obstruction behind both the soft palate and the tongue (type III). Yet up to now, this topodiagnosis has not assisted in raising the success rate of soft-palate surgery significantly above 50% [20]. Obviously this theoretical approach was too mechanistic, and has been replaced by the multiple-level obstruction concept [23].

Therefore various surgical techniques addressing the hypopharyngeal and retrolingual site of obstruction were introduced within the following years. The Stanford Group was the first to introduce a multiphase concept to treat OSA [18]. Phase 0 consisted in rhinosurgery if thought to be necessary. In phase 1, the authors combined an UPPP with tonsillectomy with genioglossus advancement and hyoid suspension. Nonresponders were offered maxillomandibular advancement as phase 2. Following this algorithm, the authors describe a success rate of 60% after phase 1 and of 90% after phase 2; however, not many patients were willing to undergo phase 2.

Today, almost 15 years later, many new treatment modalities have been introduced into the field of sleep surgery, including various minimally invasive techniques. Inasmuch, the Stanford algorithm cannot be recommended in this form any longer.

Modern concepts do not only focus on OSA but also on primary snoring and UARS, as they regard primary snoring, on the one hand, and OSA, on the other, as different manifestations of the same pathophysiological disorder (Fig. 29.2) [15]. We agree with this conception and have made it the foundation for our therapeutic decisions.

From Fig. 29.2 two important therapy principles can be inferred. The first therapy principle correlates the aggressiveness of treatment with the severity of disease: the more severe the disease, the more aggressive the therapy. For the treatment of primary snoring, minimally invasive techniques with a low complication rate should be preferred. In the case of more severe OSA, surgery is only indicated after an unsuccessful nasal CPAP therapy. For a primary surgical treatment, an AHI of approximately 30 is considered as the threshold value [17].

The second therapy principle entails that SDB is being considered more and more as a disorder of the entire upper airway. Therefore, we now assume that this simplified classification into a retropalatal and a retrolingual site of obstruction is only applicable for primary snoring and, to a certain extent, in the case of UARS and mild OSA. Starting with moderate OSA with an AHI of approximately 20 events per hour of

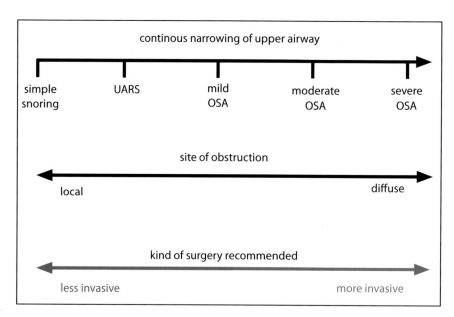

Fig. 29.2. Continuous narrowing of upper airway. *UARS* upper-airway resistance syndrome, *OSA* obstructive sleep apnea. (Modified after [15])

sleep, based on current experiences and data, one begins to consider the possibility of so-called multilevel surgery. Also in this case, the appropriate surgical technique depends upon the severity of disease and the anatomic disposition.

Figure 29.3 illustrates the indications for the surgical techniques preferred in Mannheim and Hamburg, in relationship to the severity of the SDB. The following chapters will discuss these techniques in detail.

Nasal surgery seldom affects the severity of OSA and is of use only in those patients with primary snoring [25]. Nevertheless nasal surgery is indicated as adjuvant therapy especially to facilitate a nasal ventilation therapy.

The following procedures should be limited to simple snorers as up to now there are no published data available documenting any efficiency in the treatment of OSA: laser-assisted uvulopalatoplasty, palatal implants, cautery-assisted palatal stiffening operation, and injection snoreplasty. As well, there are no sleep studies showing a reduction in AHI after radiofrequency treatment of the tonsils. Admittedly, a substantial reduction of the tonsillar volume has been documented. From knowledge that tonsillectomy is an effective treatment for OSA, there might be enough evidence to assume that radiofrequency surgery of the tonsils is effective also.

Personally, I do not recommend the transpalatal advancement pharyngoplasty and genioglossus advancement owing to lack of experience. Furthermore, tongue-base resections and tracheotomy should only be performed as a last resort, the former because of increased postoperative morbidity and the need for temporary tracheotomy [2, 3, 9], the latter because of the impairment of quality of life. Maxillofacial sur-

geries are very effective in cases of maxillofacial malformities and especially in syndromic patients [11]. In sleep apneics without malformations, maxillomandibular advancement cannot be regarded as standard procedure.

Laryngeal OSA is a rare disturbance [24]. It either occurs in newborns in the form of laryngomalacia or in elderly men presenting with a floppy epiglottis. In these cases, flexible sleep endoscopy is the diagnostic procedure of choice. The treatment strategy depends on the clinical findings.

Conclusion

In summary, the following parameters need to be kept in mind for a comprehensive treatment decision:
- Age
- Severity of disease (Fig. 29.3)
- Desire for treatment in simple snorers
- Surgical or nonsurgical treatment
- Body mass index
- Anatomic findings

In the case of pediatric SDB both conditions, namely, OSA and simple snoring, may in almost all patients be cured by adenotonsillectomy. Unsuccessful cases should be referred to specialized sleep medical centers.

In adults, I always offer a conservative treatment as first-line treatment, in other words CPAP or oral

Fig. 29.3. Indications for different surgeries depending on the severity of obstructive sleep apnea. *UARS* upper-airway resistance syndrome, *OSA* obstructive sleep apnea, *RFQ* radiofrequency surgery, *UPPP* uvulopalatopharyngoplasty, *MMA* maxillomandibular advancement, *DOG* distraction osteogenesis, combined *RFT* RFT on soft palate, tonsils and base of tongue; *nCPAP* nasally applied continuous positive airway pressure

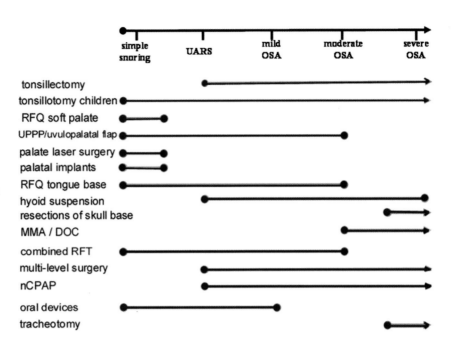

Fig. 29.4. Algorithm for treatment decisions in adult sleep-disordered breathing. *UARS* upper-airway resistance syndrome, *OSA* obstructive sleep apnea, *AHI* apnea–hypopnea index, *BMI* body mass index (kg/m^2), *CPAP* continuous positive airway pressure

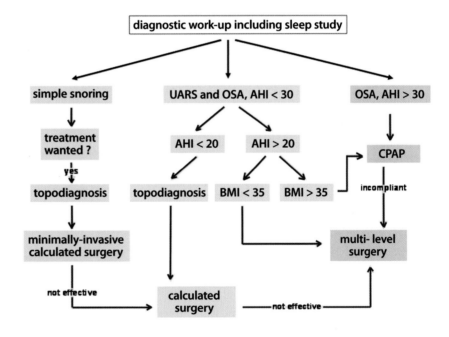

devices. As a result of daily practice over many years, I have developed the algorithm shown in Fig. 29.4, which is the basis for all my treatment decisions in cases of adult SDB.

Calculated surgery means that the surgeon makes his/her decision depending on the individual anatomic findings. For example, in patients with only palatal narrowing of the upper airway, an isolated soft-palate procedure may be sufficient, whereas multilevel surgery means that always at least one surgical procedure affecting the soft-palate and/or tonsil region is combined with at least one procedure addressing the tongue-base/hypopharynx section.

> Patients with a body mass index of more than 35 kg m^{-2} hardly meet the surgical criteria of success. This is why I do not perform surgery in these morbidly obese sleep apneics. I refer those patients to a surgical department for bariatric surgery or other therapies for weight loss.

29

References

1. American Sleep Disorders Association (1996) Practice parameters for the treatment of obstructive sleep apnea in adults: the efficacy of surgical modifications of the upper airway. Sleep 19:152–155
2. Chabolle F, Wagner I, Blumen M, Séquert C, Fleury B, de Dieuleveult T (1999) Tongue base reduction with hyoepiglottoplasty: a treatment for severe obstructive sleep apnea. Laryngoscope 109:1273–1280
3. Djupesland G, Schrader H, Lyberg T, Refsum H, Lilleas F, Godtlibsen OB (1992) Palatopharyngoglossoplasty in the treatment of patients with obstructive sleep apnea syndrome. Acta Otolaryngol Suppl 492:50–54
4. Dobrowski JM, Ahmed M (2002) Positive airway pressure for obstructive sleep apnea. In: Fairbanks DNF, Mickelson SA, Woodson BT. Snoring and obstructive sleep apnea. 3rd edition, Lippincott Williams & Wilkins, Philadelphia, pp 95–106
5. d'Ortho MP, Grillier-Lanoir V, Levy P, Goldenberg F, Corriger E, Harf A, Lofaso F (2000) Constant vs. automatic continuous positive airway pressure therapy: home evaluation. Chest 118:1010–1017
6. Ficker JH, Fuchs FS, Wiest GH, Asshoff G, Schmelzer AH, Hahn EG (2000) An auto-continuous positive airway pressure device controlled exclusively by the forced oscillation technique. Eur Respir J 16:914–920
7. Fujita S, Conway W, Zorick F (1981) Surgical correction of anatomic abnormalities in obstructive sleep apnea syndrome: Uvulopalatopharyngoplasty. Otolaryngol Head Neck Surg 89:923–934
8. Fujita S (1987) Pharyngeal surgery for obstructive sleep apnea and snoring. In: Fairbanks DNF (Eds) Snoring and obstructive sleep apnea. Raven, New York; pp 101–128
9. Fujita S, Woodson BT, Clark JL, Wittig R (1991) Laser midline glossectomy as a treatment for the obstructive sleep apnea. Laryngoscope 101: 805–809
10. He J, Kryger MH, Zorick FJ, Conway W, Roth T (1988) Mortality and apnea index in obstructive sleep apnea: Experience in 385 male patients. Chest 94: 9–14
11. Hierl T (2005) Maxillofacial surgeries. In Hörmann K, Verse T (editors). Surgery for sleep disordered breathing. Springer, Berlin, pp 91–106
12. Janson C, Nöges E, Svedberg-Brandt S, Lindberg E (2000) What characterizes patients who are unable to tolerate continuous positive airway pressure (CPAP) treatment? Resp Med 94:145–149
13. Lugaresi E, Cirignotta F, Gerardi R, Montagna P (1990) Snoring and sleep apnea: Natural history of heavy snorers disease. In Guilleminault C, Partinen M (editors): Obstructive sleep apnea syndrome: Clinical research and treatment. Raven, New York, pp 25-36
14. McArdle N, Dervereux G, Heidarnejad H, Engleman HM, Mackay TW, Douglas NJ (1999) Long-term use of CPAP therapy for sleep apnea / hypopnea syndrome. Am J Respir Crit Care Med 159:1108–1114
15. Moore K (2000) Site specific versus diffuse treatment/presenting severity of obstructive sleep apnea. Sleep Breath 4:145–146
16. Mortimore IL, Bradley PA, Murray JA, Douglas NJ (1996) Uvulopalatopharyngoplasty may compromise nasal CPAP therapy in sleep apnea syndrome. Am J Respir Crit Care Med 154:1759–1762
17. Pirsig W, Hörmann K, Siegert R, Maurer J, Verse T (1998) Guideline obstructive sleep apnea. German Society of Oto-Rhino-Laryngology, Head and Neck Surgery. [in German]. HNO 46:730
18. Riley RW, Powell NB, Guilleminault C (1993) Obstructive sleep apnea syndrome: A review of 306 consecutively treated surgical patients. Otolaryngol Head Neck Surg 108:117–125
19. Section on Pediatric Pulmonology, Subcommitte on Obstructive Sleep Apnea Syndrome. American Academy of Pediatrics (2002) Clinical practice guideline: diagnosis and management of childhood obstructive sleep apnea syndrome. Pediatrics 109:704–712
20. Sher AE, Schechtman KB, Piccirillo JF (1996) The efficacy of surgical modifications of the upper airway in adults with obstructive sleep apnea syndrome. Sleep 19:156–177
21. Souter MA, Stevenson S, Sparks B, Drennan C (2004) Upper airway surgery benefits patients with obstructive sleep apnoea who cannot tolerate nasal continuous positive airway pressure. J Laryngol Otol 118:270–274
22. Sullivan CE, Issa FG, Berthon-Jones M, Eves L (1981) Reversal of obstructive sleep apnoea by continuous positive airway pressure applied through the nares. Lancet 1:862–865
23. Verse T (2005) General aspects of surgery. In Hörmann K, Verse T (editors). Surgery for sleep disordered breathing. Springer, Berlin, pp 3–8
24. Verse T (2005) Laryngeal obstructive sleep apnea. In Hörmann K, Verse T (editors). Surgery for sleep disordered breathing. Springer Berlin, pp 107–114
25. Verse T, Pirsig W (2003) The impact of nasal surgery on obstructive sleep apnea. Sleep Breath 7:63–76
26. Verse T, Pirsig W (1997) The value of pharyngeal pressure measurements in the topodiagnosis of sites of obstruction in patients with obstructive respiratory disorders [in German]. HNO 45:898–904

Nasal Obstruction and Its Medical and Surgical Management in Sleep-Related Breathing Disorders

30

Bernard Bertrand, Philippe Rombaux, Daniel Rodenstein

Core Messages

- Although an increased nasal resistance does not always correlate with symptoms of congestion, nasal congestion typically results in a switch to mouth breathing.

- Nasal airway resistance is responsible for approximately two thirds of the total airway resistance in wakefulness.

- Nasal reflexes play an important role in modulating upper-airway patency during sleep.

- The presence of a high Mallampati score with concomitant nasal obstruction is associated with an increased risk of obstructive sleep apnea syndrome.

- Nasal obstruction secondary to allergic inflammation has an impact on sleep quality and its appropriate management seems to have a positive effect on subjective sleep quality and on polysomnographic data.

- The most common complaints with use of nasal continuous positive airway pressure are nocturnal awakenings (46% of patients) followed by dryness, congestion and sneezing (44% of patients).

Contents

Introduction

Inability to breathe through the nose is a recognized cause of disordered breathing during sleep, although the true relationship between sleep-related breathing disorders (SRBD) and nasal obstruction is still unclear. Sleep-disordered breathing can both result from and be worsened by nasal obstruction. Nasal breathing increases ventilatory drive and nasal occlusion decreases pharyngeal patency in normal subjects.

The different clinical aspects of SRBD include primary snoring, upper-airway resistance syndrome, obstructive sleep apnea-hypopnea syndrome (OSAS) and hypoventilation syndrome related to obesity [54]. The most studied form of SRBD is OSAS and its incidence is 2–4% in the general adult population [23].

In all circumstances, the nose may have a great impact on the severity of SRBD. Sensitized subjects during high allergen exposure have impaired nasal breathing and likewise everyone who has had a common cold will have experienced poor nasal breathing at night. The consequences of nasal obstruction on sleep are day-to-day discomfort, frequent complaints of poor sleep quality and daytime fatigue; they are well documented.

Risk factors for sleep-disordered breathing include central obesity, male gender, smoking habits, alcohol consumption, upper-airway obstruction and craniofacial abnormalities. Nasal obstruction must be considered to be a cofactor in the pathophysiology of SRBD.

Although an increased nasal resistance does not always correlate with symptoms of congestion, nasal congestion typically results in a switch to mouth breathing. The switch to mouth breathing that occurs with chronic nasal abnormalities is probably a common pathway for SRDB [56]. But the relationship between cause and effect remains a matter of debate.

30

Nasal Resistance

Nasal airway resistance is responsible for approximately two thirds of the total airway resistance in wakefulness [17].

Unlike the oropharyngeal segment in the upper airway which is collapsible when muscular tone decreases during sleep, the nasal airway segment has a more rigid framework, but in the valve area. The nasal valve contributes most to total nasal resistance and can be thought of as a short resistor of a few millimeters in length (Fig. 30.1). Hypotonus of dilator muscles in sleep permits the pharynx to comply with inspiratory pressures. If airflow resistances are increased by nasal disease, complete inspiratory obstructive closure of the pharynx and apnea can result from nasal breathing in sleeping subjects [8].

Tips and Pearls

- Nasal resistance is mainly under the control of the sympathetic nervous system and is dependent on the anatomical location of the nasal valve

Alar dilation muscles are synchronized with inspiration to prevent alar collapse, but their role in nasal sleep resistance is limited. The physiology of the nasal airway creates and is the result of dynamic situations where nasal resistance may vary under several circumstances and under the influence of the nasal cycle. Bilateral nasal decongestion may result from exercise and hypercapnia. On the other hand, hyperventilation with resulting hypocapnia is followed by an increase in nasal resistance.

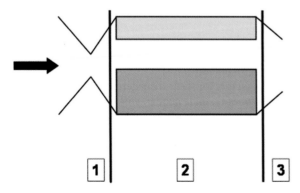

Fig. 30.1. The nasal fossa divided into three functional segments: *1* the valve area, *2* the turbinal valve, where the pink and *red areas* represent the turbinates in vasoconstriction (*pink*) and in vasodilatation (*red*), *3* the choana. Segment 2 is submitted to vasomotor activity occurring in the turbinates. The *arrow* indicates the inspiratory air stream

The influence of posture is also well recognized in that nasal resistance increases in the recumbent position owing to a hydrostatic component. This hydrostatic component contributes to the magnitude of the nasal resistive reflexes. For example, the amplitude of the nasal cycle is lower when standing up than when sleeping in the recumbent position.

Recumbency increases resistive swelling of inflamed nasal mucosa. Furthermore, in patients with normal mucosa and unilateral nasal obstruction, contralateral recumbency induces contralateral obstruction, which increases resistance to nasal breathing; and in either dorsal or lateral recumbency the congestive phase of the spontaneous nasal cycle acts in a similar way. Nasal resistive reflexes which are anatomically mediated may change the nasal resistance, and the respiratory resistors in the nasal fossae also determine the distribution of oronasal airflow [7].

This can explain the "paradoxical nasal obstruction" phenomenon. When a patient has a fixed unilateral obstruction, the nasal resistance is higher in the affected side than in the nonaffected side. When the normal side undergoes the congested phase of the nasal cycle or when the patient is sleeping on the same side as the nonaffected nostril, this results in bilateral occlusion and the patient will often attribute the problem to the normal side. Unilateral pressure on the shoulder or hip-girdle area causes ipsilateral nasal congestion and contralateral decongestion. This phenomenon is called the corporonasal reflex. All these nasal reflexes play an important role in modulating upper-airway patency during sleep.

Nasal breathing is for many reasons the preferential breathing route in wakefulness and in sleep even if resistance to airflow is high. Nasal airflow enters the nasal vestibule at the anterior nares with an air velocity of 2–3 m/s. The cross-sectional area at the anterior nares is about 90 mm^2. Where the nasal airflow crosses the nasal valve, the cross-sectional area is decreased to 30 mm^2. Owing to the Venturi effect (as a given volume of fluid moves through a conduit of decreasing diameter, the velocity of the fluid will increase), the air velocity increases to 12–18 m/s at the nasal valve level. This contributes to a higher probability of upper-airway collapse in the nasal valve area owing to the Bernoulli effect (as a fluid flows a negative pressure develops at the periphery of the flow and if the flow velocity increases so does the negative pressure). If the negative pressure increases at the interface between the airflow and the nasal valve compartment, the force to collapse increases. This is the case when compensatory forces from the alar and/or upper lateral cartilages are lacking (after surgical resection, for instance) or in case of inefficiency of the muscle dilators of the valve during inspiration (after a facial palsy, for instance). After passing the nasal valve, the airflow reaches the nasal cavity, where the cross-sectional area is greater (130 mm^2) and air velocity decreases to 2–3 mm/s. Nasal patency and SRBD are thus closely related. Although there is no strict linear relationship between the two, there is clear evidence that nasal patency must be maintained for patients with SRBD. Studies performed in normal subjects, in patients with SRBD or in patients with symptomatic nasal obstruction support the most favored pathophysiological mechanism for the role of upper-airway obstruction in the genesis of SRBD: the Starling resistor model (Fig. 30.2). In this model, the pharynx, which is the most collapsible part of the upper airway, is seen as a collapsible resistor [50].

The maximal flow rate at the pharyngeal level is related to the pressure in the upstream segment (the nasal segment) and to the transmural pressure. Once the negative transmural pressure reaches a certain level (the critical closing pressure, Pcrit), the caliber of the segment decreases and begins to either oscillate (snoring) or partly collapse (hypopnea) or totally collapse (apnea).

This single model shows that the determinants of maximal flow rate through the pharyngeal airway are:

■ The upstream resistance (i.e., the nasal resistance)
■ The transmural pressure
■ The compliance of the pharyngeal wall

The Pcrit varies between subjects (normal, snorers and apneics) and between the sleep stages. The negative intraluminal pressure and the Starling resistor model are the mechanisms which explain upper-airway obstruction during sleep and may at least partially explain why nasal patency is most important.

Nasal Patency and SRBD

Many studies have focused on the influence of nasal patency and its affect on sleep parameters and SRBD. The effects of uni(bi)lateral nasal obstruction, the effects of nasal anesthesia and the effects of nasal vasoconstriction have been studied in healthy subjects. White et al. [75] hypothesized that SRBDs in patients with nasal obstruction are secondary to a loss of afferent nasal receptors which are responsible for ventilation control.

To test the hypothesis that this respiratory dysrhythmia could result from loss of neuronal input to respiration from receptors located in the nose, they anesthetized the nasal fossae of ten normal volunteers during sleep using 4% lidocaine sprays as local anesthesia in a randomized study versus a placebo (saline solution) during the following night. Each subject spent four consecutive nights in the sleep laboratory while sleep stages, breathing patterns, respiratory effort and arterial oxygen saturation were monitored. The nasal fossae were also sprayed with a decongestant to prevent increased nasal airflow resistance resulting from mucosal swelling. On the night the placebo (decongestant plus saline) was given there were 6.4±1.8 (standard error of the mean) disordered breathing events (apneas plus hypopneas) per subject, whereas with lidocaine (plus decongestant) this increased fourfold to 25.8±7.8 events per subject ($p<0.05$). The majority of the isordered breathing events were apneas and were fairly evenly distributed between central and obstructive events. So, the administration of lidocaine increased pharyngeal obstruction, disturbed sleep, increased the number of awakenings and apnea and deteriorated the quality of sleep.

It was also demonstrated that upper-airway anesthesia reduces the phasic activity of the most important upper-airway dilating muscle during sleep, namely the genioglossus [3].

Berry et al. [3] hypothesized that stimulation of upper-airway mechanoreceptors during obstructive apnea augments upper-airway muscle activity, and that upper-airway anesthesia should reduce mechanoreceptor output and therefore upper-airway muscle activity. They studied the effect of upper-airway anesthesia on the genioglossus electromyogram and on the esophageal pressure deflection during obstructive apneas in nonrapid eye movement (non-REM) sleep in a group of six men with severe sleep apnea. After anesthesia, the mean ratio of the phasic activity of the genioglossus electromyogram to the esophageal pressure deflection decreased to 23% of the control values, suggesting that stimulation of upper-airway mechanoreceptors during obstructive apnea in non-REM sleep augments phasic genioglossus activity.

Nitric oxide is also considered to be an aerotransmitter between the nose and the lung and its role in maintaining upper-airway patency using efferent pathways has been underlined. Haight and Djupesland [21] asserted that obstructive sleep apnea

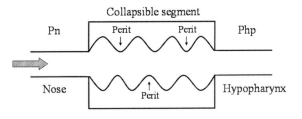

Fig. 30.2. Starling model. *Dashed arrow* inspiratory airflow, *Pn* pressure in the nose, *Php* pressure in the hypopharynx, *Pcrit* critical pressure of closure of the airways

could be described as the intermittent failure to transport the full complement of nasal nitric oxide to the lung with each breath.

Others investigators have looked at the role of experimental nasal occlusion on sleep quality in normal subjects. Use of petroleum jelly and cotton to occlude the nostrils or adhesive tapes on nostrils and polysomnographic studies with or without the devices have repeatedly shown that sleep quality worsened [34,35, 49, 66, 77].

Desaturation (SaO_2 less than 90%) occurred 27 times during control sleep compared with 255 times during obstructed-nose sleep in a study by Zwillich et al. [77] on ten normal men. These desaturation episodes occurred only during apneas. In the study of Olsen et al. [49], the subjects with the nose mechanically obstructed awoke more often, had a greater number of changes in sleep stage, had a prolongation of REM latency and spent a greater amount of time in stage I non-REM sleep (light sleep). About the same was observed by Lavie et al. [35]. Nasal obstruction caused a significant increase in the number of apneas during sleep, in the number of microarousals associated with nonapneic breathing disorders in sleep and in the amount of wake time within sleep. Surrat et al. [66] concluded that intranasal obstruction with petroleum gauze produces predominantly obstructive apneas and hypopneas during sleep.

Complete nasal packing has also induced similar effects on patients who had nasal packs after nasal polypectomy or septoplasty [67] or for treating nose bleeds [74]. These studies performed on volunteers or on subjects with no SRBD but subjected to complete nasal obstruction with nasal packing suggest that nasal obstruction may trigger the induction of sleep-disordered breathing in normal individuals and that nasal breathing increases ventilation efficiency by stimulating certain sensory trigeminal receptors in the nasal mucosa. However, the likelihood of developing SRBD after nasal resistance variation or nasal anesthesia did not concern all the volunteers.

The relationship between nasal patency and SRBD has also been studied in patients with SRBD and in patients with abnormal nasal patency. Miljeteig et al. [45] studied 683 unselected patients referred for snoring and/or apnea evaluation and assessed nasal resistance and sleep parameters.

All patients had determination of nasal resistance (performed with the patient in the seated posture during wakefulness) and nocturnal polysomnography including quantitative measurement of snoring. They found no correlation between the unilateral or bilateral increase of nasal resistance and snoring and/or apnea and no direct relation between awake seated nasal resistance and sleep parameters. This was also confirmed by others studies in which nasal obstruction was expressed as nasal airway resistance [28].

In the study by Miljeteig et al. [46] in 1993, despite the significant differences in nasal resistance, they were not reflected in the number of snores or their sound intensity, during exclusively nasal breathing.

In a study with positional anterior active rhinomanometry De Vito et al. [13] found no statistically significant differences in the degree of the apnea–hypopnea index (AHI) between 20 patients with normal positional anterior active rhinomanometry and 16 with pathologic positional anterior active rhinomanometry. Some others studies, however, suggested a relationship based on four different arguments.

Firstly, patients with a complaint of nasal obstruction and SRBD are at higher risk of developing OSAS [38, 40]. The contribution of nasal resistance to OSAS is rather weak; however, daytime nasal obstruction measured by posterior active rhinomanometry (thus including the valve area) is clearly assessed as an independent risk factor for OSAS. In the study of Losafo et al. [40] of 541 consecutive snorers, 528 underwent nasal resistance measurement by posterior rhinomanometry with a failure rate of 2.4%. Patients with OSAS (n=259) had higher nasal resistance than patients without OSAS (2.6±1.6 vs. 2.2±1.0 hPa L/s, respectively, $p<0.005$).It was found that 2.3% of the variance in the AHI was explained by nasal resistance. In a cohort study of patients referred for evaluation of SRBD, Liistro et al. [38] found a correlation between the Mallampati score (MS). In this study it was postulated that if the subjects could not breathe through the nose, the oral airway must be used, but if this airway is narrowed as well, then it could precipitate sleep-disordered breathing.

Nasal patency, MS, neck circumference and body mass index were measured in 202 subjects who were to undergo a full-night polysomnography for suspicion of SRDB. The patients were asked to open the mouth wide with voluntary protrusion of the tongue without phonation and were graded from 1 to 4, and were subjected to simple nasal examination (patients were asked to gently block one nostril and to inspire through the nonoccluded nostril, then nasal obstruction was reported if the examiner heard a noise suggesting nasal obstruction). A significant correlation was found between the MS and the AHI measured during sleep; however, the relationship between these parameters was only significant in patients with nasal obstruction [38]. Thus, the presence of a high MS with concomitant nasal obstruction is associated with an increased risk of OSAS.

Secondly, patients with SRBD, both snorers and OSAS patients, switch more frequently from nasal to mouth breathing during sleep if nasal obstruction is present. This may lead to an increase in respiratory effort and may result in alveolar hypoventilation [47, 48].

In the study by Ohki et al. [48], cotton pledgets of several sizes were inserted into the nasal vestibules in order to decrease progressively the nasal patency. Nasal respiratory resistance and nasal fraction were measured repeatedly until the subjects had to breathe through the mouth completely. Although the value of the nasal respiratory resistance in patients with complaints of snoring or sleep apnea was higher than that of normal subjects, most of the patients did not complain of a sensation of nasal obstruction. However, the switching point from nasal to mouth breathing in patients with complaints of snoring or sleep apnea was statistically higher than that in normal subjects.

Tips and Pearls

■ These results suggest that patients with complaints of snoring or sleep apnea can easily breathe through the mouth during sleep, and also that chronic nasal obstruction may induce obstructive sleep apnea [48].

Thirdly, cohort studies have demonstrated that patients with nighttime symptoms of rhinitis or with nasal congestion, and especially with nocturnal nasal obstruction, are at higher risk of developing SRBD and of snoring [42, 76].

Finally, total nasal resistance in a nonobese subgroup of patients measured in the supine position correlated with some sleep parameters. In this subgroup, Virkkula et al. [72] demonstrated a positive relationship between total nasal resistance and the AHI ($r=0.50$, $p<0.05$) and oxygen desaturation ($r=0.58$, $p<0.05$) among 41 snoring men on a waiting list for correction of nasal obstruction who underwent polysomnography, anterior rhinomanometry and acoustic rhinometry.

Tips and Pearls

■ All together, these studies suggest a weak relation between nasal resistance and SRBD for the vast majority of patients.

Nasal obstruction from any cause does augment airway collapse. It is also important to point out that this relationship may be more pronounced in a subgroup of patients if nasal resistance is measured in the supine position. Moreover, nasal obstruction appears to increase the risk of developing SRBD.

The relationship between nasal obstruction secondary to sinonasal disease and SRBD has also been evaluated. It has long been assumed that allergic rhinitis leads to daytime sleepiness and a deterioration of nocturnal sleep; some systematic studies have been conducted in this field. Allergic rhinitis (seasonal and perennial) causes daytime and nighttime nasal obstruction and is a naturally occurring model of reversible nasal obstruction. Polysomnographic studies during increased allergen exposure have shown an increase in the AHI, in excessive daytime sleepiness, in snoring and in microarousal per hours of sleep, though this increase in the AHI was not clinically relevant [36, 43, 44, 65, 76]. In patients with allergic rhinitis, obstructive sleep apneas are longer and more frequent during a period of symptomatic nasal obstruction than when symptoms are absent.

In the study by Lavie et al. [36], patients suffering from allergic rhinitis had an average of 50 "microarousals" from sleep – 10 times more than normal controls.

In the work of McColley et al. [43] in 1997, the frequency of OSAS was increased in subjects with positive radioallergosorbent test (RAST) results compared with those with negative RAST results (57 vs. 40%; $\chi^2=9.11$; $p<0.01$) in a population of pediatric patients with habitual snoring. However, in the study by Stuck et al. [65], daytime sleepiness seems to be related to the allergic condition itself rather than to an impairment of nocturnal sleep. Seasonal allergic rhinitis leads to increased daytime sleepiness, as well as to an impairment of quality of life, depending on the severity of the disease.

In patients with allergic rhinitis treated with a nasal steroid, sleep disturbances and daytime fatigue tended to improve [10].

The exact role of allergic rhinitis, however, in poor sleep quality may also be secondary to medication such as antihistamines which are frequently prescribed for this disease and are known to induce somnolence in some subjects [16].

The poor quality of sleep among patients with allergic rhinitis may be due to mechanisms other than nasal obstruction [16]. The mediators of allergic rhinitis, including histamine, leukotrienes, cytokines and prostaglandins, may play a role in sleep regulation and, thus, may be directly involved in this impairment independent of nasal obstruction. Inflammatory mediators secondary to allergic inflammation have a diurnal variation and peak during the early morning. This peak could explain the symptoms of allergic rhinitis on waking. This may result from a nighttime decrease in glucocorticoid receptor binding affinity. It is also important to point out that sympathetic tone decreases at night, producing a relative parasympathetic excess.

Tips and Pearls

■ Sleep quality may therefore decrease in patients with allergic rhinitis through different mechanisms: nasal obstruction, postural changes, clinical variations of inflammatory mediators

30

or adverse effects of antihistamine therapy especially when using the first generation of "sedating" anti-H1.

Anatomical obstruction owing to severe septal deviation or hypertrophy of the inferior turbinate may also predispose to SRBD [37, 64]. This is also true for patients with nasal polyposis [71].

Silvioniemi et al. [64] advocate that while rhinomanometry can only measure the amount of nasal resistance, acoustic rhinometry can clearly determine the exact size and location of the different stenoses in the nasal cavity that contribute to the increased nasal resistance.

Treatments for Nasal Obstruction and Their Impacts on SRBD

If nasal obstruction and increased nasal resistance may promote SRBD, it seems to be logical to study the effects of a reduced resistance on sleep parameters. This has been done in multiple ways, including medications, nasal dilators and surgical procedures.

Medications

Allergic rhinitis is classically characterized by sneezing, nasal itching, rhinorrhea and nasal obstruction. These symptoms can impair nocturnal sleep, resulting in daytime fatigue and somnolence, both of them decreasing learning capacity, work efficiency and patient quality of life. In addition, the mediators of allergic, possibly impair the quality of sleep.

Some medications that reduce nasal congestion have adverse effects on sleep. α-agonist decongestants effectively reduce nasal congestion but frequently produce stimulatory effects, palpitations and in some cases insomnia. Antihistamines reduce sneezing and pruritus, but are less effective in relieving congestion, at least during the first 3 weeks of treatment. Intranasal corticosteroids and oral leukotriene receptor antagonists effectively reduce rhinorrhea, congestion and inflammatory mediators.

Medical relief of nasal obstruction and its impact on SRDB has been studied in patients with allergic rhinitis and the effects analyzed with questionnaires or polysomnographic data.

Tips and Pearls
- Subjective sleep quality improves in patients with allergic rhinitis after treatment with intranasal steroids (Table 30.1).

This has been confirmed by two placebo-controlled studies performed with fluticasone propionate and budesonide in patients with perennial allergic rhinitis [10, 20, 27]. Often, people with perennial allergies may attribute their daytime fatigue to causes such as the side effects of medications, when in fact the fatigue may be a result of nasal congestion and associated sleep fragmentation. Decreasing nasal congestion due to allergic rhinitis with intranasal steroids may improve sleep, daytime fatigue and the quality of life of patients. Medications directed toward reversal of nasal congestion work also through suppression of inflammatory mediators and constitute a major therapy for SRBD associated with allergic rhinitis.

In seasonal allergic rhinitis, the nighttime score for fluticasone propionate was better than for the antileukotriene montelukast in a large cohort of patients consisting of 705 eligible men and women (15 years of age or older) in a randomized, double-blind, double-dummy, parallel-group study by Ratner et al. [57].

Finally, two recent studies have tried to demonstrate the objective modification of sleep parameters in patients with allergic rhinitis or in snorers with rhinitis. Both studies were performed with the topical application of fluticasone propionate. Craig et al. [9] found no difference in the polysomnographic data but an improvement in subjective sleep parameters when treating patients with perennial allergy with fluticasone propionate in an 8-week, double-blind, placebo-controlled study among 32 subjects. Fluticasone (50 mg per spray), two sprays each side every day, improved subjective sleep when compared with the placebo ($p = 0.04$); however, there was no difference in the AHI in those that were treated. Daytime sleepiness and fatigue were decreased by more than 10% in the treated group.

On the other hand, Kiely et al. [31] have demonstrated a more pronounced though slight decrease in the AHI in snorers with rhinitis treated with fluticasone propionate compared with those given a placebo.

In summary, nasal obstruction secondary to allergic inflammation has an impact on sleep quality and topical corticoid therapy seems to have a positive effect on subjective sleep quality and also on polysomnographic data in one study [9, 10, 20, 27, 31, 57].

Nasal Dilators

The ability to breath through the nose can be increased above normal by dilating the narrow nasal valve area. Nasal dilators are an attractive method of decreasing nasal resistance in the valve area and subsequently have a positive impact on snoring and/or apnea [52].

Table 30.1. **Effect of medical therapy on sleep-related breathing disorders. (Courtesy of [54] with permission)**

Authors	Medication	Number of patients	Nasal disease	Sleep parameters
Graig, 1998	Fluticasone	20	Perennial allergic rhinitis	No PSG Subjective sleep quality improvement
Hughues, 2003	Budesonide	22	Perennial allergic rhinitis	No PSG Subjective sleep quality improvement and daytime fatigue
Ratner, 2003	Fluticasone vs montelukast	705	Seasonal allergic rhinitis	No PSG Night-time symptoms score decrease FP>M
Graig, 2003	Fluticasone	32	Perennial allergic rhinitis	No difference with objective data but well with subjective ones
Kiely, 2004	Fluticasone	24	Snorers with rhinitis	Slight decrease of AHI and related to NR

PSG polysomnographic data *FP* fluticasone propionate, *M* montelukast, *AHI* apnea–hypopnea index, *NR* nasal resistance

Measurements of nasal resistance in awake subjects with the devices have shown a reduction in resistance, though not uniform, depending on the compliance of the nasal vestibule walls [51].

The dimension of the nasal valve is increased by approximately 30%. There are actually two devices commercially available as nasal dilators: Nozovent®, an internal device, and Breathe Right®, an external device. These devices have been studied in patients with polysomnographic measurements in nine studies (Table 30.2) [2, 14, 19, 24, 26, 39, 53, 61, 68].

The conclusions from these studies are that nasal dilators may reduce the subjective sensation of snoring, but the objective measurements of snoring as well as sleep parameters such the AHI reveal that nasal dilators are ineffective for the vast majority of SRBD patients. Only two studies have shown a positive effect on the AHI, but in less than 30% of the patients [26, 58]. The nasal dilators may be more effective in patients with SRDB with concomitant chronic rhinitis [53]. Djupesland et al. [14] found that Breathe Right® was an effective treatment of snoring in a subgroup of patients by morning nasal obstruction and when acoustic rhinometry revealed a minimal cross-sectional area of less than 0.6 cm². On the basis of this information, nasal dilators are ineffective for the vast majority of apneic patients but may be recommended as a trial for nonapneic snorers. Nasal dilators have no side effects and are relatively inexpensive. Patients with nasal valve stenosis and/or chronic rhinitis are the best candidates.

Nasal and Sinus Surgery

Nasal and sinus surgery are often performed to reduce nasal obstruction and their effects on SRBD may also be expected. Various surgical procedures are described to increase nasal patency: septo(rhino)plasty, turbinoplasty, radiofrequency tissue volume reduction of the inferior turbinates, functional endoscopic endonasal surgery or correction of the nasal valve.

The primary goal of these procedures is related to the nasal obstruction itself, to the improvement of SRBD, or both. Improvement of compliance with nasal continuous positive airway pressure (nCPAP) therapy by reducing nasal obstruction may also be an objective. In these procedures little attention has been paid to the nasal anterior valve, which may play a crucial role in nasal obstruction and which is dedicated to modifying the air stream penetrating the nose (Figs. 30.3, 30.4). Subjective improvement in sleep quality and reduction of snoring have been described in a study without polysomnographic data by correction of the nasal valve using a functional and aesthetic septorhinoplasty through an open approach with lateral graft cartilage insertion (modified spreader grafts) in order to enlarge the angle of the isthmus nasi (Fig. 30.5) [4]. From this study by Bertrand et al. [4], it was demonstrated that the patients recorded a significant increase in nasal patency on a visual analog scale before and 1 year after surgery, but that there is no clear-cut evidence of improvement in nasal resistances measured by anterior active rhinomanometry and posterior active rhinomanometry. The authors suggested that the decrease in snoring may be induced by changes in the direction of the nasal air-

Table 30.2. Effect of nasal dilators on sleep-related breathing disorders. (Courtesy of [54] with permission)

Authors	Nasal dilators	Number of patients	Sleep parameters and remarks
Hoijer, 1992	Nozovent	10	Improvement
Hoffstein, 1993	Nozovent	15	No change except snoring in slow wave sleep
Liistro, 1998	Breathe Right	10	No change
Todorova, 1998	Breathe Right	30	No change
Gosepath, 1999	Breathe Right	26	Reduced in 4/26
Bahamman, 1999	Breathe Right	18	No change
Schönhofer, 2000	Nozovent	21	No change
Pevernagie, 2000	Breathe Right	12	No change except snoring index in chronic rhinitis patients
Djupesland, 2001	Breathe right	18	No change except slight reduction in AHI when MCA<0.6 cm^2 (6/18)

MCA mean cross-sectional area

Table 30.3. Effect of nasal and sinus surgery on sleep-related breathing disorders. (Courtesy of [54] with permission)

Authors	Number of patients	AI before/after	AHI before/after	Results
Heimer, 1983	3			3 patients cured
Rubin, 1983	9	37.8/26.7		$p<0.5$
Dayat, 1985	6		46.8/28.2	NS
Caldarelli, 1985	23	44.2/41.5		NS
Aubert, 1989	2	47.5/48.5		NS
Séries, 1992	20		39.8/36.8	NS
Séries, 1993	14	17.8/16		NS
Utley, 1997	4		11.9/27	Worse
Verse, 2002	26		14/57.7	Worse
Friedman, 2000	50 (22 OSAS)		31.6/39.5	Worse
Verse, 2002	26		31.6/28.9	NS, 3 OSAS patients cured
Kim, 2004	21		39/29	$P=0.0001$, 4 OSAS patients cued

OSAS obstructive sleep apnea syndrome, *AI* apnea index, *NS* not significant

flow against the nasal mucosa which may produce by a reflex between mechanoreceptors of the nasal mucosa and muscles of the pharynx an increased tonus of the muscles of the pharynx.

This was also confirmed in a study examining the effects of nasal surgery on snoring where 48 of 96 patients reported complete relief of snoring after conventional nasal surgery and/or polypectomy [15].

There are objective data from preoperative and postoperative polysomnographic studies regarding the effects of nasal surgery on SRBD in 12 studies (Table 30.3) [1, 6, 11, 18, 22, 32, 37, 59, 62, 63, 69, 70]

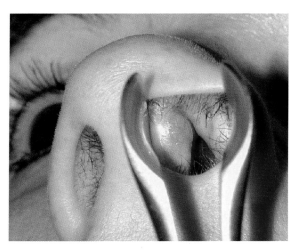

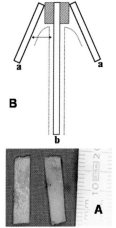

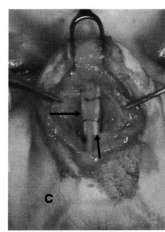

Fig. 30.3. The figure shows a closed isthmus nasi that cannot be surgically treated by common septoplasty. A surgical correction of the anterior edge of the quadrangular cartilage by an open-approach septorhinoplasty is required

Fig. 30.5. Lateral graft cartilages (modified spreader grafts) surgical technique through an open approach septorhino-plasty. **A** Small rectangular pieces of cartilage are harvested usually from the septal cartilage and shaped to the required form to be set in place in the isthmus nasi area. **B** The grafts (*hatched blocks*) are to be sutured longitudinally to the anterior edge of the nasal septum, in order to widen the angle of the isthmus nasi (*double-headed arrow*). *a* upper lateral cartilage (septolateral cartilage), *b* septal cartilage, *dotted line* nasal mucosa. **C** The two grafts are sutured along the anterior edge of the septum (*arrows*) on the left and right sides, after dissection of the mucosa and section of the junctions between the upper lateral and septal cartilages. (Courtesy of and modified from [54] with permission)

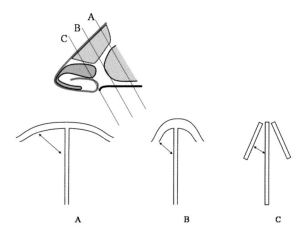

Fig. 30.4. Plane sections in *A, B* and *C* of the nasal pyramid showing the variable value of the angle (*double-headed arrows*) between the septolateral cartilage and the quadrangular cartilage. In section *C* the normal value of the angle in the valve area (isthmus nasi) is about 15°. *Dark red* skin of the nasal pyramid, *light yellow* septolateral cartilage (upper lateral cartilage), *dark yellow* alar cartilage (lower lateral cartilage), *red hatching* head of the inferior turbinate, *black* nasal floor. (Courtesy of and modified from [54] with permission)

relief may allow the patients to sleep in deeper stages of sleep. Therefore, apnea and sleep fragmentation are increased because patients sleep more comfortably. Friedman et al. have also demonstrated that nCPAP requirements are decreased after nasal surgery. The mean nCPAP titration level was 9.3 cm H_2O before surgery vs. 6.7 cm H_2O after surgery [18].

Nasal surgery, as with nasal dilators, may improve subjective snoring or daytime fatigue but cure of sleep apnea occurs only in approximately 15–20% of cases.

Tips and Pearls

■ Results of nasal surgery in patients with sleep apnea/hypopnea are therefore barely predictable.

Nasal Disease and Surgery in nCPAP Patients

Patients with moderate to severe OSAS are candidates for nCPAP, which means long-term nightly use of relatively cumbersome and expensive breathing equipment that provides CPAP via a nasal or facial mask [23]. This treatment remains the most effective for reducing snoring and morbidity related to apne-

Although some of these studies have demonstrated a slight decrease in the AHI for some patients, the success rate (as defined by an AHI reduction by at least 50% and an AHI value below 20) is very low. Verse et al. [70] reported a success rate of 15.8% (3 of 19 apneic patients) using these criteria. Friedman et al. [18] have also suggested that postoperative polysomnographic data may be worse for mild OSAS patients after nasal obstruction relief. They explain this paradoxical effect of nasal surgery by the fact that nasal obstruction

ic episodes [25]; however, it may have adverse effects, of which nasal problems are the most frequently encountered [12]. According to Hoffstein et al. [25] in a study ($n = 138$) using detailed questionnaires mailed or phoned to patients with obstructive sleep apnea, the most common complaint, voiced by 46% of the patients, was nocturnal awakenings. Nasal problems, such as dryness, congestion and sneezing, were the second most frequent complaint, present in 44% of the responders.

Tips and Pearls

- It has been demonstrated that nCPAP therapy induces nasal mucosal inflammation and promotes nasal hyperreactivity [60].

More than half of patients using nCPAP therapy present with significant nasal complaints [25]. Rhinorrhea induced by nCPAP may be treated with anticholinergic medication (ipratropium bromide), which consistently reduces watery rhinorrhea. Nasal congestion may appear after some days of nCPAP use and may be treated by topical nasal steroids or nasal vasoconstrictors for a few days. Saline nasal spray and heated humidification are commonly used to prevent problems related to nCPAP. Massie et al. [41] concluded that compliance with CPAP is enhanced when heated humidification is employed, owing to a reduction in side effects associated with upper-airway symptoms and a more refreshed feeling upon awakening and that compliance gains may be realized sooner if patients are started with heated humidity at CPAP initiation.. Corrective nasal surgery or turbinate volume reduction may help patients to tolerate nCPAP therapy [55]. When a dysfunction or weakness of the nasal valve is present, patients using nCPAP may experience alar collapse during inflation owing to the high pressure of nCPAP; this condition can be treated by surgery of the valve [4] or even by a Z-plasty of the nostrils.

Nose and Sinus Surgery and Immediate Postoperative Management of Patients with OSAS

Currently, there is no widely accepted consensus on the management of patients with OSAS undergoing nasal surgery [54]. In general, such patients should undergo a preoperative polysomnographic study and OSAS should be treated in the preoperative period with nCPAP therapy. General anesthesia during surgery should be kept to a minimum length of time and appropriate sedatives, anesthetics and analgesics should be given [23] (Table 30.4). Patients with OSAS need to be closely monitored in the postoperative pe-

riod. Although preferable, the authors do not consider a stay in intensive care mandatory. Minimum requirements, however, include nocturnal oxymetry with appropriate treatment in the event of oxygen desaturation. A crucial question when performing nasal surgery in patients with OSAS is the use of postoperative nasal packing. Nasal packing is a standard procedure after nasal surgery and is supposed to decrease postoperative bleeding and the risk of synechiae. Nasal packing, however, has many adverse effects, such as pain, discomfort, infection and obligatory mouth breathing.

Tips and Pearls

- The complete obstruction of the nostril with packing after surgery in patients with OSAS may be associated with sleep interference as the so-called nasopulmonary reflex is abolished and blood gas tension may reveal a relative hypoxemia [5, 29, 30, 58]

In a study by Buckley et al. [5] continuous digital pulse oximetry was carried out before and after submucous resection of the nasal septum in 17 otherwise healthy patients. Postoperative nasal packing produced a statistically significant change in oxygen saturation during sleep. The change was of small magnitude and is unlikely to be clinically significant. In the study by Kalogiera et al. [30] in a group of 17 patients during a 5-day period of anterior nasal packing after endonasal surgery, significant hypocapnia was observed in the early postoperative period, which was followed by significant hypoxemia within the first 2-day period after surgery, and also shortly after removal of the nasal pack. Rombaux et al. [58] recorded nocturnal oxymetry in ten otherwise healthy patients undergoing different types of nasal surgery with total nasal packing. Postoperative nocturnal oxymetry was worse than preoperative in one of six patients and judged as abnormal in four.

Other options, therefore, might be proposed in the postoperative period, such as septal suturing without nasal packing or the insertion of a nasal pack with an airway tube inside [33, 73].

Application of nCPAP therapy may sometimes be difficult and oronasal masks are in some cases essential. An oronasal mask allows the application of the positive pressure through the mouth as long as the nose is blocked. There is no absolute consensus on the length of duration of the nasal packing nor on the duration of hospitalization, but care should be taken to ensure that after removal of the packing patients will tolerate nCPAP well before being discharged (Table 30.5). After nasal surgery, the apneic patient needs to undergo a second polysomnographic study to assess the benefit of the surgical procedure. This sec-

Table 30.4. Management of nasal surgery in the OSAS patient. (Courtesy of [54] with permission)

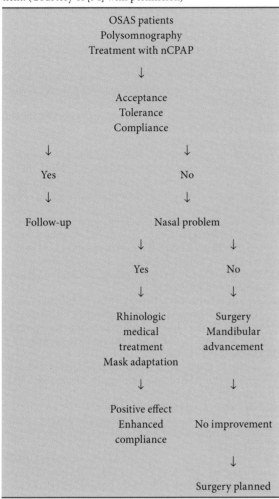

nCPAP nasal continuous positive airway pressure

Table 30.5. Management of nasal surgery in the OSAS patient. (Courtesy of [54] with permission)

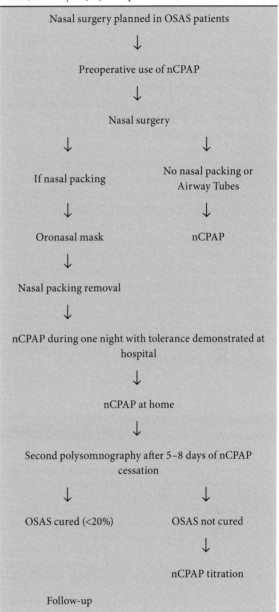

ond polysomnography should be done some days after nCPAP therapy has been stopped. An easy but not totally accepted method is to carry out the assessment in a single night using the first part of the night for the SRBD diagnosis and the second part of the night to titrate the nCPAP level if the patient fulfils the criteria for this treatment [54].

Conclusion

Nasal obstruction may trigger sleep disorders in normal subjects and make worse SRBD in patients with apnea, hypopnea, upper-airway resistance and/or primary snoring. Nasal examination by anterior rhinoscopy at least, but also through a fiberoscopy of the full nose, and measurement of nasal resistance–by anterior and posterior active rhinomanometry–are mandatory in the management of patients with SRBD. In our opinion, special attention has to be paid to the valve area of the nose. Cross sections of the valve area, which is the place where the ingoing inspiratory air stream gains its highest velocity, can be measured by acoustic rhinometry with more accura-

30

cy; unfortunately this examination is not done routinely yet.

Treatments are mainly based on topical steroid medications, nasal dilators and/or surgery. Globally, results are unpredictable in most patients. Subjective analysis with questionnaires on snoring or daytime fatigue or excessive daytime sleepiness has revealed that the treatment of nasal disorders in SRBD patients is beneficial. Objective data, however, with pretherapy and post-therapy polysomnographic studies are far less encouraging. The success rate of common nasal surgery, for instance, appears to be less than 20%, although normalization of nasal resistance is achieved in most cases. It should also be noted that nasal surgery may even worsen SRBD. In this instance, a good description of the anatomical improvement after nose surgery for septal deviation surgery is lacking in the literature. Finally, rhinologic procedures may be a consideration for patients with poor compliance with nCPAP therapy. The nasal airway segment may also be considered when a multilevel strategy is proposed to the patient with SRDB.

References

1. Aubert-Tulkens G, Hamoir M, Van Den Eeckhaut J, Rodenstein DO (1989) Failure of tonsil and nose surgery in adults with long standing severe sleep apnea syndrome. Arch Intern Med 149:2118–2121.
2. Bahamman AS, Tate R, Manfreda J, Kryger M (1999) Upper airway resistance syndrome: effect of nasal dilation on sleep stage and sleep position. Sleep 22:592–598.
3. Berry R, McNellis M, Kouchi K, Light RW (1997) Upper airway anesthesia reduces phasic genioglossus activity during sleep apnea. Am J Respir Crit Care Med 156:127–132.
4. Bertrand B, Eloy Ph, Collet S, Lamarque C, Rombaux P (2002) Effect of nasal valve surgery by open septorhinoplasty and lateral cartilage grafts (Spreader grafts) on snoring among a population of simple snorers. Acta Oto-Rhino-Laryngol Belg 56:149–156.
5. Buckley JG, Hickey SA, Fitzgerald O'Connor AF (1991) Does postoperative nasal packing cause nocturnal oxygen desaturation? J Laryngol Otol 105:109–111.
6. Caldarelli DD, Cartwright R, Lilie J (1985) Obstructive sleep apnea: variations in surgical management. Laryngoscope 95:1070–7073.
7. Cole P (1992) Nasal and oral airflow resistors. Arch Otolaryngol Head Neck Surg 118:790–793.
8. Cole P, Haight JS (1984) Mechanisms of nasal obstruction in sleep. Laryngoscope 94:1557–1559.
9. Craig TJ, Mende C, Hughes K, Kakumanu S, Lehman EB, Chinchilli V (2003) The effect of topical nasal fluticasone on objective sleep testing and the symptoms of rhinitis, sleep and daytime. Allergy Asthma Proc 24:53–58.
10. Craig TJ, Teets S, Lehman E, Chinchilli V, Zwillich C (1989) Nasal congestion secondary to allergic rhinitis as a cause of sleep disturbance and daytime fatigue and the response to topical corticosteroids. J Allergic Clin Immunol 101:633–637.
11. Dayal VS, Philipson EA (1985) Nasal surgery in the management of sleep apnea. Ann Otol Rhinol Laryngol 94:550–554.
12. Deron P, Volckaert A, Clement P (2002) Nasal patency and sleep related breathing disorders. Acta Oto-Rhino-Laryngologica Belgica 56:117–120.
13. De Vito A, Berrettini S, Carabelli A, Sellari-Franceschini S, Bonanni E, Gori S, Pasquali L, Murri L (2001) The importance of nasal resistance in obstruction sleep apnea syndrome: a study with positional rhinomanometry. Sleep Breath 5:3–11.
14. Djupesland PG, Stakvedt O, Borgersen A (2001) Dichotomous physiological effects of nocturnal external nasal dilation in heavy snorers: the answer to a rhinologic controversy? Am J Rhinol 15:95–103.
15. Elsherif I, Hussein S (1998) The effect of nasal surgery on snoring. Am J Rhinol 12: 7-79.
16. Fergusson BJ. (2004) Influence of allergic rhinitis on sleep. Otolaryngol Head Neck Surg 130:617–629.
17. Ferris B, Mead J, Opie L (1964) Partitioning of respiratory flow resistance in man. J Appl Physiol 19:653–658.
18. Friedman M, Tanyeri H, Lim J, Landsberg R, Vaidyanathan K, Caldarelli D (2000) Effects of improved nasal breathing on obstructive sleep apnea. Otolaryngol Head Neck Surg 122:71–74.
19. Gosepath J, Amedee R., Romanstschuk S, Mann W (1999) Breathe Right nasal strips and respiratory disturbance index in sleep related breathing disorders. Am J Rhinol 13:385–389.
20. Gurevich F, Glass C, Davies M, Wei W, McCann J, Fisher L, Chegini S, Mende C, Craig T (2005) The effect of intranasal steroid budesonide on the congestion-related sleep disturbance and daytime somnolence in patients with perennial allergic rhinitis. Allergy Asthma Proc 26(4):268–74.
21. Haight JS, Djupesland PG (2003) Nitric oxide (NO) and obstructive sleep apnea (OSA). Sleep Breath 7:53–62.
22. Heimer D, Scharf SM, Lieberman A, Lavie P (1983) Sleep apnea syndrome treated by repair of deviated septum. Chest 84:184–185.
23. Hoffstein V (2002) Apnea and snoring: state of the art and future direction. Acta-Oto-Rhino-Laryngol Belg 56:205–236.
24. Hoffstein V, Mateika S, Metes A (1993) Effects of nasal dilation on snoring and apneas during different stages of sleep. Sleep 16:360–365.
25. Hoffstein V, Viner S, Mateika S, Conway J (1992) Treatment of obstructive sleep apnea with nasal continuous positive airway pressure. Am Rev Respir Dis 145:841–845.
26. Höijer U, Ejnell H, Hedner J, Petrusson B (1992) The effect of nasal dilation on snoring and apnea. Arch Otolaryngol Head Neck Surg 18:281–284.
27. Hugues K, Glass C, Ripchinski M., Gurevich F, Weaver TE, Lehman E, Fisher LH, Craig TJ (2003) Efficacy of the topical nasal steroid budesonide on improving sleep and daytime somnolence in patients with perennial allergic rhinitis. Allergy 58:380–385.

28. Jessen M, Fryrsmark U (1993) Is there a relationship between the degree of nasal obstruction and the snoring ? Clin Otolaryngol 18:485–487.

29. Johannessen N, Jensen PF, Kristensen S, Juul A (1992) Nasal packing and nocturnal oxygen desaturation. Acta Otolaryngol Suppl 492:6–8.

30. Kalogjera L, Pegan B, Petric V (1995) Adaptation to oral breathing after anterior nasal packing. Acta Otolaryngol 115:304–306.

31. Kiely JL, Nolan P, McNicholas WT (2004) Intranasal corticosteroid therapy for obstructive sleep apnea in patients with co-existing rhinitis. Thorax 59:50–55.

32. Kim ST, Choi JH, Jeon HG, Cha HE, Kim DY, Chung YS (2004) Polysomnographic effects of nasal surgery for snoring and obstructive sleep apnea. Acta Otolaryngol 124:297–300.

33. Kristensen S, Bjerregaard P, Jensen PF, Juul A (1996) Postoperative nocturnal hypoxia in septoplasty: the value of nasal packing with airway tubes. Clin Otolaryngol Allied Sci 21(4):331–334.

34. Lavie P (1987) Rediscovering the importance of nasal breathing in sleep or shut your mouth and save your sleep. J Laryngol Otol 101:558–563.

35. Lavie P, Fishel N, Zomer J, Eliashar I (1985) The effects of partial and complete mechanical occlusion of the nasal passages on sleep structure and breathing in sleep. Acta Otolaryngol 95:161–166.

36. Lavie P, Gertner R, Zomer F, Podoshin L (1981) Breathing disorders in sleep associated with microarousals in patients with allergic rhinitis. Acta Otolaryngol 92:529–533.

37. Lenders H, Schaefer J, Pirsig W (1991) Turbinate hypertrophy in habitual snorers and patients with sleep apnea: findings of acoustic rhinometry. Laryngoscope 101:614–618.

38. Liistro G, Rombaux P, Belge C, Dury M, Aubert G, Rodenstein D (2003) High Mallampati score and nasal obstruction are associated risk factors for obstructive sleep apnea. Eur Respir J 21:248–252.

39. Liistro G, Rombaux P, Dury M, Pieters T, Aubert G, Rodenstein DO (1998) Effects of Breathe Right on snoring: a polysomnographic study. Respir Med 92:1076–1078.

40. Lofaso F, Coste A, D'Ortho M, Zerah-Lancner F, Delclaux C, Goldenberg F, Harf A (2000) Nasal obstruction as a risk factor for sleep apnea syndrome. Eur Respir J 16:639–643.

41. Massie CA, Hart RW, Peralez R, Richards G (1999) Effects of humidification on nasal symptoms and compliance in sleep apnea patients using continuous positive airway pressure. Chest 116:403–408.

42. Metes A, Cole P, Hoffstein V, Miljeteig H (1992) Nasal airway dilation and obstructed breathing in sleep. Laryngoscope 102:1053–1055.

43. McColley S, Carroll JL, Curtis S, Loughlin G, Sampson H (1997) High prevalence of allergic sensitization in children with habitual snoring and obstructive sleep apnea. Chest 111:170–173.

44. McNicholas W, Tarlo S, Cole P, Zamel N, Rutherford R, Griffin D, Phillipson EA (1982) Obstructive apneas during sleep in patients with seasonal allergic rhinitis. Am Rev Respir Dis 126:625–628.

45. Miljeteig H, Hoffstein V, Cole P (1993) The effects of unilateral and bilateral nasal obstruction on snoring and sleep apnea. Laryngoscope 102:1150–1152.

46. Miljeteig H, Savard P, Mateika S, Cole P, Haight JS, Hoffstein V (1993) Snoring and nasal resistance during sleep. Laryngoscope 103 918–923.

47. Nihinimaa V, Cole P, Mintz S, Shepard RJ (1980) The switching point from nasal to ornasal breathing. Respir Physiol 42:61–71.

48. Ohki M, Ushi N, Kanazawa H, Hara L, Kawano K (1996) Relationship between oral breathing and nasal obstruction in patients with obstruction sleep apnea. Acta Otolaryngol 52:228–230.

49. Olsen KD, Kern EB, Westbrook PR (1981) Sleep and breathing disturbances secondary to nasal obstruction. Otolaryngol Head Neck Surg 89:804–810.

50. Park SS (1993) Flow-regulatory function of upper airway in health and disease unified pathogenic view of sleep-disordered breathing. Lung 171:311–333.

51. Petruson B (1994) Increased nasal breathing decreases snoring and improves oxygen saturation during sleep apnea. Rhinology 32:87–98.

52. Petruson B (1990) Snoring can be reduced when the nasal airflow is increased by the nasal dilator Nozovent. Arch Otolaryngol Head Neck Surg 116:462–464.

53. Pevernagie D, Hamans E, Van Cauwenberge P, Pauwels R (2000) External nasal dilation reduces snoring in chronic rhinitis patients; an randomized controlled trial. Eur Respir J 15:996–1000.

54. Rombaux P, Liistro G, Hamoir M, Bertrand B, Aubert G, Verse T, Rodenstein D (2005) Nasal obstruction and its impact on sleep-related breathing disorders: a review. Rhinology 43(4):242–250.

55. Powell N (2001) Radiofrequency treatment of turbinate hypertrophy in subjects using CPAP: a randomized double blind placebo controlled clinical trial. Laryngoscope 111:1783–1790.

56. Rappai M, Collop N, Kemp S, deShazo R (2003) The nose and sleep-disordered breathing. What we know and what we do not know. Chest 124:2309–2323.

57. Ratner PH, Howland WC, Arastu R, Philpot EE, Klein KC, Baidoo CA, Faris MA, Richard KA (2003) Fluticasone propionate aqueous nasal spray provided significantly greater improvement in daytime and night-time nasal symptoms of seasonal allergic rhinitis compared with Montelukast. Ann Allergy Asthma Immunol 90:466–468.

58. Rombaux P, Liistro G, Hamoir M, Eloy P, Bertrand B, Collard Ph (1998) Nocturnal oxymetry in patients with total nasal packing. Acta Oto-Rhino-Laryngol Belg 52:223–228.

59. Rubin A, Eliashar I, Joachim Z, Alroy G, Lavie P (1983) Effects of nasal surgery and tonsillectomy on sleep apnea. Bull Eur Physiopathol Respir 19:612–615.

60. Rubinstein I (1995) Nasal inflammation in patients with obstructive sleep apnea. Laryngoscope 105:175–177.

61. Schönhofer B, Franklin K, Brünig H, Wehde H, Köhler D (2000) Effect of nasal valve dilation on obstructive sleep apnea. Chest 118:587–590.

62. Series F, St Pierre S, Carrier G (1992) Effects on surgical correction of nasal obstruction in the treatment of obstructive sleep apnea. Am Rev Respir Dis 146:1261–1265.

63. Series F, St Pierre S, Carrier G (1993) Surgical correction of nasal obstruction in the treatment of mild sleep apnea: importance of cephalometry in predicting outcome. Thorax 48:360–363.

64. Silvioniemi P, Suonpaa J, Sipila J, Grenman R, Erkinjuntti M (1997) Sleep disorders in patients with severe nasal obstruction due to septal deviation. Acta Otolaryngol 529:199–201.

65. Stuck BA, Czajkowski J, Hagner AE, Klimek L, Verse T, Hormann K, Maurer JT (2004) Changes in daytime sleepi-

ness, quality of life and objective signs of patterns in seasonal allergic rhinitis; a controlled clinical trial. J Allergy Clin Immunol 113:663–668.

66. Surrat PM, Turner BL, Wilhoit SC (1986) Effect of intranasal obstruction on breathing during sleep. Chest 90:324–329.

67. Taasan V, Wynne JW, Cassissi N, Block AJ (1981) The effect of nasal packing on sleep-disordered breathing and nocturnal oxygen desaturation. Laryngoscope 91:1163–1172.

68. Todorova A, Schellenberg R, Hofman H, Dimpfel W (1988) Effect of the external dilator Breathe Right on snoring. Eur J Med Res 3:367–379.

69. Utley DS, Shin EJ, Clerk AA, Terris J (1997) A cost effective and rationale surgical approach to patients with snoring, upper airway resistance syndrome or obstructive sleep apnea. Laryngoscope 107:726–734.

70. Verse T, Maurer JT, Pirsig W (2002) Effects of nasal surgery on sleep-related breathing disorders. Laryngoscope 112:64–68.

71. Verse T, Pirsig W, Kroker BA (1998) Obstructive Schlafapnoe und polyposis nasi. Laryngorhinootologie 77:150–152.

72. Virkkula P, Maasilta P, Hytonen M, Salmi T, Malmberg H (2003) Nasal obstruction and sleep-disordered breathing: the effects of supine body position on nasal measurements in snorers. Acta Otolaryngol 123:648–654.

73. Von Schoenberg M, Robinson P, Ryan R (1993) Nasal packing after routine nasal surgery–is it justified? J Laryngol Otol 107:902–905.

74. Wetmore SJ, Scrima L, Hiller FC (1988) Sleep apnea in epistaxis patients treated with nasal packs. Otolaryngol Head Neck Surgery 98:596–599.

75. White DP, Cadieux RJ, Lombard RM, Bixler EO, Kales, Zwillich CW (1985) The effects of nasal anesthesia on breathing during sleep. Am Rev Respir Dis 132:972–975.

76. Young T, Finn L, Kim H (2001) Chronic nasal congestion at night is a risk factor for snoring: in population-based cohort study. Arch Intern Med 161:1514–1519.

77. Zwillich CW, Pickett C, Hanson FN, Weil JV (1981) Disrupted sleep and prolonged apnea during nasal obstruction in normal men. Am Rev Respir Dis 124:158–160

Chapter 31

Radiofrequency of the Palate

31

Eric J. Kezirian

- Radiofrequency palatoplasty should be reserved for selected patients with a significant palatal component to primary snoring, upper airway resistance syndrome, or mild obstructive sleep apnea.

- In this procedure, radiofrequency energy is used to create thermal injury to the soft-palate musculature with possible removal of tissue. The healing process produces fibrosis to stiffen and shrink the soft palate. The most common methods of energy delivery in radiofrequency palatoplasty are temperature-controlled monopolar, bipolar, and plasma-mediated ablation.

- Treatment must be tailored to patient anatomy to minimize complications. With experience and careful attention to technique, the incidence of complications of moderate and major severity is low.

Contents

Introduction

Sleep-disordered breathing includes the spectrum of primary snoring, upper airway resistance syndrome, and obstructive sleep apnea (mild to moderate to severe). Diagnosis of these entities is based on the combination of history, physical examination, and formal evaluation with a sleep study.

Effective treatment of sleep-disordered breathing requires an accurate determination of the upper-airway structures that contribute to the disorder. For purposes of treatment, the upper airway can be artificially divided into three segments: nasal, palatal (including the palate and tonsils), and hypopharyngeal or retrolingual (actually corresponding to the portion of the oropharynx and hypopharynx posterior to the tongue base and epiglottis). In many cases, the palate plays a major role either in (1) the sound production of snoring seen in all forms of sleep-disordered breathing or (2) the airway narrowing and/or obstruction. Often there is an important difference between the structures involved in snoring sound production and the site(s) of airway obstruction; a key in evaluation and achieving successful outcomes is based on an understanding of these concepts and accurate diagnosis. Specifically, the palate may be the primary factor in the patient's condition, or it may represent only one of many structures involved.

A wide range of procedures is available to treat the spectrum of sleep-disordered breathing. A selected list of palate procedures includes the more-invasive (uvulopalatopharyngoplasty, uvulopalatal flap, lateral pharyngoplasty, transpalatal advancement pharyngoplasty, and Z-palatoplasty) and the less-invasive (radiofrequency palatoplasty, palatal implants, laser-assisted palatoplasty, injection snoreplasty, and the cautery-assisted palate stiffening operation) options. The more-invasive procedures incorporate a combination of directed tissue removal and repositioning to produce a greater change in upper-airway anatomy, while less-invasive procedures produce smaller changes in upper-airway structure and mechanics.

Among the palate procedures, radiofrequency palatoplasty is a less-invasive procedure with demonstrated success in treating patients with a significant palatal component to primary snoring, upper airway resistance syndrome, or mild obstructive sleep apnea. The procedure requires delivery of radiofrequency energy to create thermal injury to the soft-palate musculature. Three methods of radiofrequency energy delivery can be used to treat the soft palate: monopolar, temperature-controlled monopolar, and bipolar. These techniques – and the larger number of available technologies – vary in their methods of energy delivery and the information that is provided back to the surgeon; no studies have directly compared technologies or delivery methods side by side.

The advantages of radiofrequency palatoplasty are:

- Low morbidity
- Treatment can be titrated to reach the desired results
- No hospital stay required
- Lower total cost

Indications and Patient Selection

The success of radiofrequency palatoplasty depends on appropriate patient selection and an understanding of upper-airway anatomy. As described in the preceding section, the palate may be a source of sound production in snoring and/or a site of airway narrowing or obstruction; the evaluation techniques to perform this assessment are described elsewhere, but a thorough medical history, physical examination, and sleep study are critical to upper-airway assessment and formulation of an appropriate treatment plan.

There is a common misconception that all patients with primary snoring (without evidence of more-severe sleep-disordered breathing) are best treated with palate procedures alone. This is not an accurate statement. There are two aspects involved in treatment decisions: the severity of sleep-disordered breathing (determined by patient evaluation, including a sleep study) and the locations of snoring sound production and/or airway compromise (based on history and physical examination but not specifically indicated by the sleep study). Only those patients with a significant palatal component to their sleep-disordered breathing should be treated with palate procedures – either alone or with treatment of the palate as part of a multilevel upper-airway treatment plan. Once the decision has been made to treat the palate, radiofrequency palatoplasty has demonstrated effectiveness in treating selected patients with primary snoring, upper airway resistance syndrome, and mild obstructive sleep apnea. Patients with more-severe sleep-disordered breathing should not undergo radiofrequency palatoplasty, except in rare circumstances.

In choosing among the palate procedures, no studies have specifically identified factors that are associated with better outcomes after radiofrequency palatoplasty in side-by-side comparisons against alternatives. However, radiofrequency palatoplasty has the unique advantages of producing shrinkage (in addition to stiffening) of the soft-palate musculature and also avoids placement of implants into the soft palate. In this author's experience, there may be three categories of patients who may benefit from this procedure compared with certain alternatives. For patients with slightly thickened soft-palate tissues, radiofrequency palatoplasty provides some reduction in tissue bulk and may be particularly beneficial. Conversely, patients with a thin soft-palate musculature who may be considered for palatal implants may avoid the risk of a foreign-body sensation after implant placement (which may be higher in these patients) by undergoing radiofrequency palatoplasty. Finally, patients with significant webbing of the posterior tonsillar pillars may benefit specifically from lateral lesions (see discussion of technique in the following section) and a tailored treatment plan because directed treatment of this lateral muscle tissue may produce superior displacement of the posterior tonsillar pillars and a reduction in this webbing (which may or may not directly improve sleep-disordered breathing). However, these hypotheses or other factors have not been addressed systematically in any studies.

Tips and Pearls

The indications are:
- Palatal component to primary snoring, upper airway resistance syndrome, or mild obstructive sleep apnea
- (Possible) specific soft-palate anatomical features, such as a slightly thickened or thin palate as well as significant posterior tonsillar pillar webbing

The contraindications are:
- Moderate to severe obstructive sleep apnea
- No significant palatal component to sleep-disordered breathing
- Obtaining effective treatment of sleep-disordered breathing with other treatment modalities
- Significant medical comorbidities, including coagulopathies (all anticoagulants should ideally be discontinued for at least 21 days prior to the procedure and 7 days following the procedure)

Surgical Technique

A key component of patient evaluation is the assessment of the thickness and composition of the soft palate. While it is often impossible to determine the precise thickness of the soft-palate musculature, this is a critical component of the preoperative evaluation. Radiographic imaging such as the lateral cephalogram can provide a sense of overall palate thickness in the midline, although this image does not determine the thickness of the muscle itself nor does it provide a sense of the variation in muscle thickness over the surface of the soft palate. Because the soft-palate musculature is thicker in the midline owing to the presence of the musculus uvulae, there is no substitute for a careful physical examination.

Preoperative preparation may include two interventions designed to decrease the risk of infection. Oral antibiotics active against oral and pharyngeal flora can be taken approximately 30 min prior to treatment and continued for 3 days; this may decrease edema and the small risk of infection. An oral antimicrobial rinse may also decrease the oral bacterial flora.

Anesthesia can be achieved with a combination of a topical anesthesia applied to the oral surface of the soft palate in the areas of planned local anesthesia injection. Local anesthetic with a vasoconstrictive agent, approximately 2–4 ml, is then infiltrated into the muscle tissue. Patients who receive insufficient anesthesia may experience localized pain or pain referred to other areas (such as the ears or occiput) during treatment

An important advantage of submucosal radiofrequency palatoplasty is the ability to deliver energy to the muscle in order to create tissue injury without causing damage to the mucosa (Fig. 31.1).

Tips and Pearls

■ The goal, therefore, in designing a radiofrequency energy treatment plan is to deliver sufficient energy (and possible tissue removal) to produce the necessary fibrosis of the musculature without damaging the overlying oral or nasal surface mucosa

There is no clear formula for achieving this balance; with the steep learning curve associated with the use of radiofrequency, it is often better to decrease the amount of energy delivered per lesion until a surgeon is better able to tailor the treatment to the patient's underlying anatomy without complications.

Radiofrequency energy is typically delivered to the soft-palate musculature midway between the posterior nasal spine and the free edge of the soft palate in

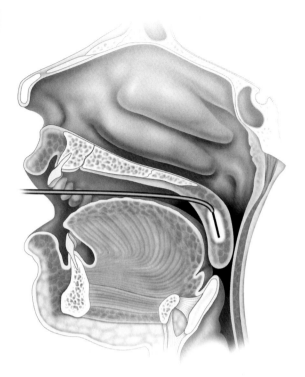

Fig. 31.1. Placement of the radiofrequency probe into soft-palate musculature midway between the posterior nasal spine and the free edge of the soft palate

midline, paramedian, or lateral locations. The midline and paramedian locations are within the thicker portion of the soft-palate musculature owing to the presence of the musculus uvulae; they can therefore tolerate larger amounts of energy than the lateral locations that include the levator veli palatini and tensor veli palatini muscles. Typically, from one to three lesions are created during each treatment session, and these can be combined as two paramedian lesions (Fig. 31.2) or a midline and two lateral lesions (Fig. 31.3). However, different lesion patterns, including a higher number of lesions per session, have been used with success; the placement and the number of lesions should be based on patient anatomy and experience.

Different radiofrequency energy delivery methods and technologies have corresponding differences in equipment settings and information available for the physician to control and monitor. The three most commonly used technologies are temperature-controlled radiofrequency (Somnus Medical Technologies, Gyrus ENT, Bartlett, TN, USA), bipolar (Celon, Olympus Corp., Tokyo, Japan) and plasma-mediated ablation, also known as Coblation® (ENTec, Arthrocare, Sunnyvale, CA, USA). This author has experience with the first and last of these because they are available in the USA, and settings for these technologies are provided as follows:

1. Temperature-controlled radiofrequency
   (a) Maximum temperature: 85 °C
   (b) Energy level for midline/paramedian lesions: 500–700 J; for lateral lesions, 300–350 J
2. Plasma-mediated ablation (Coblation®)
   (a) Power setting: 6
   (b) Time: 10-15 s per lesion

Postoperative Care

To minimize edema, patients should avoid hot (temperature) foods for 72 h and maintain their head elevated at least 30° during sleep. Routine perioperative corticosteroids are not necessary. Pain is well controlled with mild narcotics such as acetaminophen with codeine; this typically lasts 1–3 days unless there is injury to the mucosa.

The tissue injury created during the procedure heals, with the development of fibrosis, to a large extent over 6–8 weeks. Typically, more than one treatment session is necessary to achieve the desired treatment effect, and additional sessions can be performed every 6 weeks. The index for titration may be snoring or breathing patterns as observed by the bed partner, subjective complaints such as daytime somnolence, physical examination changes of the palate (which usually are minor), or, in certain cases, a repeat sleep study.

Results

Radiofrequency palatoplasty has produced decreases in snoring (measured subjectively) in 60–100% of patients – and in the majority of patients a substantial improvement – reported in several case series. [1–9, 11, 14–19] Studies which examined the effect of total energy delivery showed that there was greater improvement in snoring with a higher number of lesions and/or higher doses of radiofrequency energy delivered. [6, 7, 11, 15]

Many patients treated with radiofrequency have demonstrated improvements in daytime sleepiness, as measured by the Epworth sleepiness scale score [1, 2, 4, 6, 8–10, 14]. In those series that have objectively measured indices of sleep-disordered breathing, there has been an improvement in the maximum negative esophageal pressure (a measure of respiratory effort) [11] but no changes in other sleep study results [5, 6, 8, 9, 14].

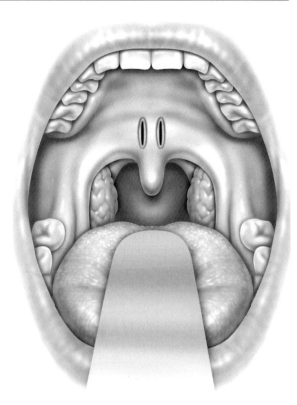

Fig. 31.2. Radiofrequency treatment pattern with two paramedian lesions

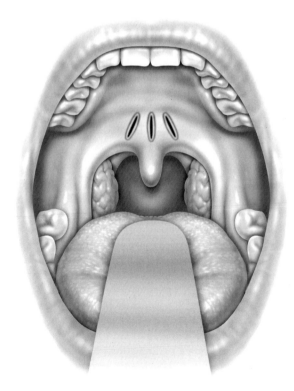

Fig. 31.3. Radiofrequency treatment pattern with one midline and two lateral lesions

Tips and Pearls

■ The benefits of radiofrequency palatoplasty may be due to changes in the intrinsic prop erties of the soft palate rather than any gross morphologic changes.

One series reported a decrease in the length of the soft palate and uvula (PNS-P distance) on a lateral cephalogram of 5.5 mm [14], but another reported no change [9]. Another study which examined patients before and after treatment with magnetic resonance imaging showed an overall change in the length of the uvula but no change in soft-palate length [2]; this study also showed imaging characteristics consistent with fibrosis of the soft palate after treatment.

One important factor to consider is the potential relapse of snoring after an initial successful result. The reported estimates of relapse within approximately 12–18 months after treatment are 11% [19] and 41% [13]. In the latter study, a single additional radiofrequency treatment restored the previous successful snoring result.

Finally, patients who demonstrate a poor response to radiofrequency palatoplasty may have significant untreated airway narrowing or obstruction at the level of the nose or hypopharyngeal regions. Several studies have specifically attempted to identify factors that may predict response to radiofrequency palatoplasty, but these efforts have been largely unsuccessful.

Complications

Complications can result from injury to the overlying soft-palate mucosa (ulceration if it involves either the oral or nasal aspect of the palate and a fistula if it involves both), infection (which may contribute to ulceration and/or fistula formation), soft-palate dysfunction producing nasal regurgitation, or velopharyngeal insufficiency.

These procedure-associated complications can be classified according to severity:

■ Minor: mucosal ulceration or injury, sloughing of the uvula
■ Moderate: hemorrhage, palatal fistula, significant dysphagia, or velopharyngeal insufficiency
■ Major: serious infection requiring drainage or other significant airway compromise

A literature review describing radiofrequency complications of the upper airway showed that the incidence of complications of minor, moderate, and major severity was 8.1% (114 in 1,443 treatment sessions), 0.5% (seven in 1,443 treatment sessions), and 0.1% (one in 1,443 treatment sessions), respectively [12].

Conclusion

▼

Radiofrequency palatoplasty is a safe, effective procedure for patients with a significant palatal component to primary snoring, upper airway resistance syndrome, or mild obstructive sleep apnea. History, physical examination, and sleep study are critical to patient selection and the tailoring of treatment to patient anatomy. Future research may identify factors which predict the therapeutic response to radiofrequency palatoplasty or enable selection among the various less-invasive palate procedures.

References

1. Back L, Palomaki M, Piilonen A, Ylikoski J. Sleep-disordered breathing: radiofrequency thermal ablation is a promising new treatment possibility. Laryngoscope 2001;111(3):464–71.
2. Back LJ, Tervahartiala PO, Piilonen AK, Partinen MM, Ylikoski JS. Bipolar radiofrequency thermal ablation of the soft palate in habitual snorers without significant desaturations assessed by magnetic resonance imaging. Am J Respir Crit Care Med 2002;166(6):865–71.
3. Blumen MB, Dahan S, Wagner I, De Dieuleveult T, Chabolle F. Radiofrequency versus LAUP for the treatment of snoring. Otolaryngol Head Neck Surg 2002;126(1):67–73.
4. Boudewyns A, Van De Heyning P. Temperature-controlled radiofrequency tissue volume reduction of the soft palate (somnoplasty) in the treatment of habitual snoring: results of a European multicenter trial. Acta Otolaryngol 2000;120(8):981–5.
5. Coleman SC, Smith TL. Midline radiofrequency tissue reduction of the palate for bothersome snoring and sleep-disordered breathing: A clinical trial. Otolaryngol Head Neck Surg 2000;122(3):387–94.
6. Emery BE, Flexon PB. Radiofrequency volumetric tissue reduction of the soft palate: a new treatment for snoring. Laryngoscope 2000;110(7):1092–8.
7. Ferguson M, Smith TL, Zanation AM, Yarbrough WG. Radiofrequency tissue volume reduction: multilesion vs single-lesion treatments for snoring. Arch Otolaryngol Head Neck Surg 2001;127(9):1113–8.

8. Haraldsson PO, Karling J, Lysdahl M, Svanborg E. Voice quality after radiofrequency volumetric tissue reduction of the soft palate in habitual snorers. Laryngoscope 2002;112(7 Pt 1):1260–3.

9. Hukins CA, Mitchell IC, Hillman DR. Radiofrequency tissue volume reduction of the soft palate in simple snoring. Arch Otolaryngol Head Neck Surg 2000;126(5):602–6.

10. Johns MW. A new method for measuring daytime sleepiness: the Epworth sleepiness scale. Sleep 1991;14(6):540–5.

11. Kania RE, Schmitt E, Petelle B, Meyer B. Radiofrequency soft palate procedure in snoring: influence of energy delivered. Otolaryngol Head Neck Surg 2004;130(1):67–72.

12. Kezirian EJ, Powell NB, Riley RW, Hester JE. Incidence of complications in radiofrequency treatment of the upper airway. Laryngoscope 2005;115(7):1298–304.

13. Li KK, Powell NB, Riley RW, Troell RJ, Guilleminault C. Radiofrequencvolumetric reduction of the palate: An extended follow-up study. Otolaryngol Head Neck Surg 2000;122(3):410–4.

14. Powell NB, Riley RW, Troell RJ, Li K, Blumen MB, Guilleminault C. Radiofrequency volumetric tissue reduction of the palate in subjects with sleep-disordered breathing. Chest 1998;113(5):1163–74.

15. Sher AE, Flexon PB, Hillman D, et al. Temperature-controlled radiofrequency tissue volume reduction in the human soft palate. Otolaryngol Head Neck Surg 2001;125(4):312–8.

16. Tatla T, Sandhu G, Croft CB, Kotecha B. Celon radiofrequency thermo-ablative palatoplasty for snoring – a pilot study. J Laryngol Otol 2003;117(10):801–6.

17. Terris DJ, Coker JF, Thomas AJ, Chavoya M. Preliminary findings from a prospective, randomized trial of two palatal operations for sleep-disordered breathing. Otolaryngol Head Neck Surg 2002;127(4):315–23.

18. Trotter MI, D'Souza AR, Morgan DW. Medium-term outcome of palatal surgery for snoring using the Somnus unit. J Laryngol Otol 2002;116(2):116–8.

19. Said B, Strome M. Long-term results of radiofrequency volumetric tissue reduction of the palate for snoring. Ann Otol Rhinol Laryngol 2003;112(3):276–9.

31

Uvulopalatal Flap

32

Chairat Neruntarat

Core Messages

- The uvulopalatal flap (UPF) is recommended as a surgical option for oropharyngeal obstruction in patients with sleep-related breathing disorders.

- The procedure is a mucosal procedure; thus, swelling and swallowing problems are moderate and transient.

- The success of the UPF depends on carefully selected patients and it is performed as a one-stage surgery.

- Patients with sleep-related breathing disorders pose a significant anesthetic risk and are generally deemed as difficult intubations. Sedating and narcotic medications pose a significant anesthetic risk. They increase the collapsibility of the pharynx and oral soft tissues, leading to additional airway obstruction. The UPF appears to be a safe and effective procedure that can be easily performed under local anesthesia on an outpatient basis with low chance of significant complications.

- There is reduction of pain and a decreased risk of wound contracture because sutures are not placed on the free edge of the palate.

- The UPF results are anatomically and clinically comparable to uvulopalatopharyngoplasty results.

- The UPF procedure is reversible since the UPF can be released in the postoperative period if necessary.

Introduction

Obstructive sleep apnea (OSA) is now seen as one end of a spectrum of sleep-related breathing disorders. It is a common event, occurring to a significant degree (more than five events per hour of sleep) in 4–9% of the population [16]. Severe disease (more than 50 events per hour) is associated with excess mortality [11] and patients present with complaints related to excessive daytime sleepiness, disturbed sleep, morning headache, impotence, and heavy snoring. In addition, OSA contributes to deficits in a number of cognitive processes, including intellectual abilities, executive functions, memory, and learning [5].

In a study by He et al. [2], the cumulative survival after 5 years in treated and untreated patients with an apnea index greater than 20 showed that cumulative survival was 100% for the continued positive airway pressure (CPAP) treated group versus about 75% for the untreated group. CPAP was demonstrated as effective in suppressing OSA, although long-term compliance remains a major problem. Many studies [3, 13, 14] report that patients with moderate to severe sleep apnea use their CPAP for only a mean of 4.7 h/night and for a mean 68% of their total sleep time. However, full-time use of CPAP is necessary to control the symptoms of OSA.

uvula is reflected back toward the soft palate and fixed into its new position with a 3-0 polyglactin suture (Vicryl) beginning with a mattress suture at the top corner and then with simple interrupted sutures (Fig. 32.1d). Tension can be varied to allow adjustment in elevating the edge of the soft palate and trimming redundant mucosa during suturing.

Tonsillectomy is performed avoiding damage to the underlying musculature. The palatopharyngeal muscle is pulled anterolaterally and sutured to the palatoglossal muscle. Several interrupted sutures are placed through the muscles between the two palatal arches. The tonsillar fossa is closed and redundant mucosa is eliminated.

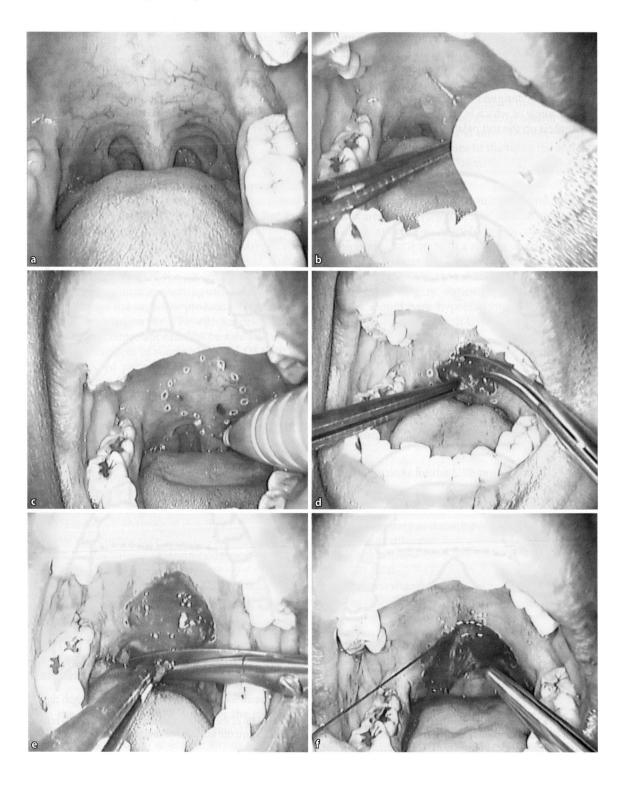

Uvulopalatal Flap Under Local Anesthesia

The UPF procedure is performed as described in the preceding section, using the modification in which the procedure is performed under local anesthesia (Fig. 32.2). The patients are given prophylactic antibiotics 1 h before surgery. Diazepam (5 mg) is administered only for patients with a significant gag reflex. The UPF procedure is performed with the patient in an upright sitting position in an examination chair. The patient is monitored with pulse oximetry during the procedure. Basic life support and emergency equipment are available in the operating room.

The soft palate is anesthetized with 10% lidocaine topical dispersion, and 5–10 ml 1% lidocaine with 1:100,000 epinephrine solution is injected submucosally into the soft palate and uvula. Adequate suction is performed to provide patient comfort. The patient is requested to relax the tongue. The patient takes a deep breath and slowly lets it out. The procedure begins 5–10 min later, after allowing the anesthetic to take effect.

Postoperative Care

The postoperative management is similar to that of tonsillectomy. Patients are placed on antibiotics, mucolytics, and analgesia for 5–7 days. They may benefit from short-term tapering doses of systemic corticosteroid. Xylocaine gel is used to relieve pain every 4 h as needed or before meals. Soft diet and avoidance of citrus and spicy foods are recommended. Patients with associated medical problems are monitored in the intensive care unit setting. Complication rates may be reduced by avoiding potent narcotic agents and other sedatives. CPAP is advised in patients with a preoperative RDI greater than 40 and lowest oxygen saturation less than 80%. Patients are seen in follow-up 7 days later and again in 4–6 weeks.

Results

Powell et al. [12] reported that the UPF procedure provided the same anatomical and clinical results as UPPP. Postoperative snoring determined by subjective measurement was similar in both procedures. A positive correlation between improved snoring and repositioned tissue was evident. UPF was performed as a one-stage surgery for snoring. In one study [10], the UPF success rate for snoring was 88% (49 of 56 patients). This demonstrated a significant improvement in the snoring index (245.8 versus 42.5 events per hour) and the percentage of sleep time spent in loud snoring (10.2 versus 3.8%). It also appeared that the changes in both parameters correlated significantly with changes in the subjective perception of the disease.

The UPF results for OSA were comparable to the UPPP results. The UPF decreased the RDI by 50% or more in 19 of 36 patients (52%). The mean preoperative and postoperative RDI was 45.2 and 10.1 events per hour, respectively. There was significant reduction in the distance between the posterior nasal spine and the soft palate of 43.8 to 45.9 mm [9]. The success of UPF in conjunction with hypopharyngeal surgery for the treatment for OSA was 70–78% [7, 8], and long-term success was 65% [6].

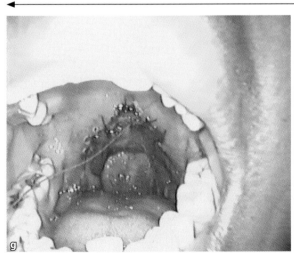
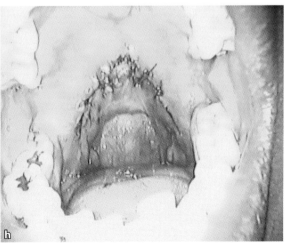

Fig. 32.2. a Before the procedure. **b** Lidocaine (1%) with epinephrine is injected. **c** Outline of the incision is performed. **d** The mucosal strip is dissected. **e** The tip of the uvula is amputated. **f** A mattress suture is placed at the top corner. **g** Simple interrupted sutures are placed. **h** After the procedure

Complications

Complications with the UPF procedure are infrequent and include [9, 12]:

- Bleeding (2%)
- Infection (2%)
- Transient VPI (4–11%)
- Wound dehiscence (2%)
- Foreign body sensation (1–4%)
- Voice change (1%)
- Transient band sensation (2%)

Airway obstruction, nasopharyngeal stenosis, and severe bleeding are not encountered.

Conclusion

The UPF procedure appears to be a safe and effective means to improve palatal obstruction. This reversible procedure can be performed as a one-stage surgery on an outpatient basis. Patients who have multilevel obstruction can undergo UPF and hypopharyngeal surgery simultaneously.

References

1. Fujita S, Conway W, Zorick F, Roth T (1981) Surgical correction of anatomic abnormalities in obstructive sleep agnea syndrome: Uvulopalatopharyngoplasty. Otolaryngol Head Neck Surg 89:923–927.
2. He J, Kryger M, Zorick F, et al (1988) Mortality and apnea index in obstructive sleep apneas. Chest 89:331–334.
3. Hoffstein V, Viner S, Mateika S, Conway J (1992) Treatment of obstructive sleep apnea with nasal continuous positive airway pressure. Patient compliance, perception of benefits, and side effects. Am Rev Resipir Dis 145:841–845.
4. Huntley TC (2000) The uvulopalatal flap. Oper Tech Otolaryngol Head Neck Sug 11:30–35.
5. Kales A, Caldwell AB, Dadiuva RJ, et al (1985) Severe obstructive sleep apnea. It associated psychopathology and psychological consequences. J Chronic Dis 38:427–434.
6. Neruntarat C (2003) Genioglossus advancement and hyoid myotomy: Short-term and long-term results. J Laryngol Otol 117:482–486.
7. Neruntarat C (2002) Genioglossus advancement under local anesthesia for obstructive sleep apnea. IMJ 9:215–219.
8. Neruntarat C (2003) Hyoid myotomy with suspension under local anesthesia for obstructive sleep apnea. Eur Arch Otorhirolaryngol 260:286–290.
9. Neruntarat C (2002) Uvulopalatal flap for obstructive sleep apnea on an outpatient basis. IMJ 9:45–49.
10. Neruntarat C (2003) Uvulopalatal flap for snoring on an outpatient basis. Otolaryngol Head Neck Surg 129:219–220.
11. Partinen M, Guilleminault C (1990) Daytime sleepiness and vascular morbidity at seven-year follow-up in obstructive sleep apnea patients. Chest 97:27–32.
12. Powell NB, Riley RW, Guilleminault C, et al (1996) A reversible uvulopalatal flap for snoring and sleep apnea syndrome. Sleep 19:593–599.
13. Rauscher H, Popp W, Wanke T, Zwich H (1991) Acceptance of CPAP therapy for sleep apnea. Chest 100:1019–1023.
14. Rolfe I, Olson LG, Saunders NA (1991) Long-term acceptance of continuous positive airway pressure in obstructive sleep apnea. Am Rev Respir Dis 144:1130–1135.
15. Strohl KP, Susan R (1996) Recognition of obstructive sleep apnea. Am J Respir Crit Care Med 154:279–289.
16. Young T, Palta M, Dempsey J, et al (1993) The occurrence of sleep-disordered breathing among middle-aged adults. N Engl J Med 328:1230–1235.

Chapter 33

Palatal Implants for Obstructive Sleep Apnea

33

Kenny P. Pang, David J. Terris

Core Messages

■ Snoring is a common social nuisance.

■ Snoring can be treated with a simple office-based technique.

■ Palatal implants are made from synthetic material, i.e., polyethylene terephthalate.

■ Palatal implants are effective for the treatment of snoring.

■ Minimal complications, including extrusion, have been documented in the literature.

Contents

Introduction

Snoring is part of a spectrum of diseases that includes upper airway resistance syndrome and obstructive sleep apnea (OSA). Snoring is due to the vibration of the structures in the oral cavity and oropharynx. It usually bothers the spouse more than the patient. Owing to poor sleep quality, fragmented sleep, intermittent nighttime hypoxemia, reduced percentage of slow-wave sleep and increased sympathetic overdrive, OSA results in daytime somnolence, morning headaches, poor concentration, loss of memory, frustration, depression and even marital discord.

Many surgical procedures of the soft palate focus on soft tissue volume reduction. The basis of each method is to create scar tissue, to incite fibrosis and to stiffen the palate, therefore resulting in reduced vibration and collapsibility of the soft palate. A new method involves the use of synthetic implants inserted into the soft palate. Palatal implants (Pillar® system, Restore Medical, St. Paul, MN, USA) are made of poly(ethylene terephthalate) (PET), a linear, aromatic polyester that was first manufactured in the late 1940s. Current medical applications for PET include sutures, surgical mesh, vascular grafts, and cuffs for heart valves [9, 11]. Extensive research on PET has demonstrated its biostability [2], promotion of tissue ingrowth [1] and a well-characterized fibrotic response [10, 12]. Each soft-palate implant is cylindrical in shape, measures 18 mm × 1.8 mm, and is made of a porous and braided PET.

Tips and Pearls

■ Palatal implantation involves the placement of three implants in the upper portion of the soft palate under local anesthesia in the office. The basic goal is to increase the rigidity of the soft palate.

There has been research showing that the implants result in a less collapsible airway by this increased rigidity [5].

Indications and Contraindications of Palatal Implant Surgery

Indications are:

■ Snorers with primary palatal snoring
■ Mallampati grade I and II
■ Small tonsils
■ Mild OSA (apnea–hypopnea index, AHI, below 15) (results may be unpredictable)
■ Moderate OSA (results may be unpredictable)

Contraindications are:

- Severe OSA (AHI > 35)
- Short soft-palate length of less than 20mm (relative contraindication)

Preoperative Workup

This involves:

- Thorough clinical history and physical examination
- Endoscopic examination of the upper airway
- Polysomnogram (sleep study)

Surgical Technique

The outpatient procedure is done with the patient under local anesthesia in the office. The patient is seated in an examination chair with the mouth open. Topical benzocaine (14%) is used to anesthetize the palatal region. A total of 3 ml of 1:100,000 epinephrine and 2% Xylocaine is injected into three sites of the soft palate (Fig. 33.1).

The midline implant is placed first, followed by two more implants that are placed approximately 2 mm to either side of the midline implant. Each palatal implant comes preloaded in the needle of a disposable delivery tool that inserts the implant into the soft palate. Ideally, the insertion site is set as close to the hard-palate and soft-palate junction as possible (Figs. 33.2, 33.3). After theprocedure, a flexible nasoendoscopy is preformed to ensure that the implant has not breached the nasal mucosal surface of the soft palate (Fig. 33.4). Hemostasis, if required, is achieved with electrocautery. All patients are prescribed anesthetic gargles and lozenges, nonsteroidal anti-inflammatory agents, narcotics or nonnarcotic analgesics.

The final result is a stiffened palate with increased rigidity and a less collapsible airway. With time, a fibrotic capsule forms around the three implants, and further stiffens the palate.

Tips and Pearls
- Careful patient selection is critical.
- Realistic patient expectation.
- Midline insertion may be hindered owing to the fibrous midline muscular raphe.
- Careful insertion is particularly prudent on the lateral sides of the soft palate, as it is thinner there and insertion of the implant may breach the nasal side of the palate.

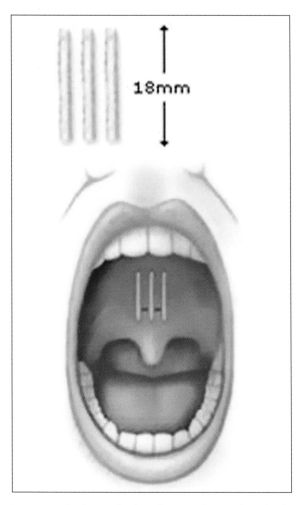

Fig. 33.1. The three palatal implants in place in the soft palate

Complications

Complications arising from this procedure are not common. The main complaint is postoperative pain; a rare patient complains of a foreign-body sensation in the throat. More severe complications like palatal fistula have not been reported. Incidents of implant extrusion have been reported.

Results/Outcomes

There is a delicate balance between the pharyngeal biomechanics and the anatomical structure that contribute to airway collapse in patients suffering from OSA. It would be rather simplistic to attribute the pathophysiology of OSA to the "small box" (craniofacial skeleton/jaw) or the crowded contents (oropharyngeal/tongue soft tissue). Nevertheless, most oto-

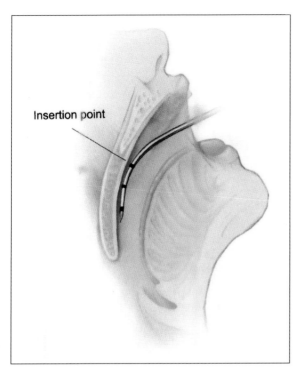

Fig. 33.2. Insertion of the implant with the implant device

laryngologists have focused attention on either removing soft tissue in the oropharynx or enlarging the jaw. The palatal implants are novel devices that do not remove soft tissue from the soft palate, but rather have been designed to stiffen and increase rigidity of the soft palate. This reduces collapsibility of the palate as well.

It was first demonstrated in 12 patients with mild OSA (AHI < 15), by Ho et al. [4] that palatal implants are safe and effective in reducing the snoring intensity and daytime sleepiness after 3 months after surgery. Nordgard et al. [7] showed in 35 patients that the mean subjective reduction in snoring intensity was 51%, with improvement in excessive daytime sleepiness as well. The longest follow-up in patients with the implants was documented at a 1-year follow-up period [6]. The authors found an encouraging reduction of snoring and daytime sleepiness; however, there was a high extrusion rate of 25% (ten out of the 40 patients) [6]. Skjostad et al. [8] revealed that stiffer implants had no advantage over the regular implants used, and that stiffer implants had higher extrusion rates than the regular implants.

The largest series was reported by Kuhnel et al. [3], in which 106 primary snoring patients showed im-

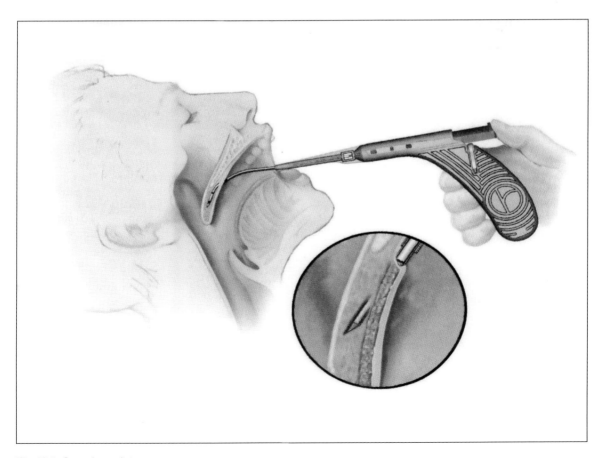

Fig. 33.3. Insertion point

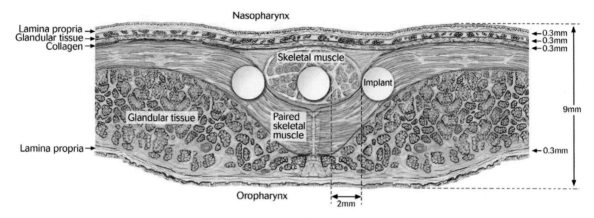

Fig. 33.4. Histology diagram of the correct position of implants

pressive subjective reduction in snoring intensity and daytime sleepiness.

Previously, surgical interventions were limited to volumetric reduction of the soft palate, and creation of scar tissue. The improvement following a reduction procedure results from a decrease in the volume of tissue as well as an increase in the stiffness of the palate secondary to scar formation. This new method of stiffening the soft palate with implants appears to be effective in the reduction of snoring intensity and daytime sleepiness. It remains premature to conclude that these implants will be effective in the treatment of sleep apnea.

References

1. Feldman D, Hultman S, Colaizzo R, et al. Electron microscope investigation of soft tissue in growth into Dacron velour with dogs. Biomaterials 1983;4:105.
2. Greenwald D, Shumway S, Albear P, et al. Mechanical comparison of 10 suture materials before and after in vivo incubation. J Surg Res 1994;56:372–77.
3. Kuhnel TS, Hein G, Hohenhorst W. Maurer JT. Soft palate implants: a new option for treating habitual snoring. Eur Arch Otorhinolaryngol 2005;262(4):277–80.
4. Ho WK, Wei WI, Chung KF. Managing disturbing snoring with palatal implants: a pilot study. Arch Otolaryngol Head Neck Surg 2004;130(6):753–8.
5. Malhotra A, Pillar G, Fogel R, et al. Upper airway collapsibility: Measurement and sleep effects. Chest 2001;120:156–161.
6. Maurer JT, Hein G, Verse T, Hormann K, Stuck BA. Long-term results of palatal implants for primary snoring. Otolaryngol Head Neck Surg 2005;133(4):573–8.
7. Nordgard S, Wormdal K, Bugten V, Stene BK, Skjostad KW. Palatal implants: a mew method for the treatment of snoring. Acta Otolaryngol 2004;124(8):970–5.
8. Skjostad KW, Stene BK, Nordgard S. Consequences of increased rigidity in palatal implants for snoring: a randomized controlled study. Otolaryngol Head Neck Surg 2006;134(1):63–6.
9. Soares B, Guidoin R, Marois Y, et al. In vivo characterization of a fluoropassivated gelatin-impregnated polyester mesh for hernia repair. J Biomed Mater Res 1996;32:293–305.
10. Tinley N, Boor P. Host response to implanted Dacron grafts, a comparison between mesh and velour. Arch Surg 1975;110:1469–72.
11. Vinard E, Eloy R, Descotes J, et al. Stability of performances of vascular prostheses retrospective study of 22 cases of human implanted prostheses. J Biomed Mater Res 1988;22:633–48.
12. Waitzova D, Kramplova M, Mandys V, et al. Biostability and morphology of tissue reaction of some synthetic polymers. Polym Med 1986;XVI:93.

Chapter 34

Injection Snoreplasty

34

Kenny P. Pang, David J. Terris

Core Messages

- Snoring is a common social nuisance.

- Snoring can be treated with a simple office-based technique.

- Injection snoreplasty is an effective method for the treatment of snoring.

- Different sclerotic agents have been used with similar results.

- Minimal complications for this procedure have been documented in the literature.

Contents

Introduction

Sleep-disordered breathing is a spectrum of diseases that includes snoring, upper airway resistance syndrome (UARS) and obstructive sleep apnea (OSA). Snoring is caused by vibration of the structures in the oral cavity and oropharynx – namely, the soft palate, uvula, tonsils, base of tongue, epiglottis and pharyngeal walls. Sleep-disordered breathing encompasses simple snorers (patients who snore without excessive daytime somnolence and with a normal apnea–hypopnea index, AHI), UARS (patients with excessive daytime somnolence but a normal AHI) and OSA (patients who snore and have both excessive daytime somnolence and an abnormal AHI).

A multitude of techniques have been introduced to treat snoring. The basis of each method is to create scar tissue, to incite fibrosis and to stiffen the palate. This decreases the vibration of the palate and diminishes snoring, with the intention of reduced collapsibility and therefore fewer apneic episodes.

Sodium tetradecyl sulfate (STS) has been used as a sclerosing agent to stiffen the palate. It has a longstanding excellent safety record for the treatment of varicose veins, and it has very low cost.

Indications and Contraindications for Injection Snoreplasty

Indications are:

- Snorers with primary palatal snoring
- Mild OSA (AHI < 15)

Contraindications are:

- Patients with a cleft palate
- Patients with velopharyngeal insufficiency
- Patients with a palatal fistula
- Patients with a thin soft palate (relative contraindication)
- Moderate and severe OSA (AHI ≥15)

Preoperative Workup

This involves:

- Thorough clinical history and physical examination
- Endoscopic examination of the upper airway
- Polysomnogram (sleep study)

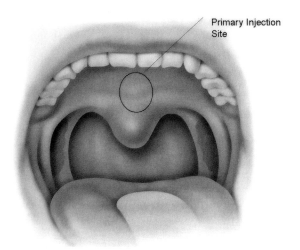

Fig. 34.1. Primary injection in the midline of the soft palate

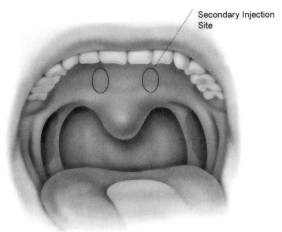

Fig. 34.2. Secondary injection sites, lateral areas of the soft palate

Surgical Technique

This 15-min outpatient procedure is done with the patient under local anesthesia in the office. The patient is seated in an examination chair with the mouth open. Topical benzocaine (14%) is used to anesthetize the palatal region. A total of 2 ml of 1:100,000 adrenaline and 2% Xylocaine is injected into the midline of the soft palate.

The primary injection site is in the midline just above the uvula (Fig. 34.1). The sclerotic agent is constituted and introduced into the soft palate by injection with a needle and syringe. A translucent bubble of fluid is seen as 2 ml of the sclerosing agent is injected within the submucosal plane. The bubble turns to a hemorrhagic color within 2–3 min of injection as the sclerosing agent takes effect. Hemostasis, if required, is achieved with electrocautery. All patients are prescribed anesthetic gargles, lozenges and narcotic or nonnarcotic analgesics.

The final result is a fibrotic palate that is retracted superiorly, with the oropharyngeal airway widened.

For the patient undergoing a repeat injection, the injection sites differ. Reinjection into the midline is usually difficult because of the already stiffened midline soft palate; therefore, the soft palate is reinjected lateral to the primary injection site, with 1 ml of the sclerosing agent on each side (Fig. 34.2). However, if the prior injected site in the midline is inadequately stiffened, reinjection there is possible.

Tips and Pearls

- Careful patient selection is crucial.
- Patient expectations should be realistic.
- Primary-site injection is made in the midline.

Secondary-site injection may be given carefully laterally, as the lateral sides of the soft palate are thinner (in order to prevent fistula formation).

Complications

There have been few reported complications from this procedure. The main patient complaint is that of postoperative pain. Most describe a "lump"-in-throat sensation, which resolves in 2–5 days. There may be mucosal breakdown over the injection site. Other complications like velopharyngeal insufficiency and palatal fistula are uncommon.

Results/Outcome

There have been a handful of articles showing fairly good results achieved with this procedure. Brietzke and Mair [1] first described this technique in 27 patients, using the sclerosant Sotradecol (STS). Twenty-five (92%) of the 27 patients reported a subjective decrease in their snoring and were satisfied. There were no significant complications documented. Levinson [5] demonstrated similar results with this procedure. Lon- term results up to 19 months were evaluated by Brietzke and Mair [2], who showed that the subjective reduction in snoring decreased from 92% at 3 months to 75% at 19 months, and the snoring relapse rate was 18%. Other sclerosants were also investigated by Brietzke and Mair [3], including ethanol, doxycycline and hypertonic saline. They observed that the

34

use of 50% ethanol as a sclerosing agent has similar results to 3% STS; however, doxycycline and hypertonic saline were not as efficacious.

There is one nonrandomized prospective study that was done on 70 simple snorers comparing the efficacy of radiofrequency ablation versus injection snoreplasty [4]. A subjective improvement was reported in 87.5% of the patients who had radiofrequency ablation and 76.7% of the patients treated with injection snoreplasty. It was concluded that the treatments were equally effective in treating snoring.

References

1. Brietzke SE, Mair EA. Injection snoreplasty: how to treat snoring without all the pain and expense. Otolaryngol Head Neck Surg 2001 May;124(5):503–10.
2. Brietzke SE, Mair EA. Injection snoreplasty: extended follow-up and new objective data. Otolaryngol Head Neck Surg 2003 May;128(5):605–15.
3. Brietzke SE, Mair EA. Injection snoreplasty: investigation of alternative sclerotherapy agents. Otolaryngol Head Neck Surg 2004 Jan;130(1):47–57.
4. Iseri M, Balcioglu O. Radiofrequency versus injection snoreplasty in simple snoring. Otolaryngol Head Neck Surg 2005 Aug;133(2):224–8.
5. Levinson SR. Injection snoreplasty. Otolaryngol Head Neck Surg 2001 Nov;125(5):579–80.

Chapter 35

Uvulopalatopharyngoplasty

35

Wolfgang Pirsig

Core Messages

- Uvulopalatopharyngoplasty (UPPP) is one surgical option to increase upper-airway diameter at the velopharyngeal level.

- UPPP as an isolated procedure does not alter enough the soft tissues of the upper airway for patients with obstructive sleep apnea. UPPP with tonsillectomy is more effective.

- The success rate of each type of velar surgery decreases with increasing follow-up period. In selected patients, long-term effectiveness of UPPP is approximately 50%. There are, however, no validated criteria to select a "velum snorer" for UPPP.

- A more radical UPPP is not more effective than a less radical UPPP but it increases the incidence of complications; therefore, there is no rationale for radical UPPP.

- A low complication rate can be achieved using some techniques of UPPP which preserve muscles and mucosa of the velum.

- A polysomnographic evaluation is necessary 1–3 years after UPPP.

Contents

Introduction

Snoring is caused by vibrations of soft tissues in constricted segments of the upper airway during respiration while asleep. It is sign of the nonsymptomatic primary snoring and of the symptomatic snoring of the upper airway resistance syndrome and of obstructive sleep apnea (OSA), all of them belonging to the subgroup of sleep-disordered breathing (SDB). To reduce excessive pharyngeal tissue for snoring patients, Ikematsu [15] introduced palatopharyngoplasty and partial uvulectomy in 1964. Fujita et al. [9] modified the technique for patients with OSA syndrome and termed it uvulopalatopharyngoplasty (UPPP) in 1981. In the meantime, several modifications of UPPP with and without tonsillectomy/tonsillotomy (T) were published and were described and illustrated in the book *Snoring and Obstructive Sleep Apnea* [6]. Newer methods of soft-palate surgery are depicted in *Surgery for Sleep-Disordered Breathing* [12].

UPPP is the most common operation performed to enlarge one segment of the upper-airway caliber for treating SDB. The amount of excised velar soft tissue varies from method to method, as does the incidence of associated complications. A more radical UPPP is not more effective than a less radical UPPP but it increases the complication rate.

Since 1986 we have preferred a UPPP technique that preserves tissue, especially the velar muscles and mucosa. From 1986 to 1990 we performed UPPP without selection criteria – none had been proposed in the literature – and since 1990 we have employed specific selection criteria [28]. In 1996 our surgical technique became more conservative based on Ikematsu's procedure from 1964 [1].

The goals of UPPP as a selective treatment in patients with SDB are:

- Significant reduction of the SDB and daytime sleepiness
- No impairment of other functions
- Highly predictable success rate

- Low complication rate
- Option for combination with other therapeutic modalities
- High long-term acceptance rate by the patient
- High acceptance rate by the sleeping partner

Unfortunately, we have not yet achieved these goals in their entirety because validated patient selection criteria are not available. Furthermore, it was shown that UPPP alone does not alter enough upper-airway soft-tissue anatomy for OSA [32].

Patient Selection and Preoperative Evaluation

UPPP can reduce or eliminate the snoring sound of the so-called velum snorer. But it is not that easy to recognize with certainty the velum snorer.

Clinically, the velum snorer displays characteristic anatomic traits of the soft palate, such as:

- Long and/or wide pendulous uvula with horizontal mucosal folds.
- Flaccid drooping and redundant posterior tonsillar pillars (webbing).
- Elongated uvula embedded in the long posterior palatal arch.
- Short distance between the soft palate and pharyngeal posterior wall.
- Formation of craniocaudal redundant mucosal folds in the posterior pharyngeal wall.
- Enlarged palatine tonsils may also add to the encroachment of the oropharyngeal caliber.

On the other hand, there are persons with typical velar webbing and hypertrophic tonsils who do not snore. This supports the argument that OSA is not only an anatomic disorder [31] but is probably initiated by neural events during sleep [34].

The velum snorer is especially distinguished by a snoring sound characterized by a base frequency of 25–50 Hz and a multitude of overtones, which results in a regular and harmonic sound pattern [30]. UPPP has no effect in the case of a "tongue base snorer," whose nighttime respiratory sounds are characterized by loud, hard, metallic, nonharmonic snoring with frequency between 1,100 and 1,700 Hz.

Examination of patients with possible velum snoring [29] involves the following: history-taking with standardized or validated questionnaires for profiling risk symptoms and daytime sleepiness; otorhinolaryngological status including orthodontic status of occlusion situation, staging after Friedman et al. [8] for tonsils and tongue position; testing the sensitivity of the soft palate, which is decreased in heavy snorers and patients with OSA [5, 22]; flexible nasopharyngeal videoendoscopy with the patient in a supine position; Finkelstein test [7] (patients are asked to drink water with their heads protruded from under a running faucet – in cases of velum sufficiency, no water enters the nose); measurement of body mass index (BMI) and neck size; measurement of nasal obstruction and/or nasal airway cross-sectional areas; portable polysomnography.

In individual cases the following are useful: lateral radiocephalogram; objective wakefulness and vigilance tests; allergy diagnosis; imaging the upper airway; tape recording of snoring noise at home. Summarizing the chances of proper patient selection for UPPP, we have to admit that this still remains a result of personal experience in many cases. The literature provides only a few prospective studies for SDB which suggest selection or exclusion criteria for UPPP.

Selection or exclusion criteria for UPPP are:

- In general, obesity is a negative selection criterion. The limit for performing UPPP alone appears to lie at a BMI between 28 and 30 kg/m2. An increased neck size, often associated with obesity, is also a negative selection criterion.
- A high apnea–hypopnea index (AHI) or oxygen desaturation index is a negative selection criterion for isolated UPPP. The "absolute" value is disputed; it seems to lie between 20 and 30 events per hour. The experience of diminishing success rates with increased initial AHI has shown that in these cases the complete upper airway is affected by the SDB. We therefore prefer a multilevel surgery concept in patients with an AHI above 25.
- The presence of large tonsils is a positive selection criterion [35]. If they still exist, we always remove tonsils in the context of UPPP for SDB.
- Retrognathia and micrognathia are negative selection criteria for isolated UPPP. In these cases the obstruction often lies behind the tongue.
- A positive Müller maneuver (provoking a collapse during inspiration against the artificially closed airway) in the context of the nasopharyngeal videoendoscopy has no predictive value; therefore, we do not employ it.
- Because of the possibility to acquire even a minimal velar insufficiency, we do not recommend UPPP to patients of certain professions: singers, speech professions, wind-instrument players and divers

35

Indications and Contraindications for Isolated UPPP

Indications are:

- Velum snorer with airway obstruction at the level of the soft palate by redundant tissue
- Velum snorer on the basis of analyzing snoring noises
- Hypertrophy of palatine tonsils
- No malocclusion in need of treatment
- BMI < 30 kg/m^2
- None or minor daytime sleepiness
- Primary snoring, mild OSA; AHI < 25
- For moderate or severe OSA as part of a multilevel surgery concept
- Contraindications are:
- Chronic heart and/or lung diseases
- Neurological/psychiatric illnesses in need of treatment
- High anesthesia risk
- Chronic alcoholism
- Soporific drug abuse
- Obesity; BMI > 30 kg/m^2; increased neck size
- Marked daytime sleepiness
- Moderate or severe OSA; AHI > 25
- Severe bite misalignment (micrognathia, retrognathia)
- Bulky, elevated base of the tongue, tongue enlargement
- Too short soft palate
- Submucous cleft palate, velopharyngeal insufficiency
- Narrow pharyngeal airway behind the tongue
- Large distance between the lower edge of the mandible to the hyoid (radiocephalogram)
- Certain craniofacial deformities
- Persons with certain professions

Ulm Procedure of UPPP

The procedure is demonstrated in Video 35.1.

On the basis of the anatomy and function of the soft palate, we markedly modified the technique of Fujita at al. [9] in 1986 [28] and returned to a more tissue-preserving technique in 1996 [1] based on Ikematsu's [15] procedure from 1964.

UPPP with or without T is performed under general anesthesia with the patient in the Rose position (supine with head hanging). After orotracheal intubation has been performed, a self-retaining mouth gag is inserted. The gag is covered with a silicone tube to protect the teeth. In case of a large tongue in a small oral cavity, intermittent decompression of the tongue may re-

duce damaging pressure and postoperative edema. The oropharyngeal structures are closely inspected to evaluate their dimensions and topography. An infiltration of the soft palate with vasoconstrictive additive and local anesthetic is not necessary, while infiltration of an anesthetic mixture in the tonsils between the tonsillar capsule and bed with a curved needle is recommended to reduce postoperative pain [27].

Step 1. Partial uvulectomy can be performed at the beginning or at the end of the operation. The uvular tip is grasped with forceps and pulled towards the tongue. This way, the muscle bellies can be clearly distinguished under the mucosa, which means that the excessive mucosa of the uvula can be adequately evaluated and removed without injuring the musculi uvulae. After bipolar cauterization of both uvular arteries, the uvula stump is sewed together with a 3-0 double Vicryl suture (Fig. 35.7). The incision into the mucosa is performed with a semicircular movement in the oral fold of the palatoglossus muscle, approximately 2 mm (!) away from the free edge, and 1 cm away from the base of the uvula (Fig. 35.2). Then, the fibers of the palatoglossus muscle are identified and preserved while

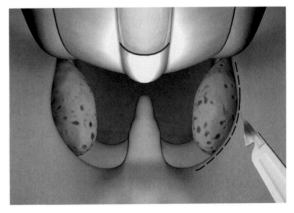

Fig. 35.1. Mucosal incision of the anterior tonsillar pillar approximately 2 mm away from the free edge

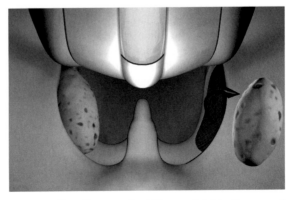

Fig. 35.2. Tonsillectomy should be restricted to the removal of lymphatic tissue and preserves the mucosa of the posterior pillar

exposing the superior pole of the tonsil by sharp dissection with scissors.

Step 2. Tonsillectomy follows, in which the posterior tonsillar pillar with its mucosa is initially preserved (Fig. 35.2). Tonsillectomy should only involve the palatine tonsil and not parts of the lingual tonsil. Bleeding is controlled by bipolar cauterization and ligature.

Step 3. The posterior tonsillar pillar (palatopharyngeus muscle with its covering mucosa and a few fibers of the superior pharyngeal constrictor muscle) is partially incised (Fig. 35.3) precisely at the site of maximum tension of the palatopharyngeus muscle as felt by pulling the posterior pillar with forceps towards the curvature of the anterior pillar. As a result, the posterior pillar opens up in a V shape, which produces a lengthened posterior pillar edge to be sewed together with the anterior pillar.

Step 4. Now the two palatal arches can be united without tension by interrupted double sutures but only in their upper parts, while the triangular inferior tonsillar fossa is left open (Fig. 35.4). This results in an anterolateral advancement of the incised superior palatopharyngeus muscles. Each interrupted double suture connects mucosa and musculature of the anterior pillar, a small muscular bundle of the lateral pharyngeal wall, and mucosa and musculature of the posterior pillar with braided, absorbable, atraumatic thread (e.g. Vicry® 2-0 SH or 2-0 SH1 or Polysorb® 2-0 X). Tightening the knots should be performed very gently to avoid ischemia of the muscles and postoperative pain. We recommend double sutures in order to prevent premature ripping of the suture during swallowing. Usually three sutures per side are sufficient (Fig. 35.5). With these sutures the posterior tonsillar pillar is moved laterally and anteriorly, thus enlarging the velopharyngeal caliber. This results in a semielliptical soft palate, which stiffens as a consequence of scarring. An identical procedure is performed on the opposite side.

In cases where the posterior pillar is very thin and the tonsillar fossa is very deep, which is mostly associated with extreme tonsillar hypertrophy, the elongation of the posterior pillar by the V-shaped incision will not be enough in order to place all sutures between the two pillars without tension. In such a case a triangle between the two sewed pillars should be left open.

Step 5. Finally, redundant mucosa of the posterior pillar on both sides of the uvula is removed (Fig. 35.6), and the mucosal folds of the anterior and posterior tonsillar pillar are sewed together. Figure 35.8 shows how the originally more Roman form of the soft palate has turned into a semielliptical one as a result of the lateralization of the posterior tonsillar pillar. Meticulous sewing results in primary wound healing in almost all patients.

35

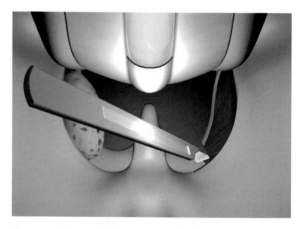

Fig. 35.3. The medial part of the palatopharyngeus muscle with its covering mucosa in the posterior pillar is partially incised to enlarge the posterior pillar

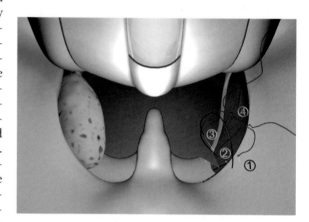

Fig. 35.4. The double suture connects mucosa and muscle of the anterior pillar (1), a muscular bundle of the lateral pharyngeal wall (2), and mucosa and muscle of the posterior pillar (3). Tightening the knots (4) should be performed very gently

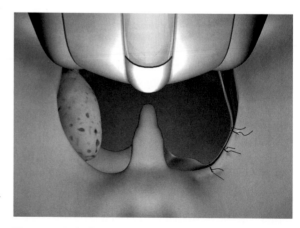

Fig. 35.5. Only the upper part of the palatal arch is sewed with interrupted double sutures

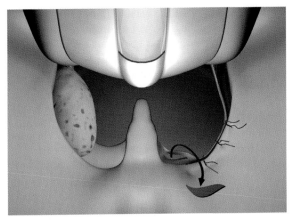

Fig. 35.6. Redundant mucosa of the posterior pillar on both sides of the uvula is removed

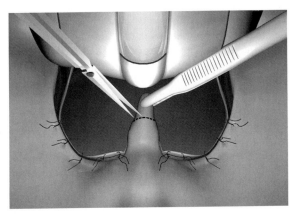

Fig. 35.7. Partial uvulectomy: excessive mucosa is resected without touching the musculi uvulae, the uvula stump is sewed

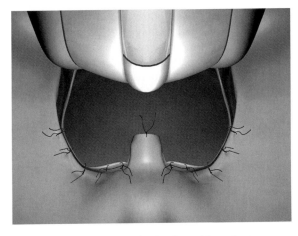

Fig. 35.8. The newly created soft palate with uvula stump

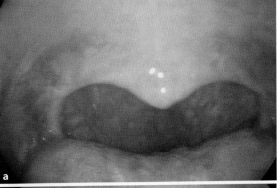

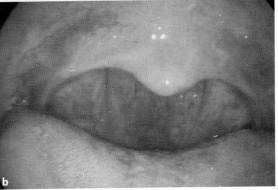

Fig. 35.9. Typical appearance of the new velum 14 months postoperatively **a** at rest and **b** in action

This Ulm procedure of UPPP with T preserves all velar muscles and sacrifices only a minimum of velar mucosa. A less vibrating new velum with a shortened uvula has been created with a lateralized upper posterior pillar and the horizontal edge of the velum more in an anterior position (Fig. 35.9). Together with the tonsillectomy, an enlargement of the upper-airway caliber on the velopharyngeal level has been achieved.

In cases where the UPPP is performed on a patient who has previously undergone tonsillectomy, one usually finds firm scarring between the remnants of the anterior and posterior tonsillar pillars, which promotes stenosis on the velopharyngeal level, especially towards the uvula. The incision is made where the caudal end of the palatoglossus muscle is assumed to be in the superior half of the tonsillar fossa. Only a small strip of scarred mucosa is excised. Underneath, the scars should be unraveled by rending them apart so that the folds of the two tonsillar pillars are well exposed again. Just as in the case of UPPP with tonsillectomy, the posterior pillar is incised at the site of its maximum tension. If the remaining tissue is scarce, small Z-plasties will enable more conducive reconstruction conditions for a semielliptical new soft palate.

In children, a conservative UPPP is performed only in exceptional cases, e.g., in neurologically im-

35

paired children [20], or those with craniofacial deformities or Down's syndrome with an underdeveloped maxilla and muscular hypotonia [13]. This procedure involves sawing of the superior parts of the tonsillar pillars after tonsillectomy and resection of the muscleless portion of the uvula.

Postoperative Care

Intraoperatively an intravenous single-shot antibiotic with 2 g cefazolin is administered; otherwise, antibiotics are only used in cases of relevant inflammatory complications. In patients with a history of oral aphthous ulcers, a virostatic is applied. The severe pain occurring in almost all of the patients in the first postoperative days is treated with diclofenac suppositories, and later with tablets. Apart from aspirin, there is no significant increased risk of postoperative bleeding for nonsteroidal anti-inflammatory drugs, as recently published in a meta-analysis [23].

In most cases, postoperatively, there is a remarkable edema of the uvula stump which can even enhance postoperative snoring. The patient should know this. During the first postoperative day, the patients are fed via infusion, and take in tea and ice cream, as in the case of a tonsillectomy. Most patients are also able to swallow liquids, albeit under pain. From the second day, they receive a special tonsillectomy diet. The sutures are removed between the tenth and 12th postoperative day. The inpatient time varies between 2 and 5 days, depending on the ability to eat and the extent of pain. Postoperative intensive care supervision is not usually necessary after isolated UPPP and T [2].

If indicated, we perform UPPP and tonsillectomy combined with rhinosurgery in the majority of patients. In these cases, the patient is forced to breathe through the mouth during the period when there is nasal packing (1–2 days). This leads to a heightened postoperative morbidity; but this is justifiable in the majority of cases. These patients need to be supervised in the recovery room immediately postoperatively (during the first 3–6 h after surgery).

Long-Term Effectiveness of UPPP for SDB

Eight groups of authors reported on long-term results after UPPP for primary snoring in 868 patients with follow-ups between 1.5 and 10 years [12]. No snoring was found in 29.8% of patients, reduced snoring in 43.1%, no change in 29.4% and worse snoring in 8.1%. Combining the values for "snoring reduced" and "no snoring" results in a long-term success rate of 73%

for isolated UPPP in the treatment of primary snoring. But these data have to be considered with caution, owing to the fact that the diverse evaluation criteria are extremely heterogeneous. Accordingly, the success rates vary in the cited studies between 44 and 91%. Six of the eight studies were retrospective, one evidence-based medicine (EBM) grade II-2 and one EBM grade II-3.

There are only a few prospective studies covering long-term results of up to 9 years after UPPP for OSA [12]. As with the other techniques, the comparability of these data is problematic owing to varying success criteria. Almost unanimously, all authors find a discrepancy between adequate subjective improvement of the symptoms and nearly unchanged objective sleep parameters after UPPP; therefore, polysomnographic postoperative evaluation is necessary after 1–3 years.

Every surgeon should study the excellent survey by Sher et al. [33]. The authors used as success criteria AHI < 20 and a reduction of the AHI of at least 50% (or analogously apnea index of less than 10 and a reduction of the apnea index of less than 50%). For the nonselected patient pool this meta-analysis yielded a surgery success rate of 40.7%. In the selected group with clinically suspected obstruction solely on the level of the soft palate, a success rate of 52.3% was found. For the most part, these data are based on short-term results.

If one combines data from four studies [14, 16, 24, 25] that use the success criteria of Sher et al. [33], this yields a long-term success rate of 49.5% for isolated UPPP including tonsillectomy in the treatment of OSA. This long-term success rate of approximately 50% also corresponds to our own results for selected patients within the last 19 years; therefore, one can rightly assume a positive long-term effect of isolated UPPP, possibly in connection with a tonsillectomy.

In accordance with these results, in a group of 400 patients with SDB who had received a UPPP or a laser uvulopalatoplasty, no increase in mortality was found in comparison with a control group comprising 744 persons [26]. These data may indicate a positive survival effect of UPPP surgery. Keenan et al. [19] contacted their OSA patients treated with either UPPP (*n*=149) or nasal continuous positive airway pressure (*n*=126) over a 6-year period to compare long-term survival rates between these two treatment options. There was no difference between the two treatment groups. Furthermore, UPPP for SDB turned out to improve the patients' stimulated long-term driving performance [10] and decreased the number of car accidents within a 5 year period after surgery [11].

Complications

Postoperative edema and respiratory depression enhance the risk of reintubation or emergent tracheotomy within the first few hours after surgery [4, 17]. The incidence of lethal complications is given as 0.03–0.2% [3, 21]. Serious cardiopulmonary complications other than death occur in 1.5% of the cases [21]. Among the early post-UPPP complications, transient velopharyngeal insufficiency, wound dehiscence, hemorrhage and wound infection are described in order of frequency in the literature [18].

UPPP as described in this chapter has been performed in Ulm and Mannheim on more than 600 patients with primary snoring and OSA. Although our patients experienced postoperative pain, especially during swallowing, we did not observe nasal regurgitation or hypernasal speech.

Despite the use of interrupted double sutures, wound dehiscence in the region of the inferior tonsillar fossa mostly occurred within the first postoperative days. Therefore, in recent years, we stopped sewing the anterior and posterior pillars in the inferior tonsillar fossa and leave the wound to heal by secondary intention.

As with any tonsillectomy, postoperative bleeding during the healing phase is a possibility. In the author's series there is approximately 1% incidence in post-UPPP/T bleeding. Oral aphthous ulcers are rare since we have begun using antibiotics only perioperatively, or administering a virostatic in patients with a history of oral aphthous ulcers. Also, the fetid mouth odor observed on the third postoperative day, which is so typical for tonsillectomy without a mucous membrane, is usually absent in our patients.

Katsantonis [18] has classified the late-term complications after UPPP in order of frequency as follows:

- Pharyngeal discomfort, dryness, tightness
- Postnasal secretion
- Dysphagia
- Inability of initiating swallowing
- Prolonged angina
- Taste disorders
- Speech disorders
- Numbness of tongue
- Permanent velopharyngeal insufficiency
- Nasopharyngeal stenosis

None of our patients developed velopharyngeal insufficiency. For approximately 10% of our patients a follow-up nasal continuous positive airway pressure therapy was necessary because UPPP and T were not enough to cure OSA for the long term. In none of these cases was the ventilation therapy impaired by an oral air leakage. Furthermore, we did not observe the problems with speech which are published as sequels of uvulectomy. Several patients who had received a tonsillectomy with UPPP reported of a positive change in timbre and resonance of their voice. In addition, our patients did not experience an increased mucous production in the pharynx because the remaining uvula stump with the undisturbed ciliated epithelium of the nasal surface transports the nasal mucous into the hypopharynx.

Nasopharyngeal stenosis is a dreaded complication, and is extremely difficult to correct. The following are considered as risk factors for the development of nasopharyngeal stenosis: aggressive posterior pillar resection, extension of surgery to the lateral pharyngeal walls, excessive mucosa destruction, electrocautery, postoperative wound infection and acromegaly [18]. As a result of lateralization of the upper posterior tonsillar pillar and forward relocation of the horizontal edge of the velum, no nasopharyngeal stenosis has been observed in our patients in connection with our UPPP procedure.

Conclusion

The Ulm procedure of UPPP with T preserves all velar muscles and sacrifices only a minimum of velar mucosa. A less vibrating new velum with a shortened uvula has been created with a lateralized upper posterior pillar and the horizontal edge of the velum more in an anterior position. Together with the tonsillectomy an enlargement of the upper-airway caliber on the velopharyngeal level is achieved.

Acknowledgement

The author thanks David Nagel from Immenstadt, Germany, for preparing Figs. 35.1–35.8.

References

1. Brosch S, Matthes C, Pirsig W, et al (2000) Uvulopalatopharyngoplasty changes fundamental frequency of the voice – a prospective study. J Laryngol Otol 114:113–118
2. Burges LP, Derderian SS, Morin GV, et al (1992) Postoperative risk following uvulopalatopharyngoplasty for obstructive sleep apnea. Otolaryngol Head Neck Surg 106:81–86

3. Carenfelt C, Haraldsson PO (1993) Frequency of complications after uvulopalatopharyngoplasty. Lancet 341:437.

4. Connolly LA (1991) Anesthetic management of obstructive sleep apnea patients. J Clin Anesth 3:461–469

5. Dematteis M, Lévy P, Pépin J-L (2005) A simple procedure for measuring pharyngeal sensitivity: a contribution to the diagnosis of sleep apnoea. Thorax 60:418–426

6. Fairbanks DNF, Fujita S (eds) (1994) Snoring and Obstructive Sleep Apnea, 2nd edn. Raven Press, New York, pp 136–145

7. Finkelstein Y, Talmi Y, Zohar Y (1988) Readaptation of the velopharyngeal valve following the uvulopalatopharyngoplasty operation. Plast Reconstr Surg 82:20–27

8. Friedman M, Tanyeri H, La Rosa M, et al (1999) Clinical predictors of obstructive sleep apnea. Laryngoscope 109:1901–1907

9. Fujita S, Conway W, Zorick F (1981) Surgical correction of anatomic abnormalities in obstructive sleep apnea syndrome: uvulopalatopharyngoplasty. Otolaryngol Head Neck Surg 89:923–934

10. Haraldsson PO, Carenfelt C, Persson HE, et al (1991) Simulated long-term driving performance before and after uvulopalatopharyngoplasty. ORL J Otorhinolaryngol Relat Spec 53:106–110

11. Haraldsson PO, Carenfelt C, Lysdahl M, et al (1995) Does uvulopalatopharyngoplasty inhibit automobile accidents? Laryngoscope 105:657–661

12. Hörmann K, Verse T (2005) Surgery for Sleep-Disordered Breathing. Springer, Berlin Heidelberg New York

13. Hultcrantz E, Svanholm H (1991) Down syndrome and sleep apnea – A therapeutic challenge. Int J Pediatr Otorhinolaryngol 21:263–268

14. Hultcrantz E, Johansson K, Bengtson H (1999) The effect of uvulpalatopharyngoplasty without tonsillectomy using local anaesthesia: a prospective long-term follow-up. J Laryngol Otol 113:542–547

15. Ikematsu T (1964) Study of snoring. 4th report. Therapy (in Japanese). J Jpn Otol Rhinol Laryngol Soc 64:434–435

16. Janson C, Gislason T, Bengtsson H, et al (1997) Long-term follow-up of patients with obstructive sleep apnea treated with uvulopalatopharyngoplasty. Arch Otolaryngol Head Neck Surg 123:257–262

17. Johnson JT, Braun TW (1998) Preoperative, intraoperative, and postoperative management of patients with obstructive sleep apnea syndrome. Otolaryngol Clin North Am 31:1025–1030

18. Katsantonis GP, Limitations, pitfalls, and risks management in uuvulopalatopharyngoplasty. In: Fairbanks DNF, Fujita S (eds) (1994) Snoring and Obstructive Sleep Apnea. 2nd edn. Raven Press, New York, pp 147–162

19. Keenan SP, Burt H, Ryan CF, et al (1994) Long-term survival of patients with obstructive sleep apnea treated by uvulopalatopharyngoplasty or nasal CPAP. Chest 105:155–159

20. Kerschner JE, Lynch JB, Kleiner H, et al (2002) Uvulopalatopharyngoplasty with tonsillectomy and adenoidectomy as a treatment for obstructive sleep apnea in neurologically impaired children. Int J Pediatr Otorhinolaryngol 62:229–235

21. Kezirian EJ, Weaver ME, Yueh B, et al (2004) Incidence of serious complications after uvulopalatopharyngoplasty. Laryngoscope 114:450–453

22. Kimoff RJ, Sforza E, Champagne V, et al (2001) Upper airway sensation in snoring and obstructive sleep apnea. Am J Respir Crit Care Med 164:250–255

23. Krishna S, Hughes LF, Lin SY (2003) Postoperative hemorrhage with nonsteroidal anti-flammatory drug use after tonsillectomy. Arch Otolaryngol Head Neck Surg 129:1086–1089

24. Larsson LH, Carlsson-Nordlander B, Svanborg E (1994) Four-year follow-up after uvulopalatopharyngoplasty in 50 unselected patients with obstructive sleep apnea syndrome. Laryngoscope 104:1362–1368

25. Lu SJ, Chang SY, Shiao GM (1995) Comparison between short-term and long-term post-operative evaluation of sleep apnea after uvulopalatopharyngoplasty. J Laryngol Otol 109:308–312

26. Lysdahl M, Haraldsson PO (2000) Long-term survival after uvulopalatopharyngoplasty in nonobese heavy snorers: a 5- to 9-year follow-up of 400 consecutive patients. Arch Otolaryngol Head Neck Surg 126:1136–1140

27. Naja MZ, El-Rajab M, Kabalan W, et al (2005) Pre-incisional infiltration for pediatric tonsillectomy: A randomized double-blind clinical trial. Int J Pediatr Otorhinolaryngol 69:1333–1341

28. Pirsig W, Schäfer J, Yildiz F, et al (1989) Uvulopalatopharyngoplasty without complications: a Fujita modification (in German). Laryngo-Rhino-Otol 68:585–590

29. Pirsig W, Hörmann K, Siegert R, et al (1999) ENT Medicine and Otolaryngology Guidelines of the German Society of Otorhinolaryngology – Head and Neck Surgery. Primary snoring, obstructive sleep apnea (OSA) and obstructive snoring/upper airway resistance syndrome (UARS) Sleep Breath 3:63–64

30. Schäfer J (1989) How can one recognize a velum snorer? (in German). Laryngo-Rhino-Otol 68:290–294

31. Schwab RJ (2003) Pro: Sleep apnea is an anatomic disorder. Am J Respir Crit Care Med 168:270–273

32. Sher AE (2002) Upper airway surgery for obstructive sleep apnea. Sleep Med Rev 6:195–212

33. Sher AE, Schechtman KB, Piccirillo JF (1996) The efficacy of surgical modifications of the upper airway in adults with obstructive sleep apnea syndrome. Sleep 19:156–177

34. Strohl KP (2003) Con: Sleep apnea is not an anatomic disorder. Am J Respir Crit Care Med 168:271–273

35. Verse T, Kroker B, Pirsig W, et al (2000) Tonsillectomy as a treatment of obstructive sleep apnea in adults with tonsillar hypertrophy. Laryngoscope 110:1556–1559

35

Chapter 36

Z-palatoplasty

Michael Friedman, Paul Schalch

36

Core Messages

- Classic uvulopalatopharyngoplasty (UPPP) sometimes causes narrowing of the palatal arch, with an ensuing decrease in the size of the oropharyngeal inlet.

- Patients with previous tonsillectomy are poor candidates for classic UPPP, owing to scarring or absence of the posterior pillar.

- Appropriate selection criteria are mandatory in order to identify patients with higher likelihood for cure using Z-palatoplasty (ZPP).

- The goal of ZPP is to widen the space between the palate and the posterior pharyngeal wall and the tongue base, and to maintain or widen the lateral dimensions of the retropalatal pharynx.

- The key elements are the removal of the anterior mucosa, the splitting of the soft palate in the midline, cutting the palatoglossus muscle, and the sewing of the posterior palatal mucosa to the anterior resection margin.

- The midline is retracted anterolaterally, which widens the retropharyngeal airway.

- ZPP is performed simultaneously with tongue-base radiofrequency reduction.

- There is always risk of temporary as well as permanent velopharyngeal insufficiency after ZPP.

- This procedure should be reserved for patients with moderate to severe obstructive sleep apnea–hypopnea syndrome, with significant symptoms.

Contents

Introduction

Owing to its limited success in curing obstructive sleep apnea–hypopnea syndrome (OSAHS) [1], many adjunctive procedures and modifications were proposed after the introduction of the classic uvulopalatopharyngoplasty (UPPP) by Fujita et al. [2] in 1981. However, its role as part of a comprehensive treatment plan remains solidly accepted in most situations in which the palate, with or without the tonsils, is contributing to airway turbulence and obstruction. The goal of UPPP is to widen the airspace in three areas: (1) the retropalatal space; (2) the space between the tongue base and the palate; and (3) the lateral dimensions. This is accomplished through two components: (1) the palatoplasty component, which involves palatal shortening with closure of mucosal incisions; and (2) the pharyngoplasty component, which comprises a classic tonsillectomy with pharyngeal closure. These goals, however, are not always achieved with classic UPPP. In spite of our best efforts, patients may end up with an extremely narrow palatal arch, in which the diameter of the oropharyngeal inlet is decreased owing to a forward approximation of the posterior palatal mucosa. The resulting new shape of the free edge of the palate is triangular, rather than square (Fig. 36.1). Further contraction of the wound occurs owing to scarring secondary to the resection of the posterior tonsillar pillars, and additional narrowing is caused, which further affects long-term results [3]. Additionally, patients who previously underwent tonsillectomy are poor candidates for classic UPPP, owing to scarring or absence of the posterior pillar from the previous tonsillectomy. These patients have an already narrowed space between the soft palate and the posterior pharyngeal wall, and often do not have any redundant pharyngeal folds. Important modifications of the classic UPPP proposed by Fairbanks, [4] in which the posterior pillar is advanced lateral cephalad in order to widen the retropalatal space, are, hence, not possible. It is well known that when UPPP fails, the severity of obstruction may actually worsen [5]. It became apparent that appropriate selection criteria needed to be implemented in order to identify patients with a higher likelihood of cure after UPPP. A staging system introduced by Friedman et al. [6] determined that patients with anatomic stage I disease (Friedman tongue position, FTP, I and II), with large tonsils, have a better than 80% chance of success; whereas patients with stage II and III disease (FTP III and IV) are less than ideal candidates, and should therefore undergo a combined procedure that addresses both the palate and the hypopharynx (Table 36.1). The Z-palatoplasty (ZPP) technique was developed as a more aggressive technique for patients with stage II and III disease. This includes all

Table 36.1. Friedman staging system based on Friedman tongue position, tonsil size, and body mass index (*BMI*). (Reprinted from Friedman et al. [6] copyright 2004 The American Laryngological, Rhinological and Otological Society)

Modified Staging System for Patients with Obstructive Sleep Apnea/Hypopnea Syndrome			
Stage	Friedman Palate Position	Tonsil Size	BMI
I	1	3, 4	<40
	2	3, 4	<40
II	1, 2	1, 2	<40
	3, 4	3, 4	<40
III	3	0, 1, 2	<40
	4	0, 1, 2	<40
IV	1, 2, 3, 4	0, 1, 2, 3, 4	>40

All patients with significant craniofacial or other anatomic deformities.

patients who have had previous tonsillectomy, as well as patients with small tonsils, and those with unfavorable tongue positions.

Tips and Pearls

- The goal of ZPP is to widen the space between the palate and the posterior pharyngeal wall, to widen the space between the palate and the tongue base, and to either maintain or widen the lateral dimensions of the pharynx

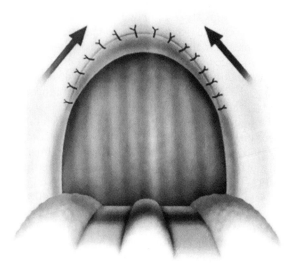

Fig. 36.1. After traditional uvulopalatopharyngoplasty, an anteromedially directed pull eventually causes narrowing of the retropalatal airspace in the lateral dimension. (Reprinted from Friedman et al. [7] copyright 2004, with permission from the American Academy of Otolaryngology – Head and Neck Surgery Foundation)

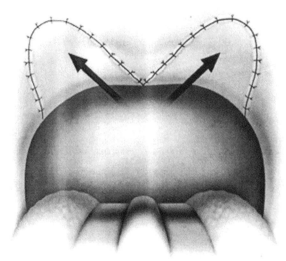

Fig. 36.2. After Z-palatoplasty, the anterolateral direction of pull on the soft palate widens the retropalatal space. (Reprinted from Friedman et al. [7] copyright 2004, with permission from the American Academy of Otolaryngology – Head and Neck Surgery Foundation)

This is accomplished by changing the scar contracture tension line to an anterolateral vector, and by widening the anteroposterior and lateral oropharyngeal air spaces at the level of the palate. By splitting the soft palate and retracting it anterolaterally, an effective anterolateral pull is created, which actually continues to widen the airway as healing and contracture occur (Fig. 36.2). None of the palatal musculature is resected, in spite of the aggressive palatal shortening, thereby addressing and minimizing the risk for permanent velopharyngeal insufficiency (VPI). This procedure is performed with adjunctive tongue-base reduction by radiofrequency (TBRF), which addresses the hypopharyngeal airway.

Tips and Pearls

- ZPP widens the retropalatal space by creating an anterolateral pull after splitting the soft palate.
- No palatal musculature is resected; the resection is limited to the anterior mucosa.
- The pharyngeal airway continues to widen as healing and contracture occur.

Patient Selection and Preoperative Evaluation

General guidelines for surgical intervention include significant symptoms of snoring and daytime somnolence; documented failure in continuous positive airway pressure (CPAP) trials; and documented failure of conservative measures, such as dental appliances, changes in sleeping position, and sleep hygiene in general. Apparent obstruction at the level of the soft palate must be determined by fiberoptic nasopharyngolaryngoscopy, and Müller maneuver or sleep endoscopy. Adequate medical clearance and a thorough review with the patient of the procedure, its implications, and potential outcomes and complications are essential components of the preoperative workup.

Specific criteria for ZPP include patients classified as stage II or III, according to Friedman's anatomic staging system (Table 36.1). ZPP is an aggressive procedure because it produces a significant widening of the retropalatal space, and it is associated with significant temporary VPI and the risk for permanent VPI. It should be reserved for patients with moderate to severe OSAHS, with moderate to severe symptoms. It is not a surgical option for snoring alone. Additionally, Friedman described a technique for revision in patients who previously underwent UPPP and subsequently failed. This technique involves principles similar to ZPP; taking into account the modified, postoperative anatomy of the pharyngeal airway [2].

Tips and Pearls

- UPPP may result in persistent or worsening retropalatal obstruction or nasopharyngeal stenosis that may worsen OSAHS.
- Appropriate patient selection using Friedman's anatomic staging system significantly improves outcomes.
- Patients need to be informed of the risk of temporary and permanent VPI before undergoing the procedure.
- All patients with FTP III or IV have obstruction at the retrolingual airway, in addition to any retropalatal obstruction. This area must be treated as well.

Indications/Contraindications

ZPP is indicated in:

- Patients with significant symptoms of snoring and daytime somnolenc
- Documented failure of CPAP trials.
- Documented failure of conservative measures
- Patients appropriately selected based on FTP and tonsil size, as detailed in the "Patient Selection and Preoperative Evaluation" section

ZPP should not be performed

- In patients with snoring but no documented OSAHS
- In patients with Friedman stage I disease, who do well with classic UPPP
- In patients classified as Friedman stage IV, based on a body mass index above 40, or significant craniofacial abnormalities
- In patients unwilling to accept the risk of VPI, and postoperative symptoms

Surgical Technique

The procedure is demonstrated in Video 36.1.

Candidates eligible to undergo a modified UPPP technique can be divided into patients with intact tonsils and patients after tonsillectomy.

The key points of ZPP are the removal of the anterior mucosa only and the splitting of the soft palate in the midline, cutting the palatoglossus muscle, and the sewing of the posterior palatal mucosa to the anterior resection margin, which retracts the midline anterolaterally and widens the retropharyngeal area.

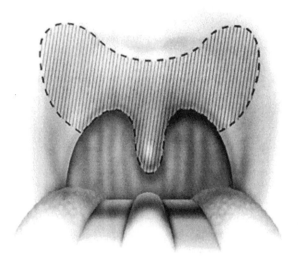

Fig. 36.3. Outline of the palatal flaps, marked before incision. (Reprinted from Friedman et al. [7] copyright 2004, with permission from the American Academy of Otolaryngology – Head and Neck Surgery Foundation)

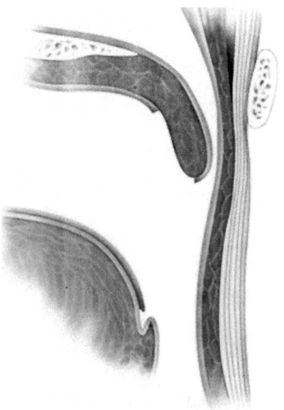

Fig. 36.5. Lateral view of the soft palate and uvula after excision of the anterior mucosa. The uvula and palate hang close to the posterior pharyngeal wall, narrowing the retropharyngeal space. (Reprinted from Friedman et al. [7] copyright 2004, with permission from the American Academy of Otolaryngology – Head and Neck Surgery Foundation)

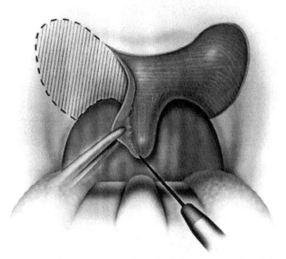

Fig. 36.4. The mucosa over the palatal flap is removed and the palatal musculature is exposed. (Reprinted from Friedman et al. [7] copyright 2004, with permission from the American Academy of Otolaryngology – Head and Neck Surgery Foundation)

The surgical technique for the modified ZPP is illustrated in Figs. 36.3–36.10.

Two adjacent flaps are outlined in the palate (Fig. 36.3). The anterior midline margin of the flap is halfway between the hard palate and the free edge of the soft palate, and the distal margin corresponds to the free edge of the palate and uvula. The lateral extent is posterior to the midline, and extends to the lateral edge of the palate. The mucosa from only the anterior aspect of the two flaps is subsequently removed (Fig. 36.4). Figure 36.5 illustrates how the preoperative uvula and

palate hang close to the posterior pharyngeal wall, narrowing the retropharyngeal space. The two flaps are then separated from each other by splitting the palatal segment down the midline (Fig. 36.6), extending them laterally in a butterfly fashion (Fig. 36.7), and dividing the palatoglossus muscle. A two-layer closure is then performed, which brings the midline all the way to the anterolateral margin of the palate (Figs. 36.8, 36.9). The primary closure is performed at the submucosal level, which enables a tension-free closure of the mucosa. A distance of at least 3–4 cm between the posterior pharynx and the palate is created [7]. Figure 36.10 illustrates the widening of the nasopharynx after the midline palatoplasty. The lateral dimension of the palate is usually increased to approximately 4 cm.

TBRF is adjunctively performed in all patients, by administering 3,000 J (rapid lesion technique by Gyrus™, Gyrus ENT, Memphis, TN, USA), which is distributed to ten points along the midline of the tongue behind the circumvallated papillae. This initial treatment is followed by monthly sessions, as needed. The addition of TBRF has shown significantly better sub-

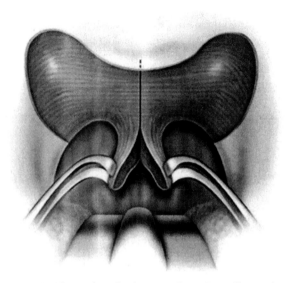

Fig. 36.6. The uvula and palate are split in the midline with a cold knife. (Reprinted from Friedman et al. [7] copyright 2004, with permission from the American Academy of Otolaryngology – Head and Neck Surgery Foundation)

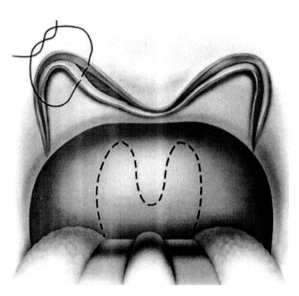

Fig. 36.8. Two-layered closure of the palatal flaps. The submucosal layer is approximated first with 2-0 Vicryl™ (Ethicon,, Somerville, NJ, USA). (Reprinted from Friedman et al. [7] copyright 2004, with permission from the American Academy of Otolaryngology – Head and Neck Surgery Foundation)

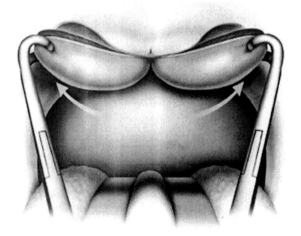

Fig. 36.7. The uvular flaps, along with the soft palate, are reflected posteriorly and laterally over the soft palate. (Reprinted from Friedman et al. [7] copyright 2004, with permission from the American Academy of Otolaryngology – Head and Neck Surgery Foundation)

Table 36.2. Comparison of complications between Z-palatoplasty (ZPP) and classic uvulopalatopharyngoplasty (UPPP), based on a series of 25 matched patients who underwent each procedure. (Modified from Friedman et al. [7])

	ZPP (n=25)	UPPP (n=25)
Tongue-base infection	1 (4%)	2 (8%)
Bleeding	0	0
Postnasal drip	3 (12%)	4 (16%)
Dysphagia	1 (4%)	11 (44%)*
Foreign body sensation	11 (44%)	17 (68%)
Temporary VPI	12 (48%)	7 (28%)
Permanent VPI	0	0

VPI velopharyngeal insufficiency
*p<0.001

jective and objective improvement in stage II and III patients undergoing UPPP, when compared with patients who undergo UPPP only [9].

Postoperative Management and Complications

As with any intervention that involves resection of the soft palate, significant morbidity is observed in the first 24–72 h postoperatively, in the form of significant pain and dysphagia. The ability of the patient to tolerate at least a liquid diet, oral pain medications, antibiotics, and steroids determines the moment when the patient can be safely discharged. While discharge could in theory be on the same day as the surgery, most patients will need 1 or 2 days of intravenous fluids and medications before they can start an oral diet. Prior to discharge, patients are prescribed acetaminophen with codeine elixir, as needed for pain. Pain medication requirements average 6.5 days; the same goes for the pro-

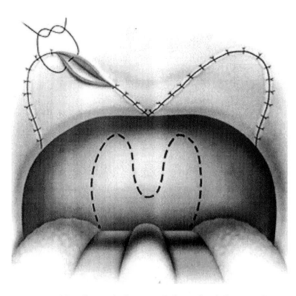

Fig. 36.9. Two-layered closure of the palatal flaps with 3-0 chromic suture. (Reprinted from Friedman et al. [7] copyright 2004, with permission from the American Academy of Otolaryngology – Head and Neck Surgery Foundation)

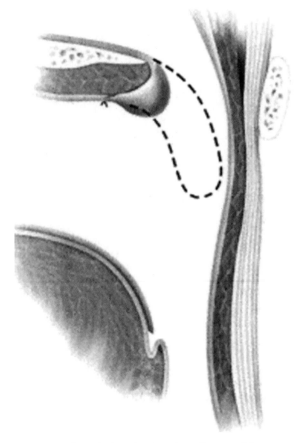

Fig. 36.10. Lateral view showing the widening of the nasopharynx after Z-palatoplasty. (Reprinted from Friedman et al. [7] copyright 2004, with permission from the American Academy of Otolaryngology – Head and Neck Surgery Foundation)

gression from liquid or soft diet, to regular diet. Postoperative antibiotics and steroids are also recommended, for a total of 7 days. Additional TBRF sessions may be necessary, depending on the improvement of symptoms in each individual patient.

Complications of the procedure are comparable to those of classic UPPP (Table 36.2). Bleeding is always a potential complication, and the risk is again comparable to that of classic UPPP. Typically, patients can eat a regular diet after 2 weeks. Mild VPI may manifest when drinking quickly, and may persist for up to 3 months. After 3 months, patients have normal deglutition. The severity of VPI symptoms diminishes with time, and is expected to progressively resolve. Permanent VPI is a potential complication that must be considered by every patient. Additional morbidity of the procedure is usually related to throat discomfort symptoms, including globus sensation, mild dysphagia, dry throat, and the inability to clear the throat. These symptoms are almost universal after any form of UPPP.

Other complications are related to the adjunctive procedures performed. Tongue-base infection is related to TBRF and requires antibiotic treatment. In rare cases, it may lead to tongue-base abscess formation, which may require incision and drainage.

Outcomes: Subjective and Objective Symptom Elimination

Subjective success is based on comparative improvement in snoring level, daytime sleepiness, and overall well-being. Patients who underwent ZPP were compared with patients who had previously undergone UPPP for the treatment of OSAHS. The results achieved were far superior with ZPP, particularly with adjunctive TBRF. Quality-of-life scores improved significantly more often after ZPP than after UPPP [4]. When focusing on objective success, ZPP showed considerable improvement over UPPP. Objective cure rates for stage II patients treated with ZPP and TBRF were close to 70%, compared with about 30% for classic UPPP with TBRF.

Limitations of this technique include a higher risk of temporary VPI, owing to a more aggressive modification of the palatal anatomy even though the resection is limited to the mucosa. While VPI is usually temporary, should permanent VPI ensue, ZPP is probably not reversible. There are also no clear anatomic landmarks to assist in describing the size of the flaps, and ultimately the guidelines outlined in this chapter do not substitute for the surgeon's judgment. The procedure is significantly more difficult technically, and it takes longer to perform. A learning curve, as with any other procedure, leads to progressively better results.

36

The treatment, like any other, may fail. Failure can be defined as a persistence of symptoms, which demands additional treatment. Failure also occurs when symptoms of snoring and daytime sleepiness are eliminated, but polysomnography scores still indicate persistent disease. Typically, patients who fail will show a pattern of elimination of apneas, with persistent hypopneas. Failure in achieving satisfactory results may in some cases convince the patient to accept CPAP therapy. When CPAP is not accepted by the patient, further evaluation and treatment are essential. The first step should be a thorough investigation in order to identify the site of failure. Sleep endoscopy evaluation may be a valuable test at this point. If the level of obstruction continues to be retropalatal, a transpalatal advancement pharyngoplasty can be considered [10]. If the persistence of obstruction is at the tongue base or hypopharyngeal level, genioglossus advancement alone or in combination with thyrohyoid suspension could be an option [11]. Bimaxillary advancement should be kept in mind as a second-line procedure as well, if the above interventions fail. This procedure will correct failures both at the retropalatal and the retrolingual levels [12].

Conclusion

▼

No single procedure is effective in treating all OSAHS patients. Treatment should be tailored to the anatomy of each patient. Rerouting the uvula together with the soft palate laterally improves airway characteristics by enlarging the retropalatal space, which is a distinct advantage over traditional UPPP. This acquires even more importance when addressing the obstruction at the level of the palate in patients without tonsils.

References

1. Sher AE, Schechtman KB, Piccirillo JF (1996) The efficacy of surgical modifications of the upper airway in adults with obstructive sleep apnea syndrome. Sleep 19:156–177
2. Fujita S, Conway W, Zorick F, Roth T (1981) Surgical correction of anatomic abnormalities in obstructive sleep apnea syndrome: uvulopalatopharyngoplasty. Otolaryngol Head Neck Surg 89:923–934
3. Friedman M, Landsberg R, Tanyeri H (2000) Submucosal uvulopalatopharyngoplasty. Oper Tech Otolaryngol Head Neck Surg 11:26–29
4. Fairbanks DN (1999) Operative techniques of uvulopalatopharyngoplasty. Ear Nose Throat J 78:846–850
5. Senior BA, Rosenthal L, Lumley A, Lumley A, Gerhardstein R, Day R (2000) Efficacy of uvulopalatopharyngoplasty in unselected patients with mild obstructive sleep apnea. Otolaryngol Head Neck Surg 123:179–182
6. Friedman M, Ibrahim H, Joseph N (2004) Staging of obstructive sleep apnea/hypopnea syndrome: a guide to appropriate treatment. Laryngoscope 114:454–459
7. Friedman M, Ibrahim HZ, Vidyasagar R, Pomeranz J (2004) Z-palatoplasty (ZPP): a technique for patients without tonsils. Otolaryngol Head Neck Surg 131:89–100
8. Friedman M, Duggal P, Joseph NJ (2006) Revision uvulopalatoplasty by Z-palatoplasty. Otolaryngol Head Neck Surg (in press)
9. Friedman M, Ibrahim H, Lee G, Joseph NJ (2003) Combined uvulopalatopharyngoplasty and radiofrequency tongue base reduction for treatment of obstructive sleep apnea/hypopnea syndrome. Otolaryngol Head Neck Surg 129:611–621
10. Woodson BT, Toohill RJ (1993) Transpalatal advancement pharyngoplasty for obstructive sleep apnea. Laryngoscope 103:269–276
12. Li KK, Riley RW, Powell NB, Guilleminault C (2000) Maxillomandibular advancement for persistent OSA after phase I surgery in patients without maxillomandibular deficiency. Laryngoscope 110:1684–1688
11. Powell NB, Riley RW, Guilleminault C (1994) The hypopharynx: Upper airway reconstruction in obstructive sleep apnea syndrome. In: Fairbanks DNF, Fujita S (eds) Snoring and obstructive sleep apnea. 2nd edn. Raven Press, New York

Chapter 37

Transpalatal Advancement Pharyngoplasty

37

B. Tucker Woodson

Core Messages

- Palatal advancement pharyngoplasty is a segmental pharyngeal procedure indicated to structurally enlarge the retropalatal and retromaxillary airway in patients with obstructive sleep apnea syndrome.

- The procedure enlarges the proximal pharyngeal isthmus, which is inaccessible by other techniques other than maxillary advancement.

- Advancement may be performed in patients with uvulopalatopharyngoplasty failures who have adequate swallow, sufficient palatal length, and normal lateral wall movement with swallow.

- The procedure enlarges the retropalatal airway at the expense of narrowing the oropalatal airway and often requires treatment of tongue base associated airway.

- The procedure may be performed primarily with or without combined conservative distal pharyngoplasty procedures.

- Clinical success is dependent on treating all areas of upper-airway obstruction, including the epipharynx, oropharynx, and hypopharynx.

- Technical success is dependent on adequate mobilization and closure of the soft palate. The tensor aponeurosis and fascia is released to advance the palate and incorporates the closure of the tensor aponeurosis to prevent a fistula.

Contents

Introduction

The purpose of segmental pharyngeal procedures to treat obstructive sleep apnea syndrome is to increase airway size and decrease collapsibility. Procedures also reduce total airway resistance and sites of flow limitation and choke point during sleep. Surgically the challenge is to improve ventilatory structure while maintaining other normal functions of speech and swallowing. Palatal advancement pharyngoplasty is a method of enlarging the retromaxillary and retropalatal airspace by removing a posterior portion of midline hard palate (maxilla and palatine bone) and advancing the soft palate anteriorly into the defect. Conceptually this has similarities to maxillary advancement, but does not require altering or moving dentition (Fig. 37.1).

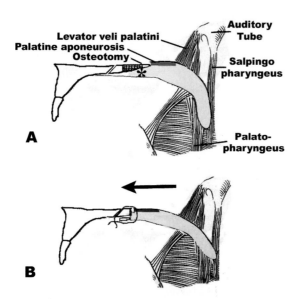

Fig. 37.1. A Midsaggital depiction of the palate and lateral walls demonstrating palatal advancement. An osteotomy is created at the posterior palate. Bone is removed proximally (*crosshatched*). Drill holes are placed anterior to bone removal and leaving a strong rim of bone to support sutures. The palatal flap that is advanced is thicker than the original mucosa (*asterisk*). Flap mucosa is preserved to cover the thicker flap. Some fibroadipose tissue may also be carefully trimmed to reduce the thickness of the soft-tissue flap. **B** Following bone removal, sutures are placed submucosally through the drill holes around the bony osteotomy fragment and the soft palate is advanced

37

The pharyngeal isthmus is the narrowest and most compliant portion of the upper airway and is the most common segment of obstruction in the obstructive sleep apnea sydnrome [1]. Although tongue-base narrowing and collapse has been blamed for failure palatal procedures such as uvulopalatopharyngoplasty (UPPP), objective airway evaluation after surgery demonstrates that persistent retropalatal collapse occurs in many surgical failures [2]. Persistent obstruction is common and occurs in the retropalatal airway proximal to the site of prior palatopharyngoplasty. This collapse has been associated with inadequate increases in airway size [3].

Proximal collapse may be primary or secondary. Primary narrowing of the pharyngeal isthmus may result from posterior maxillary constriction and a narrow pharyngeal isthumus occurs during facial growth and development. Narrowing is suggested by maxillary retrusion, an Angle class III occlusion, a narrow facial depth, and a high arched palate. The airway shape when observed endoscopically is often narrow in an anterior to posterior direction. Secondly, narrowing may be secondary to hypertrophy of muscle, soft tissue, obesity, or trauma (surgery). Lateral pharyngeal wall hypertrophy and collapse may be observed with some secondary causes. Scar from prior surgery may narrow the velopharyngeal inslet. In 1990, Woodson and Toohill described a technique of removing midline bone of the palate and advancing the soft palate into the defect. This procedure advanced the palate medially and was combined with mucosal advancement flaps along the lateral border of the soft palate to improve the lateral airway. Significant improvement was seen in some patients who had failed prior UPPP and subsequent studies demontrated marked improvements in airway size and collapsibility after the procedure. The initial method to mobilize the soft palate was to fracture the hamulus. Unfortunately in some patients this resulted in otitis media with effusion. Subsequently the procedure was modified to mobilize the soft palate by incising the tensor aponeurosis and leaving the hamulus intact. Better mobilization resulted in improved airway size and reduced lateral pharyngeal wall collapse but also an increased oropalatal fistula rate. Subsequently it was appreciated that this dehiscence resulted partly from failure to adequately close the palatine aponeurosis, which was exposed to the repeated forces of swallowing (and particularly gag). Although anteriorly anchored strongly to bone, sutures were anchored only to soft fibroadipose tissues of the palate, which in some cases was inadequate. To address this, the procedure was modified so that separation of the hard palate and the soft palate was not done at the junction of bone and soft tissues, but a small osteotomy was performed just anterior to the junction. This left a small osteotomized rim of bone strongly attached via periosteal ligaments and tendons to the soft palate to prevent soft-tissue seperation and sutures from tearing through the tissues. Additionally, better understanding of palatal anatomy and the position of the fibrous tendon (Fig. 37.2) improved in the lateral closure to allow precise identification and suturing of the tensor aponeurosis. Combined, these reduce the opportunities for an oronasal fistula.

Palatal advancement enlarges the pharyngeal isthmus. It potentially narrows the oropalatal airway. For this reason most patients require tongue-base treatment (i.e., glossectomy, tissue oblation, genioglossus advancement, or tongue suspension).

Tips and Pearls

The advantages of the palatal advancement procedure include:

- Theproximal retropalatal airway is enlarged.
- Muscle function is maintained with reduced requirements for soft-tissue excision of the distal palate.
- There is no alteration or movement of maxillary dentition.

Fig. 37.2. View of the dorsal (nasopharyngeal) surface of the soft palate. Anterior and lateral soft-tissue attachments to the hard palate and hamulus have been released. A thin layer of nasopharyngeal mucosa has been removed exposing the tensor apponeurosis (*large white arrow*) which lies immediately underneath. The levator palatini muscle is intact (*small white arrow*). The anterior belly of the levator palatini muscle is partially enveloped in fascia and needs to be released to adequately mobilize the palate (*black arrow*)

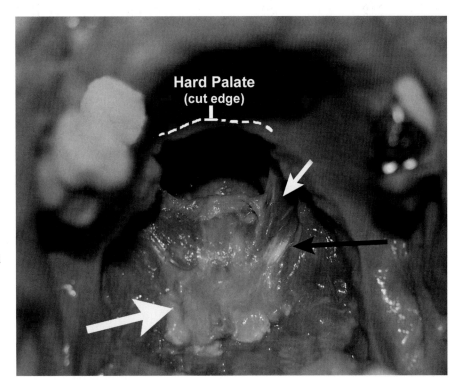

- There is less pain than with traditional tonsillectomy, UPPP.
- It may be added to other pharyngeal procedures and pharyngoplasty.
- The methods and technique of closure are important.

Indications and Patient Selection

Surgery for obstructive sleep apnea syndrome is indicated following failure, ineffectiveness, or noncompliance of more conservative treatments for obstructive sleep apnea syndrome. Patients should have an understanding of available reconstructive procedures and likely outcomes and that multiple surgical steps may be required. Surgical candidates should have undergone an appropriate sleep evaluation and objective testing to address associated sleep and medical problems.

Palatal advancement is indicated when narrowing of the proximal pharyngeal isthmus (retropalatal airway) is present. The most common method of identifying this narrowing is during sitting and supine endoscopic evaluation (Video 37.1). Although narrowing may be identified by an experienced examiner, identification of persistent narrowing may only be appreciated following failed UPPP. It is the author's bias that the best candidates for palatal advancement are those with a pattern of narrowing primarily in an anterior to posterior dimension. Although the procedure enlarges the lateral wall, those patients with marked lateral wall hypertrophy and collapse may not be ideal candidates for limited pharyngeal procedures of any type. Although obesity is not an absolute contraindication, morbidly obese patients with severe obstructive sleep apnea syndrome who have been recalcitrant to weight loss should be considered for possible bimaxillary advancement, bariatric surgery, or tracheotomy. Surgeons who perform palatal advancement techniques should be aware that the potential exists following the procedure for a reduction in blood flow to the maxilla caused by disruption of soft-tissue attachments to the maxilla. Such a loss may potentially reduce blood flow to the maxilla. Normally, this would be of no significance; however, in cases of complicated maxillary surgery with bilateral disruption of greater palatine arteries, maxillary necrosis could theoretically be augmented. For this reason, individuals at high likelihood of requiring maxillofacial surgery should have this procedure prior to palatal advancement if possible.

Preoperative Evaluation

As part of the preoperative evaluation the surgeon should do the following.

Polysomnography is appropriate in patients with sleep-disordered breathing, including mild to moderate or severe obstructive sleep apnea syndrome undergoing airway reconstruction. Since successful clinical outcomes of surgery cannot be guaranteed, maximal attempts at more conservative treatments are appropriate. Additionally, the sleep study provides information on the severity of disease and the nadir of oxygen desaturation and helps to identify those who warrant postoperative care and observation. Individuals at higher general surgical risk also include those with severe obesity, severe sleepiness, difficult intubation, or severe pharyngeal tissue redundancy. Individuals with preexisting speech or swallowing disorder should be identified and warned that pharyngeal surgery may worsen symptoms or problems with dysphagia, mucociliary function, mouth dryness, and aspiration.

Cephalometric upper-airway evaluation is optional. No specific measures are available that select surgical patients for this procedure. The main method of evaluation is endoscopy. Endoscopy is performed in a sitting and supine body position. Size, shape, areas of collapse, and pharyngeal swallow are evaluated. During endoscopy when the nasopharynx is visualized, close attention is focused on the size of the proximal pharyngeal isthmus. Narrowing of the airway proximal to any level of palatal excision with traditional palatopharyngoplasty should be noted. The position of the levator muscle in the soft palate and the size of the associated airway should be assessed. The levator muscle can be identified by visualizing the torus tubarius. The position of the anterior fold is the torus levatorious, with the posterior fold the salpingopharyngeus muscle. A more posteriorly placed levator muscle in close approximation to the posterior pharyngeal wall cannot be addressed by traditional palatopharyngoplasty without aggressive excision of the levator muscle. During endoscopy, swallow is performed and lateral wall motion assessed. Finally, the oral cavity and oropalatal airway is assessed. An oropalatal airway that allows oral ventilation without deformation of the tongue may not require treatment. Evidence of oropalatal collapse manifested by "tongue grooving" or a midline deformation of the posterior tongue indicates relative macroglossia and the need for treatment of this segment.

Indications and Contraindications for Palatal Advancement Pharyngoplasty

Indications are:

- The patient understands available medical, reconstructive, and other therapeutic options.
- Retropalatal narrowing proximal to the free margin of the soft palate.
- Retropalatal narrowing following failed UPPP.
- Approach to benign midline nasopharyngeal masses (with or without sleep apnea).
- Choanal narrowing.
- Combined with other procedures to enlarge the retropalatal airway for cases of nasopharyngeal stenosis.

Contraindications are:

- Partial or complete cleft palate
- Large torus palatinus (requires removal first)
- Maxillary advancement surgery (relative)
- Impaired palatal blood flow such as with radiation therapy or severe palatal scarring
- Impaired swallow
- Velopharyngeal insufficiency
- Obligate mouth breather (may worsen oral ventilation)
- Surgeon has inadequate resources to address an oronasal fistula

Surgical Technique

The procedure is demonstrated in Video 37.2

Palatal advancement pharyngoplasty is an evolving technique that advances the soft palate forward to enlarge the pharyngeal isthmus. The procedure may be divided conceptually into steps including (1) incision, (2) flap elevation, (3) palatal osteotomy, (3) tendinolysis, (4) palate advancement, (5) wound closure, and if needed (6) distal palatopharyngoplasty or tonsilectomy.

The procedure is performed under general anesthesia delivered oroendotracheally. Patients are placed supine in the Rose position, and operative exposure is obtained with a Dingman mouth gag (Pilling Instrument Co., Philadelphia, PA, USA). The Dingman mouth gag facilitates handling of multiple sutures during closure. All patients are administered perioperative antibiotics (1–2 g cephazolin and 500 mg metronidazole) and 10 mg dexamethasone. For homeostasis, 1% lidocaine with 1:100,000 epinephrine is infiltrated into the greater palatine foramen and the incision sites prior to the procedure. Injection includes the junction of the hard palate and and soft palate, the tissues over the hamulus and lateral soft palate, and the line of incision of the mucosal flap over the hard palate. Oxymetazoline-soaked pledgets are placed along the floor of the nose to reduce bleeding from the nasal mucosa when placing drill holes and sutures.

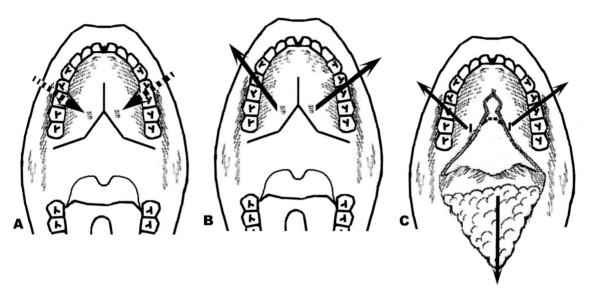

Fig. 37.3. Procedure of transpalatal advancement pharyn-goplasty. **A** The Ω-shaped incision is outlined medial to the greater palatine foramen and flared laterally over the hamulus. **B** Lateral flaps are elevated (*arrows*). **C** The tip of the midline flap is planned to be 5 mm anterior to bone removal (*dotted line*). The midline flap is elevated just to the junction of the hard palate and the soft palate. Care is taken to not separate the tendon attachments to the hard palate. Elevation is exaggerated in the figure to depict anatomy

Incision, Flap Elevation, and Mobilization

A palatal incision is outlined beginning at the central hard palate posterior to the alveolus (Fig. 37.3a). The tip should extend 5–10 mm anterior to the planned osteotomy. The incision is outlined immediately medial to the greater palatine foramen. At the junction of the hard palate and the soft palate, it is flaired laterally over the hamulus. This results in a curvilinear "Ω-arch" appearance. Anteriorly, a midline vertical incision is extended up the midline of the hard palate ("T" incision). The mucosa lateral to the "T" incision is elevated providing greater exposure to the hard palate (Fig. 37.2b). This reduces the need for a longer midline flap and reduces risk of tip necrosis. The midline mucoperiosteal flap is elevated back to the junction of the hard palate and the soft palate (Fig 37.3c). During elevation, the central mucosa is usually thin and care must be taken to avoid tearing it. Laterally, the flap is thicker and the fibroadipose tissue is bluntly dissected to avoid damage to the greater palatine vessels (a small mastoid currette with both a curved blunt surface and a sharp edge works well). Posteriorly, lesser palatine vessels and nerves may be transected. Elevation of the flap beyond the border of the soft palate and the hard palate to expose of the soft palate is not necessary. Care must be taken not to dissect the tendon and periosteal attachments of the soft palate from the posterior edge of the hard palate. Flap elevation must remain superficial to the tensor aponeurosis.

Several methods of division of the soft palate and the hard palate have been described. Initially, electrocautery separated the soft and hard palates at the the posterior junction of the hard palate and exposed the nasopharynx. Sutures in fibroadipose tissue, however, were inadequate to support closure when the distraction forces applied to the palate with speech and swallowing are applied. An oronasal fistula was noted in 10% or more of patients. To address this an "osteotomy technique" was developed. Although this technique created more work in seperating the hard and soft palates, it significantly decreased the work required to close the wound using multiple difficult figure-of-eight soft-tissue sutures.

The current technique separates the hard and soft palates using a distal transverse osteotomy of the posterior hard palate. With this, the tensor apponeurosis remaines solidly attached to bone and oronasal fistulas are significantly reduced. A 1–2-mm margin of posterior hard palate bone is left attached to the soft palate (Fig. 37.4a). The osteotomized segment is then released by cutting it from the palate and alveolus as far laterally as possible and by cutting the attached posterior septum. The septal cut may be done with a smalll rotary burr, a small saggital saw, or heavy sissors.

After the distal osteotomy has been performed, a posterior 0.5–1.0-cm margin of the hard palate (palatine bone) is removed to provide space to move the soft palate anteriorly. Bone removal may be performed with either a small angled sagittal saw or a ro-

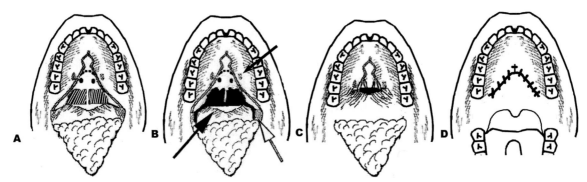

Fig. 37.4. Procedure of transpalatal advancement pharyngoplasty (continued). **A** A posterior osteotomy is performed leaving a 1–2-mm rim of bone. Nasal mucosa is preserved at this point (*crosshatched*). Proximal drill holes are placed. **B** The soft palate and the hard palate are separated exposing the nasopharynx. The osteotomy is separated from the posterior nasal septum (*larger black arrow*) and lateral tendinolysis is performed (*white arrow*). A solid rim of bone remains between the osteotomies and palatal drill holes **C** Sutures are placed through palatal drill holes and around the palatal osteotomy. Sutures are placed into the tensor aponeurosis laterally. Posterior traction is used to advance the flap and sutures are tied **D** Mucosa is approximated with multiple interrupted sutures

tary drill. Mucosa of the floor of the nose is initially preserved if possible.

Leaving the nasal mucosa intact allows for easier backwards elevation of the nasal mucosa off the floor of the nose. This elevation allows for the transpalatal sutures to remain submucosal. If they are not submucosal, there is a small risk of nasal granuloma in the postoperative period. Palatal drill holes are placed at 45° to the palate, extending from the oral surface of the palate into the nasal cavity (see also Fig. 37.1). A strong segment of bone must be left between these drill holes and the excised bony margin.

Tendonolysis

In the first reports of the procedure, mobilization of the soft palate was done by fracturing the hamulus in order to release stress on the tensor tendon. The occasional complication of serous otitis media with effusion was observed and new techniques were developed. The hamulus is now left undisturbed, and mobilization is achieved by bilaterally cutting and freeing the tensor tendon just medial to the hamulus. Complete incision of the tensor tendon medial to the hamulus markedly increased the amount of palate advancement achieved. The current technique incises the tensor tendon as well as the facial bands of the anterior belly of the levator palatini muscle (Fig. 37.4b). This provided almost unlimited potential for advancement. Tendonolysis is performed by first cutting the nasal mucosa (with electrocautery) proximal to the osteotomy. Additionally, nasal mucosa lateral to the osteotomy needs to be released. The nasopharynx is now visualized. Visualizing the nasopharynx is important to identify the lateral nasopharyn-

geal walls and avoid dissection into the lateral wall of the nasopharynx. Although, tendonolysis was initially, approached from the ventral surface of the palate, it is now approached from the dorsal (nasopharyngeal) surface. With blunt, sharp, or judicious electrocautery dissection, the tensor tendon is identified and cut.

Advancement

A free needle is then used to pass suture (braided, long duration) through the drill holes into the nasopharynx. Sutures are now placed in a simple fashion from the nasopharyngeal side around the osteotomy into the tensor tendon and out the oral cavity. Additional absorbable sutures are placed in the lateral tendon to reapproximate the tensor tendon to the lateral walls and the tissues around the hamulus. Identifying and placing accurate sutures in the aponeurosis is important (Fig. 37.2). Sutures are tied while an assistant pulls the palate forward with a curved retractor or blunt-tipped Jankar suction (Fig. 37.4c).

Closure

Excess or redundant tissue of the palate is present after advancement. Mucosa is preserved since the posterior flap is thicker than the original hard-palate mucosa and extra mucosa is needed to cover and broach this difference. Fibroadipose tissue may be trimmed as required. The anterior flap is closed with interrupted long-lasting absorbable sutures (Fig. 37.4d). An arched hard palate may make flap closure difficult. A soft diet is begun on the first day. The use of an upper denture is avoided for at least 4 weeks, or until healing is completed. If wound breakdown is noted, an upper palatal splint (even if only partially occlusive) may be easily fashioned (dentist, dental laboratory, other) and worn until healing has been achieved. Closure may be expedited by placing temporary sutures which will last for several days and will relieve tension on the wound. These can be replaced as needed.

Distal Palatopharyngoplasty

In a patients with an anatomically normal palate and uvula, no surgery of the uvula and distal palate is required. In patients with redundant palate, pillar mucosa, uvula, or tonsils, conservative surgery to tighten or remove this tissue may be needed with or without a tonsillectomy. In many patients, it may be performed after UPPP failure. In cases of pharyngeal stenosis after surgery or trauma, scar release may be needed with or without additional procedures.

Postoperative Care

Postoperative care includes:

- Perioperative antibiotics
- Avoiding dentures or other soft-tissue compression
- A soft diet for 2 weeks to avoid undoing stress on the closure with swallow and gag
- Close observation for a fistula (early use of oral splint if one is identified)

Results and Complications

Published data on transpalatal advancement pharyngoplasty includes case series and studies of airway mechanics [4–6]. Early experience observed significant reductions in the apnea–hypopnea index (AHI) and the apnea index. A 67% successful response rate with a respiratory disturbance index (RDI) of less than 20 events per hour was observed in patients who only underwent transpalatal advancement. The RDI in the responder group decreased from 52.8 to 12.3 events per hour. Seven of 11 patients (64%) had the RDI reduced to less than 20 events per hour. This group was skewed by several individuals with massive redundant nasopharyngeal lymphoid tissue that when removed likely contributed to such marked improvement. Subsequent studies on subjects without lymphoid blockage demonstrated improvement in the AHI, although these studies primarily evaluated upper-airway structure. Increased retropalatal size and decreased compliance were observed. Photographic evaluation demonstrated an increased velopharyngeal anterior–posterior dimension and enlargement of the lateral pharyngeal ports.

More recently a controlled study compared a cohort of patients with palatal advancement to a matched historical group of UPPP patients all of whom were categorized as Friedman stage 3. This group would be predicted to have an 8% success rate with UPPP alone. The palatal advancement group demonstrated significant improvement over UPPP. The odds ratio of success using palatal advancement over UPPP was 5.77 (95% confidence interval of 1.80–17.98) when controlling for body mass index, tongue-base surgery, age, and presurgical AHI.

Postoperatively, velopharyngeal insufficiency has been rare. One case following aggressive UPPP is known to have occurred and resolved with partial suture release. Clinical success also occurred. This is similar to maxillofacial surgery where velopharyngeal insufficiency is rare even following UPPP. As with UPPP, transient symptoms of mild nasopharyngeal reflux may occur immediately postoperatively. Dysphagia may occur for several weeks postoperatively. Increased pharyngeal volume, UPPP effects, or other factors may decrease afferent triggering of swallow or may decrease bolus pressures and contribute to delayed pharyngeal clearance. As with all palatopharyngoplasty techniques, sensation of globus, mucocilliary dysfunction, dry throat, excessive salivation, and increased aspiration may occur. In isolated palatal advancement, these complaints seem to be rare and less common than with traditional UPPP techniques. Rarely, palatal flap necrosis and a subsequent oronasal fistula may occur. All have closed with conservative treatment including the creation and wearing of an upper palatal prosthesis for 1–6 weeks. No fistula has required an operative procedure to close secondarily. Gentle tissue technique, careful hemostasis, perioperative antibiotics, and placement of the site of incision to minimally overlap the bone removal are recommended to lessen this complication. Smokers may be particularly prone to poor healing and fistula.

References

1. Morrison DL, Launois SH, Isono S, et.al. Pharyngeal narrowing and closing pressures in patients with obstructive sleep apnea. Am Rev Respir Dis 148:606–611, 1993.
2. Shepard JW, Thawley SE. Localization of upper airway collapse during sleep in patients with obstructive sleep apnea. Am Rev Respir Dis 141:1350-1355, 1990.

346

3. Caballero P, Alvarez-Sala R, Garcia-Rio F. CT in the evaluation of the upper airway in healthy subjects and in patients with obstructive sleep apnea syndrome, Chest 113:111–116, 1998.

4. Woodson BT, Toohill RJ. Transpalatal advancement pharyngoplasty for obstructive sleep apnea. Laryngoscope 103:269-276, 1993.

5. Woodson BT. Retropalatal Airway Characteristics in UPPP Compared to Transpalatal Advancement Pharyngoplasty. Laryngoscope 107:735–740, 1997.

6. Woodson BT. Acute Effects of Palatopharyngoplasty on Airway Collapsibility. Otolaryngol Head Neck Surg 121:82–6, 1999.

37

Chapter 38

Tongue-Base Suspension

Adam M. Becker, Christine G. Gourin

38

Core Messages

- Tongue-base suspension should be considered in patients who are suitable candidates for uvulopalatopharyngoplasty with an apnea–hypopnea index above 20 and documented moderate tongue-base obstruction on clinical examination.

- The addition of hyoid myotomy and suspension to tongue-base suspension may further improve the retrolingual airway.

- Overcorrection can result in tongue thrusting, dysarthria, and dysphagia, which may not resolve.

- Tracheostomy rather than tongue-base suspension should be offered to patients with severe tongue-base obstruction or to patients with severe cardiopulmonary comorbidity or apnea-related cardiac events.

Contents

Introduction

As early as 1981, Fujita et al. [1] recognized that patients with obstructive sleep apnea (OSA) often have multiple levels of obstruction. The tongue base and hypopharynx have been found to be the major sites of obstruction in up to 50% of patients [2]. Although uvulopalatopharyngoplasty (UPPP) remains the cornerstone of surgical therapy for OSA, failure to address additional sites of obstruction can significantly limit the effectiveness of surgical intervention. In their series, Sher et. al. [3] demonstrated cure rates with UPPP alone of only 40% in nonselected patients and 5–10% in patients with type II/III airway collapse. Riley et. al. [4] concluded that the tongue base was the cause of persistent obstruction in patients who failed UPPP.

Many techniques have been developed to address obstruction in the hypopharynx and tongue base and include midline glossectomy, lingualplasty, radiofrequency tongue ablation, hyoid suspension, mandibular osteotomy with genioglossus advancement, and maxillary-mandibular advancement. Many of these treatments are associated with significant morbidity, including mental nerve anesthesia, dental trauma, and the potential to change the facial appearance. Most recently, a minimally invasive tongue-base suture suspension procedure has been developed and has been shown in many series to be a safe and effective means of addressing obstruction at this level. This technique utilizes a submucosal suture that is anchored to the genial tubercle to prevent the tongue from occluding the pharynx when muscle activity is reduced during sleep.

DeRowe et. al. [2] conducted a phase 1 study including 16 patients with a respiratory disturbance index (RDI) between 12.5 and 70 who underwent isolated tongue-base suspension. Data was collected retrospectively with preoperative and postoperative comparisons. Two patients required suture removal for complications and were excluded from the analysis. The RDI improved from 35 ± 16.5 to 17 ± 8 (a 51.4% reduction, $p=0.001$). Although a validated questionnaire was not used, the remaining 14 patients all noted improvement in snoring.

Thomas et. al. [5] examined 17 patients with severe OSA and Fujita type II collapse in a prospectively enrolled, randomized crossover trial examining genioglossus advancement and Repose (Influ-ENT Medical, Concord, NH, USA) tongue suspension. Patients were over 21 years of age and exhibited moderate OSA with failure of conservative therapy. Retropalatal and retrolingual collapse was demonstrated by Müller maneuvers. Patients underwent UPPP with either genioglossus advancement or Repose tongue suspension. Nine patients underwent Repose tongue suspension with Epworth scores decreasing from 12.1 ± 7.2 to 4.1 ± 3.4 ($p=0.007$). The RDI improved from 35 ± 16.5 to 17 ± 8 (51.4% reduction) ($p=0.001$). Airway collapse as measured by Müller's maneuver improved by 64% at the palate and 83% at the tongue base ($p=0.0006$ and 0.0003, respectively). In four of nine patients, snoring questionnaire scores fell from 9.3 ± 1.0 to 3.3 ± 2.1 ($p=0.02$). Seven of the nine patients had postoperative sleep studies, and a surgical response was achieved in four of them (57%). In the tongue-advancement group, Epworth scores fell from 13.3 ± 4.5 to 5.0 ± 3.5 ($p=0.002$). Airway collapse improved by 31% at the palate and 75% at the tongue base ($p=0.1$ and 0.03, respectively). In four of eight patients, snoring questionnaire scores went from 9.3 ± 1.0 to 5.0 ± 0.6 ($p=0.04$). Four patients underwent postoperative polysomnography, two of whom achieved a surgical response (50%). It was concluded that Repose tongue suspension was slightly more effective in improving daytime somnolence and snoring.

Woodson [6] investigated polysomnographic and subjective outcomes 2 months following Repose tongue suspension in 43 patients. The study included snorers with an apnea–hypopnea index (AHI) below 15 and OSA patients with AHI > 15 who demonstrated tongue-base obstruction on Müller's maneuver. Patients were excluded for AHI > 60, average desaturation less than 80%, and body mass index above 34. The RDI improved from 35.4 ± 13.7 to 24.5 ± 14.5 in the OSA group ($p=0.009$), however only a small number were definitively treated. There was significant improvement in OSA symptoms but no significant difference in snoring.

Miller et. al. [7] performed a retrospective analysis of 19 patients who underwent UPPP with Repose tongue suspension. The RDI declined from 38.7 ± 12.3 to 21.0 ± 7.4 (46%) ($p<0.05$) with a surgical cure rate of 20%.

Kühnel et. al. [8] performed a study of 28 male patients with sleep-disordered breathing. The RDI improved from 41 to 38 at 3 months and to 31 at 12 months after surgery. Epworth scores improved from 12 to 9 at 3 months and to 9 at 12 months after surgery. In nine cases, Epworth scores were worse after 1 year. Endoscopy findings did not reveal a significant difference between preoperative and postoperative data. Lateral cephalometric analysis was performed to evaluate changes of the posterior airway space (PAS), defined as the distance between the tongue base and the posterior wall of the pharynx at the level of the line connecting the supramental point and gonion. The PAS increased from 10.6 ± 3.5 to 12 ± 3.8 ($p=0.0056$) for a difference of 2 mm. However, when patients in whom the uvula constituted the rostral boundary of the PAS were excluded, the difference was reduced to only 1.3 mm. It was concluded that a marked improvement in symptoms could be achieved in some patients who do not respond to conservative therapy.

Indications/Contraindications

The extent of surgical treatment of sleep apnea is determined by patient motivation, the severity of symptoms, the severity of disease as determined by polysomnography, and the site of obstruction as well as the medical and psychological fitness of the patient. General recommendations for the surgical treatment of sleep apnea are as follows [9, 10]:

- AHI of more than 15
- Oxyhemoglobin desaturation of less than 90%
- AHI of more than 5 and less than 14, with excessive daytime sleepiness
- Upper airway resistance syndrome, preferably with objective improvement of neurocognitive dysfunction using medical therapy (continuous positive airway pressure, CPAP)
- Significant cardiac arrhythmias associated with obstruction
- Unsuccessful or inability to tolerate medical therapy

The type of surgery performed is dependent on the severity of OSA and the site of obstruction. Most patients with significant OSA will require UPPP. Multilevel pharyngeal surgery consisting of UPPP, hyoid myotomy, and surgery to address the tongue base is generally offered to patients with a RDI greater than 20 [11]. An attempt is made to identify the site of obstruction, and tongue surgery is advocated when tongue-base collapse is greater than 50% of the cross-sectional area of the airway.

Preoperative Workup

It is important to consider that patients with OSA often suffer from concurrent depression, reflux laryngopharyngitis, hypertension, chronic obstructive pulmonary disease, reactive airway disease, and coronary artery disease. Up to 40% of patients seeking surgery for sleep apnea have a history of cardiovascular disease [12]. Preoperative assessment therefore should include an electrocardiogram, chest X-ray, complete blood count, and a thorough general medical evaluation to assess the risks of cardiopulmonary complications and the need for medical referral. Stress testing and pulmonary function testing should be considered for those patients with significant histories. Preoperative flexible laryngoscopy is useful to assess the ease of intubation for surgery and also to rule out an occult lesion as the source of airway obstruction. The addition of Müller's maneuver assists in determination of areas of collapse. Upper-airway imaging, including lateral cephalometric radiographs, fluoroscopy, CT, and MRI, is usually unnecessary, but may aid in identification of the site of collapse.

Tracheostomy rather than tongue-base suspension should be offered to patients with severe tongue-base obstruction or patients with severe cardiopulmonary comorbidity or apnea-related cardiac events. Such patients are unsuitable candidates for multilevel airway surgery and require definitive control of apnea.

Technique

Tongue-base approaches range from radiofrequency ablation to reduce tongue-base volume, to genioglossus advancement, which entails mandibular osteotomies to reposition the genial tubercle, and thus the genioglossus muscle, anteriorly. A recent advance is the development of the Repose lingual suspension procedure for genioglossus advancement. This is the authors' preferred approach to tongue-base suspension and is performed using commercially available instrumentation (Influ-ENT Medical) (Fig. 38.1). If palatal surgery is being performed in conjunction with tongue-base suspension, palatal surgery is performed first.

After establishment of general nasotracheal anesthesia, the mouth is held open with a bite block. A 2-0 silk suture is placed in the anterior tongue in the midline to facilitate retraction. Local anesthetic containing epinephrine is injected into the floor of mouth and a blade is used to make a small incision in the floor of the mouth in the midline, posterior to Wharton's duct orifices. Dissection is carried down between the ducts to the genial tubercle of the mandible using a fine hemostat. The periosteum overlying the genial tubercle is elevated using a Cottle elevator. The screw inserter is preloaded with a small bone screw with a loop of permanent 1-0 polypropylene suture attached to the end of the screw, which is housed within the screw-inserter handle. The screw inserter is placed such that the screw is inserted through the incision in the floor of the mouth in the midline (Fig. 38.2). The screw is pressed perpendicularly against the genial tubercle of the mandible, well below the tooth roots, and the inserter is activated until the screw completely penetrates the mandible (Fig. 38.3). Once the screw has engaged the mandible, upward traction on the screw-inserter handle facilitates advancement of the screw through the mandibular cortex. When the screw has been inserted, the screw-inserter handle disengages and is removed. This leaves the screw attached to the genial tubercle with the attached loop of permanent polypropylene suture exiting through the floor of the mouth incision. The loop of permanent suture is cut directly in the middle, leaving two equal ends attached to the screw and exiting from the incision. The ends are tagged with small hemostats.

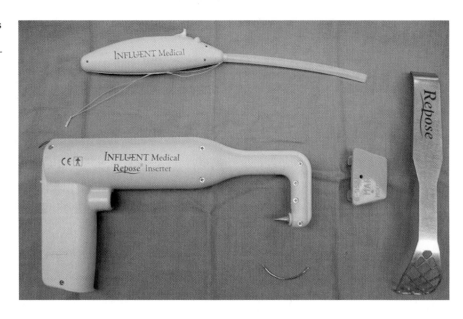

Fig. 38.1. The components of the Repose genioglossus advancement and stabilization procedure (Influent Medical, Concord, NH, USA) set include a bone screw inserter, suture passer, bite block and tongue retractor

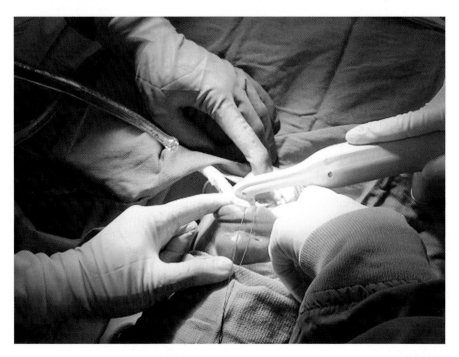

Fig. 38.2. After incising the floor of mouth mucosa posterior to Wharton's ducts, the periosteum is elevated over the genial tubercle and the screw inserter is placed through the incision

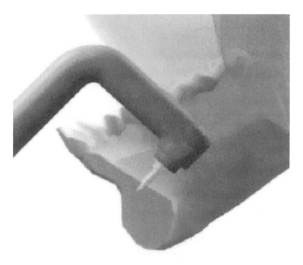

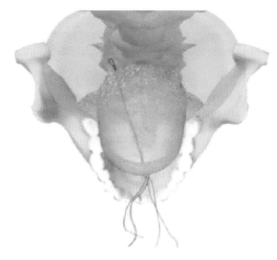

Fig. 38.3. The screw-inserter handle is positioned perpendicular to the angle of the mandible: the screw should abut the mandible at 90°. (Used with the express written permission of Influent Medical)

Fig. 38.4. The suture passer containing a preloaded temporary suture loop is inserted through the floor of the mouth incision to exit the tongue base posterior to the circumvallate papillae, and 1–1.5 cm lateral to the midline. (Used with the express written permission of Influent Medical)

The suture passer is preloaded with a temporary surgical loop suture (Fig. 38.1). The suture passer is then inserted through the floor of the mouth incision to exit the tongue base 2 cm posterior to the circumvallate papillae, and 1–1.5 cm lateral to the midline (Fig. 38.4). If the suture passer exits less than 1 cm from the midline, inadequate suspension results; if it is passed more than 1.5 cm lateral from the midline, injury to the neurovascular bundle can result. The temporary suture is then released from the su-

ture passer and the passer is removed, which results in a looped suture protruding from the tongue base. One of the mandibular screw's polypropylene suture ends is then loaded into the empty suture passer and is passed through the floor of the mouth incision in a similar manner to exit the contralateral tongue base (Fig. 38.5) This permanent suture is then loaded onto a Mayo needle and passed submucosally from the exit point of that suture in the tongue base to the exit point of the contralateral suture loop (Figs. 38.6, 38.7). The

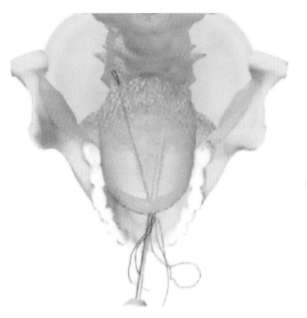

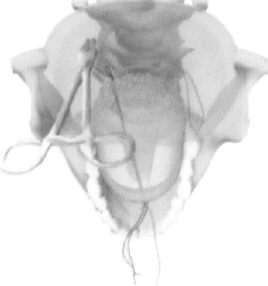

Fig. 38.5. A polypropylene suture attached to the mandibular screw is loaded into the empty suture passer and is passed through the floor of the mouth incision to exit the contralateral tongue base, 1–1.5 cm lateral to the midline. (Used with the express written permission of Influent Medical)

Fig. 38.6. The permanent suture is loaded onto a Mayo needle and passed submucosally from the exit point of the suture to the exit point of the contralateral temporary suture loop. (Used with the express written permission of Influent Medical)

Fig. 38.7. The tongue retractor openings facilitate passage of the tongue-base suture while allowing tongue-base retraction

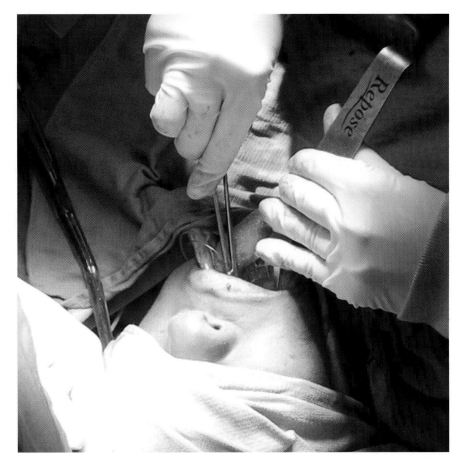

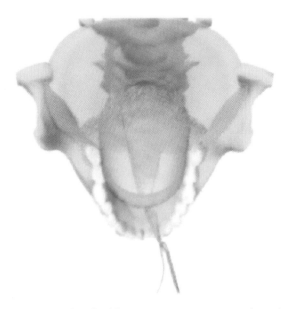

Fig. 38.8. Both ends of the permanent suture now exit through the floor of the mouth incision. The sutures are tied to suspend the tongue anteriorly. (Used with the express written permission of Influent Medical)

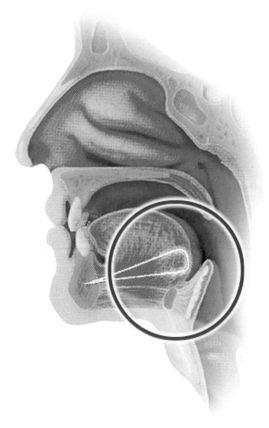

Fig. 38.9. Adequate suspension creates a palpable dimple in the base of the tongue and just lifts the base of the tongue off the posterior hypopharyngeal wall. (Used with the express written permission of Influent Medical)

needle is removed and the permanent suture is then passed through the suture loop. The looped suture is pulled anteriorly, which pulls the permanent suture anteriorly to exit through the floor of mouth incision (Fig. 38.8).

The sutures are tied with a surgeon's knot to create an amount of tension that results in a palpable dimple in the base of the tongue. Adequate suspension is ascertained by placing a finger over the tongue base and determining that tightening of the suture just lifts the base of the tongue off the posterior hypopharyngeal wall (Fig 38.9). Overcorrection should be avoided as this may acutely result in strangulation of tissue with heightened degrees of pain and swelling, and may result in dysarthria and dysphagia from tongue thrusting which may not resolve.

After securing the permanent suture, the ends are trimmed to bury the suture and copious irrigation is used. The floor of the mouth incision is closed with several interrupted absorbable sutures.

Tips and Pearls

- Screw engagement with the mandibular cortex is difficult if inadequate soft tissue or periosteum has been elevated from the genial tubercle.
- Once the screw abuts the mandible, screw placement is facilitated by upward traction on the screw inserter sufficient to just lift the patient's head off the table. This prevents the screw from slipping while the cortex is engaged.
- Perioperative steroids greatly ameliorate tongue-base and floor-of-mouth edema resulting from manipulation of these areas during tongue suspension.
- All patients should be admitted for overnight observation with pulse oximetry following tongue-base suspension.

Complications

Complication rates from tongue suspension range from 15 to 26% [1, 6–8]. Common complications include local infection, pain, odynophagia, and dysarthria. These generally resolve within 1–2 weeks. Less commonly, hematoma, persistent globus sensation, sialoadenitis, tongue hypesthesia, delayed infection, suture extrusion, and suture breakage may occur. Ideally, tongue-base suspension suspends the tongue such that the patient is unaffected while awake, but retrolingual prolapse is prevented during sleep: overcorrection may result in tongue thrusting, dysarthria, and dysphagia. Careful attention to tongue placement during suture suspension is required to avoid this complication. An advantage of suture suspension of

38

the tongue base over more complex procedures is the ready reversibility of the procedure in such instances with minimal patient morbidity and inconvenience. Tooth loss and mental nerve anesthesia are common complications of genioglossus advancement using mandibular osteotomies, which are avoided with the use of the suture suspension technique.

Postoperative Care

It is important to recognize that surgical intervention of OSA may result in a temporary exacerbation of airway obstruction. The tongue suspension procedure, in particular, involves manipulation of the floor of the mouth and the base of the tongue, which often results in temporary edema with the potential for respiratory embarrassment; therefore, the authors advocate overnight hospitalization with pulse oximetry monitoring for all patients undergoing tongue suspension. Admission to an intensive care setting should be considered when severe comorbidity is present. Patients with severe OSA should continue CPAP in the perioperative period. Narcotic pain medications are used judiciously, recognizing that the use of these medications may worsen the severity of OSA. Patients are treated with broad-spectrum antibiotics; perioperative steroids ameliorate discomfort and edema from tongue and floor-of-mouth manipulation. Patients are suitable for discharge once pain has been controlled and adequate oral fluid intake has been demonstrated. Polysomnography is repeated 3–4 months postoperatively to determine the response to surgery.

References

1. Fujita S, Conway W, Zorick F, et al: Surgical correction of anatomic abnormalities in obstructive sleep apnea syndrome: uvulopalatopharyngoplasty, Otolaryngol Head Neck Surg 89:923–934, 1981

2. DeRowe A, Gunther E, Fibbi A, et al: Tongue-base suspension with a soft tissue-to-bone anchor for obstructive sleep apnea: preliminary clinical results of a new minimally invasive technique. Otolaryngol Head Neck Surg 122:100–103, 2000

3. Sher A, Schectman K, Piccirillo J: The efficacy of surgical modifications of the upper airway in adults with obstructive sleep apnea syndrome. Sleep 19:156–177, 1996

4. Riley R, Guilleminault C, Powell N, et al: Palatopharyngoplasty failure, cephalometric roentgenograms, and obstructive sleep apnea. Otolaryngol Head Neck Surg 93:240–244, 1985

5. Thomas A, Chavoya M, Terris D: Preliminary findings from a prospective, randomized trial of two tongue-base surgeries for sleep-disordered breathing. Otolaryngol Head Neck Surg 129:539–546, 2003

6. Woodson T: A tongue suspension suture for obstructive sleep apnea and snorers. Otolaryngol Head Neck Surg 124:297–303, 2001

7. Miller F, Watson D, Malis D: Role of the tongue base suspension suture with the repose system bone screw in the multilevel surgical management of obstructive sleep apnea. Otolaryngol Head Neck Surg 126:392–398, 2002

8. Kühnel T, Schurr C, Wagner B et al: Morphological changes of the posterior airway space after tongue base suspension. Laryngoscope 115:475–480, 2005

9. Riley R, Powell N: Maxillofacial surgery and obstructive sleep apnea syndrome. Otolaryngol Clin North Am 23:809, 1990

10. Riley R, Powell N, Guilleminault C: Obstructive sleep apnea syndrome: a review of 306 consecutively treated surgical patients, Otolaryngology head Neck Surg 108:117–125, 1993

11. Terris DJ: Multilevel pharyngeal surgery for obstructive sleep apnea: indication and techniques. Oper Tech Otolaryngol Head Neck Surg 11:12–20, 2000

12. Riley R, Powell N, Guilleminault C, et al: Obstructive sleep apnea surgery risk management and complications. Otolaryngol Head Neck Surg 117:648–652, 1997

Chapter 39

Hyoid Suspension

39

Karl Hörmann, Alexander Baisch

Core Messages

■ Hyoid suspension prevents the hypopharyngeal collapse of the tongue musculature, which relaxes during sleep.

■ The modified hyoid suspension is indicated for mild obstructive sleep apnea (OSA) with retrolingual obstruction.

■ For moderate to severe OSA, the hyoid suspension should be a part of a multilevel surgery concept.

■ The modified hyoid suspension uses a single wire and the procedure is easy to perform without division of the stylohyoid ligaments.

■ The majority of patients reported reduction of their snoring and tolerated the discomfort and side effects associated with the modified hyoid suspension procedure.

Contents

Introduction

Many surgical procedures were developed to treat airway obstruction, with one being the hyoid suspension, which addresses hypopharyngeal constriction. The idea to prevent the hypopharyngeal collapse of the tongue musculature, which relaxes during sleep, with the help of a suspension of the hyoid bone is not new. In 1986 a new therapy concept was presented for the treatment of the hypopharyngeal constriction: the inferior sagittal osteotomy of the mandible with hyoid myotomy suspension [7], which attempts to move the hyoid bone cranial and anterior. The procedure involved a medial mandibular osteotomy with genioglossus advancement and suspension of the hyoid to the mandible using homologous fascia lata strands after myotomy of the infrahyoidal musculature. In 1994, this technique was modified first by Riley et al. [8], who no longer fixated the hyoid bone on the mandible but on the upper edge of the thyroid cartilage. The resulting movement of the tongue base towards anterior and caudal increases and stiffens the upper airway. Access is achieved via a 3–4-cm-wide horizontal skin incision along the relaxed skin tension lines at the level of the hyoid bone. A portion of the body of the hyoid is isolated in the midline. The inferior body of the hyoid bone is cleanly dissected. The stylohyoid ligaments are sectioned from the lesser cornu, but the remaining suprahyoid musculature is left intact. A subcutaneous vertical incision is made to allow exposure of the thyroid notch and superior thyroid lamina. Ticron no. 1 sutures (Davis & Geck, American Cyanamid Co., Danbury, USA) are placed through the superior portion of the thyroid cartilage and around the hyoid bone.

This method was modified [2, 3] by Hörmann, who avoids cutting the stylohyoid ligaments and does not perform a myotomy of the suprahyoidal and infrahyoidal musculature in order to be less invasive and more effective.

Indications and Contraindications

We recommend an extensive clinical evaluation pre-operatively with the help of rigid endoscopy and polysomnography. We see no primary indication for the hyoid suspension for primary snoring except in cases where the snoring problem is severe or an alternative operation did not succeed or in cases with an endoscopic diagnosed retrolaryngeal stenosis.

In the case of mild obstructive sleep apnea (OSA) with a suspected retrolingual collapse, hyoid suspension is an alternative to radiofrequency therapy of the tongue base. We primarily choose the radiofrequency procedure owing to the lower invasiveness and postoperative morbidity, and offer hyoid suspension secondarily, after failed radiofrequency surgery. But for mild OSA and diagnosed retrolaryngeal stenosis, we often choose the hyoid suspension in combination with radiofrequency therapy of the tongue base.

In the case of moderate OSA, the cure rate of radiofrequency therapy decreases. For this situation, hyoid suspension is superior to radiofrequency therapy. Therefore, we consider moderate OSA (apnea–hypopnea index, AHI, from 20 to 40) as a primary indication for the hyoid suspension procedure. If the obstruction site is suspected to lie solely in the retrolingual segment, an isolated hyoid suspension presents itself as an option.

For more severe forms of OSA (AHI>40), we increasingly assume that the complete airway is affected.

For severe OSA, respiratory therapy is to be preferred in general; but when conservative therapy fails, surgery becomes an option. Since severe OSA most often involves multilevel obstruction, an isolated hyoid suspension is often not sufficient. When severe OSA is present, we recommend a multilevel surgery concept which combines the hyoid suspension with procedures at the soft palate and the tongue base.

Tips and Pearls

Indications for hyoid suspension are:
- Mild OSA and diagnosed retrolaryngeal stenosis
- Moderate OSA (AHI from 20 to 40)
- Isolated retrolingual segment obstruction
- As part of a multilevel surgery concept in cases with severe OSA, which combines the hyoid suspension with procedures at the soft palate and the tongue base

Procedure

The procedure is demonstrated in Video 39.1

We prefer to perform hyoid suspension under general anesthesia with intubation; however, the

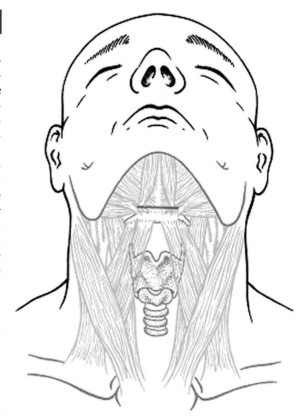

Fig. 39.1. The *red line* shows the skin incision

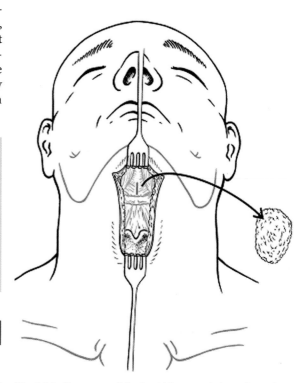

Fig. 39.2. Exposure of the hyoid bone and thyroid cartilage. Resection of subplatysmal fat

39

procedure can also be performed under local anesthesia [6] with intravenous sedation. The patient receives an intraoperative single shot of 2 g cefazolin. The patient is then placed on the operating table with a slightly reclined head. The skin of the throat between the chin and the sternum is prepared with antiseptic solution and isolated with sterile drapes. Prilocaine (1%) with 1:200,000 epinephrine solution is injected in the skin to minimize intraoperative bleeding. The skin incision is placed above the hyoid bone along the relaxed skin tension lines (Fig. 39.1).

The upper and lower skin flaps are elevated to expose the subplatysmal fat and muscles. For cosmetic reason, some of the mobilized subplatysmal fat is resected (Fig. 39.2). Failure to do so will, as a result of the advancement of the hyoid, create an unattractive supralaryngeal wrinkle with a turkeylike appearance.

In contrast to the originally described method, our new modification of the technique requires only one triangular suture, which passes (bilaterally) through the paramedial thyroid cartilage and medially around the hyoid. For the suture, a monofilamentous grade 3 steel wire (Ethicon, Hamburg, Germany) is used. For this, first the suprahyoidal musculature is vertically separated precisely in the midline (Fig. 39.2, red line), until a Langenbeck retractor can be applied. The fascia in the midline between each sternohyoid muscle is incised using electrocautery until the plane of the thyroid cartilage is reached. The muscles on both sides are retracted to expose the lateral parts of the thyroid cartilage.

Tips and Pearls

- The blood supply to the thyroid cartilage is provided by the blood vessels of the perichondrium. Unnecessary elevation of the perichondrium should, therefore, be avoided to reduce the risk of necrosis.

Now, starting caudally, a sharp needle is pierced through the cartilage without drilling. A steel wire is fixed at the end of the needle, which is pierced out on the contralateral side of the thyroid cartilage from behind (Fig. 39.3, left). No further alteration of the cartilage is needed to fixate the wire, which is now placed near the thyroid notch.

Tips and Pearls

- It must be emphasized that the level of the surgical placement of the wire should be near the thyroid notch in order to prevent damage to the vocal cords.

Then the hyoid body is encircled with the wire ligature until the tip of the needle appears at the top of the Langenbeck retractor (Fig. 39.3, center). In order to prevent an accidental opening up of the pharynx by the needle, the assistant elevates the hyoid with a Joseph retractor. In order to prevent a tearing of the wire, the distance to the free upper edge of the thyroid cartilage should be at least 5 mm. Especially in men, ossifications of the thyroid cartilage may complicate the piercing of the cartilage with the ligature,

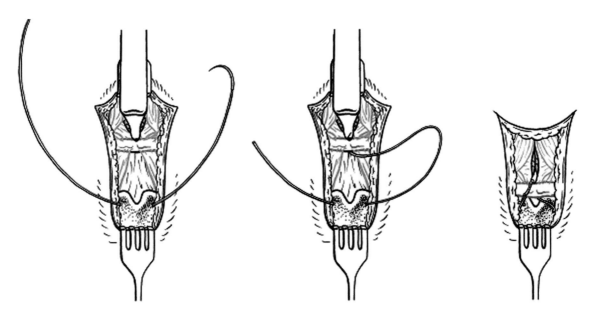

Fig. 39.3. Technique of hyoid suspension. *Left*: Transfixing the thyroid cartilage with steel wire suspension. *Center*: Undermining the hyoid bone. *Right*: Completion of suspension

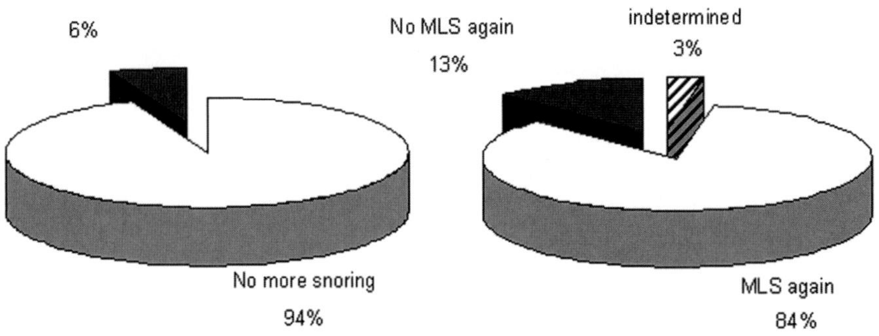

Fig. 39.6. *Left*: 94% of all patients (*n*=102) reported a sufficient reduction of snoring. *Right*: 84% of the patients would undergo the same surgery once again. *MLS* multilevel surgery

they had to start all over again, and 94% reported a successful reduction of their snoring (Fig. 39.6).

Cocnlusions

Nearly all patients tolerated the discomfort and side effects of hyoid suspension in the context of multilevel surgery for the treatment of OSA. The majority of the patients reported reduction of their snoring, and despite the associated discomfort and temporary speech difficulties they would consider undergoing this procedure if they had to start all over again. Further studies are needed to estimate long-term success rates of hyoid suspension used alone or in the context of multilevel surgery.

References

1. Baisch A, Hein G, Goessler U, Stuck BA, Maurer JT, Hörmann K. (2005) Subjective outcome after multi-level surgery in sleep-disordered breathing [in German]. HNO; 53:863–868.
2. Hörmann K, Baisch A. (2004) How I do it: the hyoid suspension. Laryngoscope; 114:1677–1679.
3. Hörmann K, Hirth K, Erhardt T, Maurer JT, Verse T. (2001) Modified hyoid suspension for therapy of sleep related breathing disorders. operative technique and complications [in German]. Laryngo-Rhino-Otol; 80:517–521.
4. Hörmann K, Maurer JT, Baisch A. (2004) Snoring/sleep apnea – The success of surgery [in German]. HNO; 52:807–813.
5. Li KK. (2003) Hyoid suspension/advancement. In: Fairbanks DNF, Mickelson SA, Woodson BT (Eds). Snoring and obstructive sleep apnea. Lippincott Williams & Wilkins, Philadelphia; 3rd edition; pp. 178–182.
6. Neruntarat C. (2003) Hyoid myotomy with suspension under local anesthesia for obstructive sleep apnea syndrome. Eur Arch Otorhinolaryngol; 260:286–290.
7. Riley RW, Powell NB, Guilleminault C. (1986) Inferior sagittal osteotomy of the mandible with hyoid myotomy-suspension: a new procedure for obstructive sleep apnea. Otolaryngol Head Neck Surg; 94:589–593.
8. Riley RW, Powell NB, Guilleminault C. (1994) Obstructive sleep apnea and the hyoid: a revised surgical procedure. Otolaryngol Head Neck Surg; 111:717–721.
9. Verse T, Baisch A, Hörmann K. (2004) Multi-Level surgery for obstructive sleep apnea. Preliminary objective results [in German]. Laryngo-Rhino-Otol; 83:516–522.

39

Chapter 40

Genioplasty (Genoid Advancement) for Obstructive Sleep Apnea Syndrome

40

Jean M. Bruch, Nicolas Y. Busaba

Core Messages

- Manipulation of chin position aims at increasing the hypopharyngeal airway and preventing its collapse by advancing the genial tubercle and genioglossus muscle.

- Genioplasty is indicated for the treatment of patients suffering from obstructive sleep apnea syndrome with a respiratory disturbance index above 15 per hour of sleep and oxyhemoglobin desaturation to less than 87% that failed conservative management.

- Genioplasty aims at widening the posterior airway space in the region of the hypopharynx–tongue base.

Contents

Introduction

Obstructive sleep apnea is a common, but not a new disorder. Health care providers are becoming increasingly aware of the entity and its health impact. Up to 24% of men and 9% of women meet the polysomnography criteria to diagnose obstructive sleep apnea. When the polysomnography data are combined with symptoms of sleep apnea (obstructive sleep apnea syndrome, OSAS), the prevalence rate is around 4 and 2% in men and women, respectively [12].

The airway collapse leading to OSAS commonly occurs at multiple levels and thus complicates the surgical treatment of the disorder. Nasal and palatopharyngeal surgery are the most frequently performed procedures to treat OSAS, but their failure rate can be higher than 50%. Most of the failures of palatopharyngeal surgery are due to persistent airway collapse at the level of the hypopharynx–tongue-base region.

There are numerous surgical procedures designed to deal with the hypopharyngeal airway, but none have been consistently successful and most have a relatively high morbidity. Manipulation of chin position aims at increasing the hypopharyngeal airway and preventing its collapse by advancing the genial tubercle and genioglossus muscle. This places the genioglossus muscle under tension, thereby restricting posterior collapse of the tongue during sleep and resulting in relative forward fixation of the pharyngeal dilators. This operation may be performed in conjunction with palatopharyngeal surgery, or at a later time in the event of palatopharyngeal surgery failures.

The sliding genioplasty (Fig. 40.1) involves advancement of the chin and a portion of the inferior mandibular border with attached muscles. This results in forward movement of the genioglossus, geniohyoid, anterior digastric, and mylohyoid muscles and places anterosuperior traction on the hyoid bone with subsequent increase in posterior airway space. The pedicle tends to be well vascularized; however, there is risk of injury to the mental nerves, damage to tooth roots, symphyseal fracture, and poor esthetic result secondary to advancement of the chin point or shortening of height of the lower face [3].

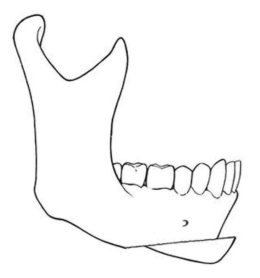

Fig. 40.1. A sliding genioplasty showing the mandible, site of osteotomy, and the mandibular segment that was advanced. This results in the advancement of the chin and a portion of the inferior mandibular border with attached muscles, which in turn leads to forward movement of the genioglossus, geniohyoid, anterior digastric, and mylohyoid muscles and places anterosuperior traction on the hyoid bone with subsequent increase in posterior airway space

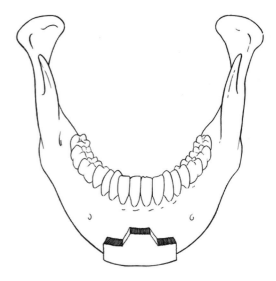

Fig. 40.3. A mortise genioplasty showing osteotomy circumscribed about the genial tubercle along with a small portion of the adjacent anterior inferior border of the mandible which allows for advancement of some additional musculature with the advancement of the genioglossus muscle

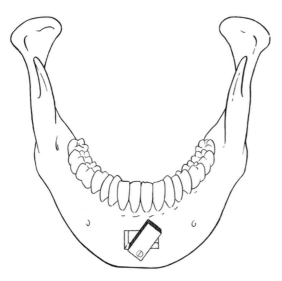

Fig. 40.2. A geniotomy (or genioglossus advancement) showing the mandible, osteotomy in the genoid tubercle area creating a window of bone that encompasses the genial tubercle, and then the advancement and rotation of the bony window with the genial tubercle that is fixed in this anterior position, and thus leading to advancement of the genioglossus muscle

40

Geniotomy, or genioglossus advancement (Fig. 40.2), which involves a limited rectangular osteotomy around the genial tubercle, can be performed to minimize the risks encountered with sliding genioplasty. The isolated genial tubercle is then advanced with the attached genioglossus and there is no movement of the other anterior mandibular muscles or change in position of the chin point. A variation of this technique, the trephine osteotomy approach, involves creation of a circular osteotomy centered over the genioglossus insertion using a standardized system of instruments, trephine, and drill guide. Advantages of this technique may include reduced operative time, less bleeding, and decreased risk to the canine roots secondary to the circular shape of the bone cuts [2, 5, 8].

A hybrid of the sliding genioplasty and geniotomy techniques, the so-called mortise genioplasty (Fig. 40.3), incorporates an osteotomy circumscribed about the genial tubercle along with a small portion of the adjacent anterior inferior border of the mandible so that advancement of some additional musculature can occur with advancement of the genioglossus. Multiple variations of this technique have been developed; however, most have been abandoned in favor of the geniotomy approach [3].

Clinical Evaluation

History and Physical Examination

The first step in evaluating individuals suspected of having OSAS is a detailed medical history. In addition to the typical medical history pertaining to OSAS, the surgeon needs to address issues that are of particular relevance for genioplasty.

The physical examination may be divided into general and upper-airway-specific examination. The general examination aims at detecting findings that predispose to or are associated with OSAS. Weight, height, and neck circumference are recorded and body mass index is calculated.

The upper-airway examination aims at determining the cause and site of airway narrowing and detecting anatomic abnormalities that are amenable to surgical correction. Fiberoptic transnasal endoscopy provides valuable information and is an essential component of the physical examination. Greater than 30–40% narrowing of the airway at the level of the tongue-base–hypopharynx during a Müller maneuver suggests a poor outcome with uvulopalatopharyngoplasty [1, 7]. This latter subset of patients may be candidates for genioplasty.

A few patients with significant OSAS are thin and have no apparent anatomic abnormalities on physical examination, and their oropharyngeal inlet appears widely patent.

Imaging

The role of imaging in the workup of patients suspected of having OSAS is controversial. Imaging studies are not routinely done because of their cost and the fact that they frequently do not add to the airway assessment by the physical examination. However, imaging studies are useful in the workup of patients with OSAS who have no apparent anatomic abnormalities on physical examination, who have failed palatopharyngeal surgery, or for whom maxillofacial surgery is planned.

Cephalometry is the most commonly performed imaging study for this purpose. It offers both bone and soft-tissue measurements, and is used for surgical planning and predicting outcome. Its main drawback is lack of normative data, especially for soft-tissue measurements. Findings that correlate with the diagnosis of sleep apnea are low hyoid bone position, long and thick soft palate, diminished size of the posterior airway space, increased distance from the tip of the tongue to the base of the vallecula, and facial skeletal abnormalities (such as micrognathia) [4, 11].

Dental radiographs, including periapical and panoramic views, can be obtained to evaluate the overall health and periodontal status of the dentition, as osteotomies near the apices of the teeth risk compromise to the neurovascular supply traversing this area. These films also enable assessment of the relative length of the tooth roots and the height of bone inferior to the root apices, which may be helpful in planning the location and configuration of the genioplasty osteotomy. Additionally, they may be used to estimate the site of genioglossus insertion, since there is often an area of increased bone density visible in the midline symphysis region corresponding to the genial tubercle.

Computed tomography (CT) has excellent airway and bone resolution. It offers accurate determination of upper-airway cross-sectional area and volume and is helpful in evaluating the efficacy of dental appliances and maxillomandibular advancement in patients with sleep apnea. Spiral CT provides direct three-dimensional volumetric reconstruction of the images [6].

Magnetic resonance imaging (MRI) offers superior soft-tissue resolution, multiplanar imaging, three-dimensional reconstruction, ultrafast imaging techniques, and lack of radiation exposure. MRI is useful in evaluating the efficacy of soft-tissue surgery, but not in predicting surgical outcome in sleep apnea patients [9].

However, both MRI and CT are not routinely used in the clinical evaluation of patients with sleep apnea because of cost, supine imaging, poor prediction of surgical outcome, and the additional risk of radiation exposure with CT.

Polysomnography

Polysomnography (sleep study) is essential for the diagnosis of sleep apnea. It serves to confirm the presence of sleep apnea and exclude other causes of excessive daytime somnolence such as narcolepsy, insufficient amount of sleep, and periodic limb movement disorder. Moreover, polysomnography determines the severity of the sleep apnea since the information obtained from the medical history and physical examination in any particular patient is a poor indicator of the level of the disease severity [10]. In addition, polysomnography allows for continuous positive airway pressure (CPAP) titration and initiation of CPAP therapy.

Indications for Genioplasty

Genioplasty is indicated for the treatment of patients suffering from OSAS with a respiratory disturbance index above 15 per hour of sleep and oxyhemoglobin desaturation to less than 87% that failed CPAP or are unwilling to use CPAP on a long-term basis. Documentation of hypopharyngeal airway obstruction contributing to OSAS based on the physical examination (including fiberoptic laryngoscopy) and/or imaging (typically cephalometry) is needed. The operation may be performed as a same-stage operation with palatopharyngeal surgery or a second stage for failures of palatopharyngeal surgery. In addition, the operation may be performed as the sole procedure to address the hypopharyngeal airway or in combination with other procedures that deal with the same region of the airway, such as hyoid myotomy and suspension, or radiofrequency reduction of the tongue base.

Surgical Technique

Sliding Genioplasty

The lower lip is stretched taut. Infiltration of local anesthesia with epinephrine is used for hemostasis. The mucosal incision is made from premolar to premolar. The incision is placed approximately 1–1.5 cm anterior to the depth of the gingivolabial sulcus. The mucosa is incised perpendicular to the surface; the blade angle is then changed so that it is tangential to the mucosa and perpendicular to the bone. The mentalis muscle is incised down to bone; the blade angle is perpendicular. The periosteum is dissected in a subperiosteal plane to expose the osteotomy site (Fig 40.4). The mental nerves are identified and preserved. A vertical mark is scored in the osteotomy segment for reference. A reciprocating saw is used to make the horizontal osteotomy below the dental apices and mental foramina and is carried posteriorly to the molar region bilaterally. The bony segment is advanced on its soft-tissue pedicle and fixed into position with a lag screw or plate(s) (Fig. 40.1). The soft tissue is closed in layers, with reconstruction of the mentalis. A drain can be placed, but is not often necessary. A pressure dressing can be applied.

Tips and Pearls

- Labial branches of the mental nerves can often be visualized superficially under the mucosa; these should be identified and preserved.
- Placement of the incision should allow an adequate cuff of mucosa for closure of the wound. Placement of the incision too close to the attached gingiva will make suturing difficult as well as cause potential injury to the gingiva.
- Changing the angle of the blade allows clean incisions through both mucosa and mentalis and helps avoid perforation of the lip.
- Leave adequate cuffs of mentalis to reconstruct and avoid extensive stripping from the bone.
- Avoid excessive stripping of the periosteum when possible. Widely degloving the chin point can result in ptosis of the soft-tissue chin pad.
- Extending the osteotomy far enough posteriorly positions the inevitable step at the inferior border under cover of thicker soft tissue and

will be less noticeable. It also flattens the angle of the osteotomy, minimizing unwanted vertical shortening of the lower facial height with advancement of the chin.
- Failure to reconstruct the mentalis muscle can result in ptosis of the chin and lower-lip insufficiency with unsightly exposure of the lower teeth.
- Watertight closure minimizes the risk of infection, wound breakdown, and exposure of hardware. A pressure dressing can help reduce hematoma formation.

Geniotomy

The incision is as for sliding genioplasty, except that it extends from canine to canine (Fig. 40.4). Subperiosteal dissection is only enough to expose the osteotomy site (Fig. 40.4). A rectangular bicortical osteotomy, approximately 2 cm × 1 cm, is made with an oscillating saw and is centered over the genial tubercle. It should be approximately 5 mm or more below the root apices. The horizontal cuts should be parallel; however, they may be angled slightly upward to fully encompass the superior attachment of the genioglossus muscle. The bone segment with attached genioglossus is advanced until the lingual (inner) cortex of the fragment is anterior to the labial (outer) cortex of the mandible. The bone segment is rotated until bone overlap is achieved (20–90°); the outer cortex and marrow are removed with a saw or rongeur (Fig. 40.2). The fragment is fixed with one or two lag screws. Wound closure and dressing are as described for sliding genioplasty.

Tips and Pearls

- Bimanual palpation of the floor of the mouth can aid with estimation of the depth of the genioglossus attachment.
- If the bone window is too small, there will be limited incorporation of genioglossus fibers; if it is too large, there is increased risk of dental injury and symphyseal fracture.
- Leave an adequate strut of bone at the inferior mandibular border, approximately 6–8 mm.
- If there is excessive bleeding, the bone fragment can be pushed toward the floor of the mouth and hemostasis achieved.
- A temporary screw can be placed in the center of the osteotomy fragment to facilitate manipulation of the fragment.
- Overrotation of the bone fragment can result in avulsion of the muscle attachments or torsion/strangulation of the pedicle.

40

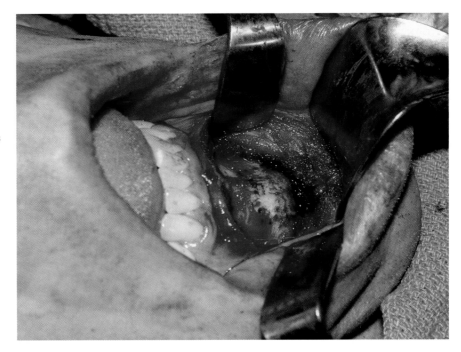

Fig. 40.4. Intraoperative view of the transoral excision and surgical exposure. The periosteum of the anterior mandible is elevated. Retractors are positioned to provide the exposure necessary to perform a sliding genioplasty, geniotomy (or genioglossus advancement), or mortise genioplasty

Complications

Complications are:

- Mandibular fracture
- Floor of mouth hematoma
- Edema of tongue and floor of mouth
- Injury to teeth/roots; devitalization of teeth
- Sensory changes in the labiomental region
- Wound dehiscence
- Necrosis of bone segment
- Infection

Conclusion

In conclusion, the therapy of OSAS is multidisciplinary and involves behavioral, medical, and surgical interventions. Surgery is typically reserved for CPAP failures. Genioplasty is one such surgery that aims at widening the posterior airway space in the region of the hypopharynx–tongue base. Genioplasty is technically simple; surgical outcome is not consistent, but can be improved with appropriate patient selection.

References

1. Katsantonis GP, Maas CS, Walsh JK: (1989) The predictive efficacy of the Muller maneuver in uvulopalatopharyngoplasty. Laryngoscopy 99:677.
2. Lee NR: (2002) Genioglossus muscle advancement techniques for obstructive sleep apnea. Oral Maxillofacial Surg Clin North Am 14:377.
3. Lee NR, Woodson T: (2000) Genioglossus muscle advancement via a trephine osteotomy approach. Operative Techniques Otolaryngol Head Neck Surg. 11:50.
4. Petri N, Suadicani P, Wildschiodtz G, Bjorn-Jorgensen J: (1994) Predictive value of Muller maneuver, cephalometry, and clinical features for the outcome of uvulopalatopharyngoplasty: Evaluation of predictive factors using discriminant analysis in 30 sleep apnea patients. Acta Otolaryngol (Stockh) 114:565.
5. Riley RW, Powell, NB, Guilleminault, C: (1986) Inferior sagittal osteotomy of the mandible with hyoid myotomy suspension: A new procedure for obstructive sleep apnea. Otolaryngol Hean Neck Surg. 94:589.
6. Ryan CF, Lowe AA, Li D, Fleetham JA: (1991) Three-dimensional upper airway computed tomography in obstructive sleep apnea. Am Rev Respir Dis 144:428.
7. Sher AE, Thorpy MJ, Shprintzen RJ et al: (1985) Predictive value of Muller maneuver in selection of patients for uvulopalatopharyngoplasty. Laryngoscope 95:1483.
8. Silverstein, K, Costello BJ, et al: (2000) Genioglossus muscle attachments: An anatomic analysis and the implications for genioglossus advancement. Oral Surg Oral Med Oral Pathol Oral Radiol Endod 90:686.
9. Sudo Y, Matsuda E, Noue Y, Suzuki T, Ohta Y: (1996) Sleep apnea syndrome: comparison of MR imaging of the oropharynx with physiologic indices. Radiology 201:393.

10. Viner S, Szalai JP, Hoffstein V: (1991) Are history and physical examination a good screening test for sleep apnea? Ann Intern Med 115:356.
11. Woodson BT, Conley SF: (1997) Prediction of uvulopalatopharyngoplasty response using cephalometric radiographs. Am J Otolaryngol 18:179.
12. Young T, Palta M, Dempsey J, Skatrud J, Weber S, Dadr S: (1993) The occurrence of sleep-disordered breathing among middle-aged adults. N Engl J Med 328:1230.

Chapter 41

Maxillomandibular Advancement in Sleep Apnea Surgery

41

Kasey K. Li

Core Messages

- Maxillomandibular advancement is the most effective procedure in the management of obstructive sleep apnea.

- Maxillomandibular advancement achieves enlargement of the pharyngeal and hypopharyngeal airway by physically expanding the skeletal framework.

- Maxillomandibular advancement can be effective in obstructive sleep apnea patients with or without facial skeletal deficiency.

- Although the facial esthetic is altered by maxillomandibular advancement, compromise in facial esthetics is uncommon.

- When properly performed, maxillomandibular advancement results in minimal adverse effects.

Contents

Introduction

Since the first tracheotomy performed by Kuhlo [8] for the treatment of upper-airway obstruction in a "Pickwickien" subject, multiple operations have been developed for the treatment of obstructive sleep apnea (OSA). Ironically, tracheotomy still remains the most effective procedure for OSA. However, owing to the associated morbidity with tracheotomy, patient acceptance is extremely poor. Of the remaining surgical procedures, maxillomandibular advancement (MMA) has been shown to have the best outcome. Initially, MMA was recommended in patients with significant maxillomandibular deficiency, which is a major risk factor and a well-recognized predictor for OSA. It has been recognized that maxillomandibular deficiency results in diminished airway dimension, which leads to nocturnal obstruction [7].

Tips and Pearls

- MMA achieves enlargement of the pharyngeal and hypopharyngeal airway by physically expanding the skeletal framework.

In addition, the forward movement of the maxillomandibular complex improves the tension and collapsibility of the suprahyoid and velopharyngeal musculature. Moreover, MMA improves lateral pharyngeal wall collapse [12], which has been shown to be a major contributor in OSA [17, 18, 20].

Although MMA has been primarily recommended in OSA patients with significant maxillomandibular deficiency, this operation is currently also advocated for the treatment of OSA in patients with relatively "normal" maxillofacial features as well. It appears that despite alteration of facial esthetics following MMA, only a minority of patients feet that their appearances are compromised [13, 14]. The explanation is such that since most patients with OSA are middle-aged adults with some soft-tissue sagging and facial aging, MMA "augments" the support of facial soft tissues, reducing soft-tissue sagging, which enhances the facial esthetics. Indeed, approximately half of patients feel that they appear more youthful following surgery; therefore, the majority of patients can be considered for MMA for the treatment of OSA [13, 14].

Preoperative Evaluation

Preoperative evaluation consists of a thorough head and neck evaluation combined with radiography (lateral cephalometric and panoramic radiographs) and fiberoptic pharyngolaryngoscopy. Fiberoptic airway assessment is helpful to assess the extent of tongue base/lateral pharyngeal wall collapse (Fig. 41.1). The lateral cephalometric radiograph provides information on the skeletal and airway dimension (Fig. 41.2). The panoramic radiograph is essential to evaluate the maxillary and mandibular anatomy, the dentition, as well as the position of the inferior alveolar neurovascular bundles. A thorough understanding of the anatomy will minimize the potential of injury to vital structures intraoperatively.

Patient Consideration

The majority of the surgeons consider MMA as "the procedure of last resort" and only recommend this surgical option when other "less invasive" procedures have been ineffective in sufficiently improving OSA. Clearly, this "staged" surgical concept is the most accepted practice. However, there is sufficient evidence demonstrating that MMA should be considered as the first and only surgical option in some patients.

Indications for MMA are:

- Patients with severe OSA without significant pharyngeal tissue redundancy
- Patients with significant maxillomandibular deficiency
- Young patients who require long-term resolution of OSA
- Patients who desire the most effective single-stage surgery [1].

41

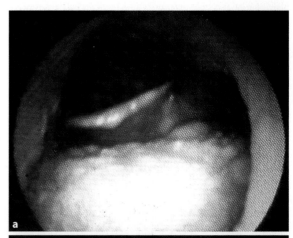

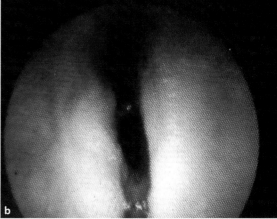

Fig. 41.1. Fiberoptic evaluation. **a** Obstructed hypopharyngeal airway. **b** Lateral pharyngeal wall collapse during Müller's maneuver

Maxillomandibular Advancement Procedure

The MMA procedure has been used for many years to correct skeletal facial deformities for malocclusion and is well described in the maxillofacial surgical literature. However, it must be emphasized that MMA for the treatment of OSA is quite different from the conventional orthognathic procedure. Furthermore, bone grafting in the region of the osteotomies is often necessary because of the significant extent of skeletal advancement.

Since the occlusion must be preserved while the maxilla and the mandible are advanced the same distance, either arch bars or orthodontic bands are required prior to the osteotomies.

The surgical steps for MMA are as follows.

A Le Fort I maxillary osteotomy is performed above the apices of the teeth. The maxilla is downfractured after pterygomaxillary separation. The descending palatine arteries are identified and are pre-

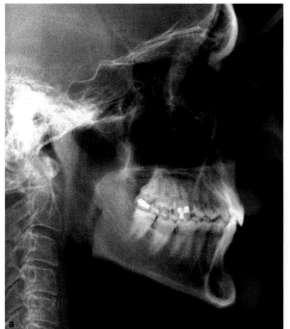

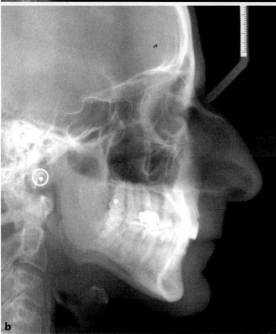

Fig. 41.2. Cephalometric radiograph. **a** Normal cephalometric radiograph. **b** Abnormal cephalometric radiograph; note the maxillomandibular deficiency and the reduced upper-airway dimension

ing four plates and the bone grafts are placed in the osteotomy sites. The alignment of the maxilla in relation to the mandible, dentition, and the face is crucial to ensure acceptable occlusion and aesthetics. The use of a prefabricated intermediate splint can improve the positioning and fixation of the maxilla in the advanced position. Mandibular osteoeotomy is performed via the sagittal split technique. The medial and lateral cortex of the mandible is separated at the ramus region while preserving the inferior alveolar nerve. The dentated mandibular segment is advanced the same distance as the maxilla; thus, occlusion is restored. Rigid fixation is achieved with three positional screws on each side (plates are often used to bridge the osteotomy sites to further ensure rigidity) after the mandible has been stabilized via intermaxillary fixation (Figs. 41.3, 41.4). Bone grafts are sometimes used at the osteotomy sites to promote ossification.

Perioperative Management

It is well known that patients with OSA have an increased risk for perioperative airway compromise; therefore, anesthesia induction and intubation are especially critical for OSA patients. A fiberoptic intubation or tracheotomy with the patient awake should be considered in difficult airway situations, especially in obese patients with an increased neck circumference and associated skeletal deformities (significant mandibular deficiency and low hyoid bone). The use of an arterial line for blood pressure monitoring should be considered. Although autologous blood transfusion can be used, it is not mandatory in the majority of the patients when there is a sufficient preoperative hemoglobin level.

All patients are extubated awake in the operating room with intermaxillary fixation in place immediately following surgery. Although some surgeons prefer wire fixation for intermaxillary fixation, the use of elastic fixation allows the patients to open their mouth if sufficient mouth-opening force is generated, thus reducing the risk of aspiration or airway obstruction. Wire cutters accompany the patients at all times. All patients are monitored in the intensive care unit for the first postoperative day. The use of narcotics should be closely monitored owing to the increased potential of airway compromise. The control of hypertension is important to reduce edema. Humidified oxygen (35%) via a face tent provides some relief for thickened airway secretions; thus, it is used throughout the hospitalization.

The patients are transferred from the intensive care unit after the first day. When there is significant facial edema, fiberoptic airway evaluation should be con-

served if possible. The mobilized maxilla is manipulated and advanced approximately 10–14mm. During the mobilization, the integrity of the descending palatine artery must be observed. If excessive tension is noted, the artery should be clipped and divided to prevent excessive bleeding due to tearing of the vessels. The maxilla is stabilized with rigid fixation us-

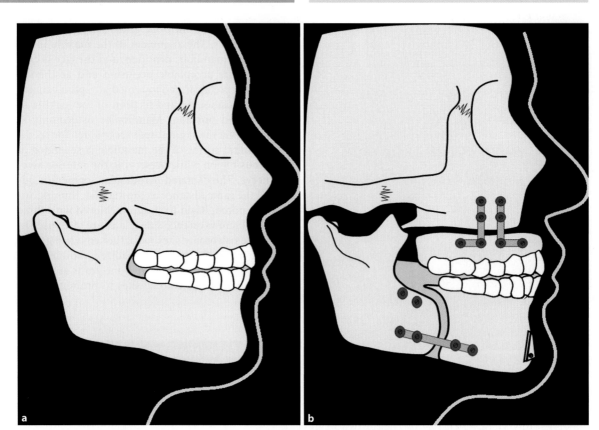

Fig. 41.3. Maxillomandibular advancement. **a** Before surgery. **b** After surgery

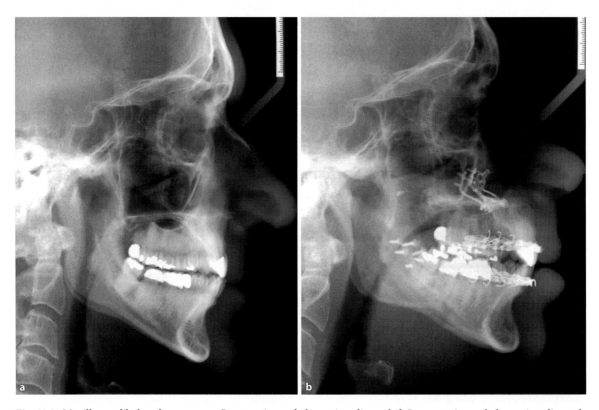

Fig. 41.4. Maxillomandibular advancement. **a** Preoperative cephalometric radiograph. **b** Postoperative cephalometric radiograph

sidered to monitor the airway. Perioperative steroid coverage can be considered to limit the extent of edema. Upon transfer to the regular ward, all patients are encouraged to ambulate and begin a liquid diet. The majority of patients are discharged on the second day. Discharge criteria include a stable airway, adequate oral intake of fluids, and satisfactory pain control. Fiberoptic airway assessment is usually performed prior to discharge. The rigidity of intermaxillary fixation is reduced over the ensuing 4 weeks. A liquid diet is maintained for 4 weeks and a soft diet begins at the fifth week. A regular diet is resumed in 4–5 months.

Surgical Outcomes

As stated already, MMA is a highly effective surgical treatment for OSA. The success rate is usually between 75 and 100% [1, 3–6, 9, 15, 16, 19], with a long-term success rate approaching 90% [10, 11]. In addition, patient perception of the surgical outcome has been very favorable [2]. Although MMA is considered a fairly invasive procedure, the associated surgical risks are low. Potential complications include bleeding, infection, malocclusion, and permanent numbness. The data from the literature support the findings from a recent review by the author. Three hundred and twenty consecutive patients underwent MMA in a 12-year period. Three hundred and five patients had sufficient preoperative and postoperative data for analysis. The mean age was 45±9.5 years. The mean pretreatment body mass index (BMI) was 32.7±6.7 kg/m^2 and the posttreatment BMI was 32.0±6.0 kg/m^2. The mean pretreatment respiratory disturbance index (RDI) and the lowest oxygen saturation (LSAT) were 63.6±26.7 events per hour and 71.7±15.1%, respectively. The RDI improved to 10.5±10.0 events per hour ($p<0.0001$) and the LSAT improved to 86.9±6.7% ($p<0.0001$) after treatment. Two hundred and seventy-two patients (89%) achieved successful results objectively and subjectively. There were no differences between the successful group and the incomplete responder group in terms of age, RDI, and LSAT; however, the mean BMI was greater in the incomplete responder group (32.4±6.6 vs. 35.0±7.2 kg/m^2).

Cocnlusions

MMA is an effective treatment for OSA and even though it is considered a fairly invasive procedure, it is generally well accepted, and when properly performed, it results in minimal complications.

References

1. Bettega G, Pepin J, Veale D, et al. (2000) Obstructive sleep apnea syndrome: Fifty-one consecutive patients treated by maxillofacial surgery. Am J Respir Crit Care Med: 162:641–649.
2. Conradt R, Hochban W, Brandenburg U, Heitmann J, Peter JH. (1997) Long term results after surgical treatment of obstructive sleep apnea by maxillomandibular advancement. Eur Respir J;10:123–128.
3. Conradt R, Hochban W, Heitmann J, Brandenburg U, Cassel W, Penzel T, Peter JH. (1998) Sleep fragmentation and daytime vigilance in patients with OSA treated by surgical maxillomandibular advancement compared to CPAP therapy. J Sleep Res;7:217–223.
4. Dattilo DJ, Drooger SA. (2004) Outcome assessment of patients undergoing maxillofacial procedures for the treatment of sleep apnea: comparison of subjective and objective results. J Oral Maxillofac Surg;62:164–168.
5. Hendler BH, Costello BJ, Silverstein K, Yen D, Goldberg A. (2001) A protocol for uvulopalatopharyngoplasty, mortised genioplasty, and maxillomandibular advancement in patients with obstructive sleep apnea: an analysis of 40 cases. J Oral Maxillofac Surg;59:892–897.
6. Hoekema A, de Lange J, Stegenga B, de Bont LG. (2006) Oral appliances and maxillomandibular advancement surgery: an alternative treaetment protocol for the obstructive sleep apnea-hypopnea syndrome. J Oral Maxillofac Surg;64:886–891.
7. Jamieson A, Guilleminault C, Partinen M, Quera-Salva MA. (1986) Obstructive sleep apneic patients have craniomandibular abnormalities. Sleep;9:469–477.
8. Kuhlo W, Doll E, Frank MD. (1969) Erfolgreiche Behandlung eines Pickwick-syndroms durch eine Dauertrachealkanule. Dtsch Med Wochenschr;94:1286–1290.
9. Lee NR, Givens CD Jr, Wilson J, Robins RB. (1999) Staged surgical treatment of obstructive sleep apnea syndrome: a review of 35 patients. J Oral Maxillofac Surg;57:382–385.
10. Li KK, Powell NB, Riley RW, Troell RJ, Guilleminault C. (2000) Long-term results of maxillomandibular advancement surgery. Sleep Breathing;4:137–139.
11. Li KK, Riley RW, Powell NB, Gervacio L, Troell RJ, Guilleminault C. (2000) Obstructive sleep apnea surgery: Patients' perspective and polysomnographic results. Otolaryngol Head Neck Surg;123:572–575.
12. Li KK, Riley RW, Powell NB, Guilleminault C. (2002) Obstructive sleep apnea and maxillomandibular advancement: An assessment of airway changes using radiographic and nasopharyngoscopic examinations. J Oral Maxillofac Surg;67:27–33.
13. Li KK, Riley RW, Powell NB, Guilleminault C. (2000) Maxillomandibular advancement for persistent OSA after phase I surgery in patients without maxillomandibular deficiency. Laryngoscope;110:1684–1688.
14. Li KK, Riley RW, Powell NB, Guilleminault C. (2001) Patient's perception of the facial appearance after maxillomandibular advancement for obstructive sleep apnea syndrome. J Oral Maxillofac Surg;59:377–380.
15. Li KK, Riley RW, Powell NB, Troell RJ, Guilleminault C. (1999) Overview of Phase II surgery for obstructive sleep apnea syndrome. ENT J;78:851–857.
16. Prinsell JR. (1999) Maxillomandibular advancement surgery in a site-specific treatment approach for obstructive sleep apnea in 50 consecutive patients. Chest;116:1519–1529.

17. Schwab RJ, Gefter WB, Hoffman EA, Gupta KB, Pack AI. (1993) Dynamic upper airway imaging during respiration in normal subjects and patients with sleep disordered breathing. Am Rev Respir Dis;148:1385–1400.

18. Schwab RJ, Gupta KB, Gefter WB, Metzger LJ, Hoffman EA, Pack AI. (1995) Upper airway and soft tissue anatomy in normal subjects and patients with sleep-disordered breathing. Significance of lateral pharyngeal walls. Am J Respir Crit Care Med;152:1673–1689.

19. Smatt Y, Ferri J. (2005) Retrospective study of 18 patients treated by maxillomandibular advancement with adjunctive procedures for obstructive sleep apnea syndrome. J Craniofac Surg;16:770–777.

20. Suratt PM, Dee P, Atkinson RL, Armstrong P, Wilhoit SC. (1993) Fluoroscopic and computer tomographic features of the pharyngeal airway in obstructive sleep apnea. Am Rev Respir Dis;127:487–492.

41

Chapter 42

Maxillomandibular Widening in Sleep Apnea Surgery

42

Kasey K. Li

Core Messages

- Maxillofacial skeletal deficiency in the frontal plane is a risk factor for obstructive sleep apnea.

- Maxillomandibular widening by distraction osteogenesis expands the airway and improves obstructive sleep apnea.

- When properly performed, maxillomandibular widening by distraction osteogenesis results in minimal adverse effects.

Contents

Introduction

It is well known that patients with obstructive sleep apnea (OSA) generally have a smaller airway than patients without OSA. Maxillomandibular deficiency contributes to diminished airway dimension and is a well-recognized risk factor in OSA patients [5, 9]. Currently, the most effective surgical treatment of OSA is maxillomandibular advancement (MMA). MMA enlarges the airway by physically expanding the skeletal framework.

Although the majority of emphasis in recognizing maxillomandibular deformity as well as maxillofacial surgery in managing OSA has been limited to the sagittal plane, recent data suggest that transverse deficiency of the maxilla and/or mandible is a potential risk factor in OSA patients. In a comparative study between OSA patients and control subjects by Seto et al. [15], OSA subjects were found to have narrower, more tapered and shorter maxillary arches. Kushida et al. [12] found that the intermolar distance of the maxilla is related to the presence of OSA. Cistulli et al. [3] have reported that patients with Marfan's syndrome, in which maxillary constriction is a common finding, have increased incidence of OSA and elevated nasal resistance. The relationship of nasal resistance and maxillary morphology has long been recognized. The use of distraction osteogenesis to achieve widening of the maxillomandibular complex leads to expansion of the skeletal framework and enlarges the airway, an is thus is a potential treatment of OSA.

History of Distraction Osteogenesis in the Maxillofacial Region

The advent of skeletal expansion by slow osseous distraction (distraction osteogenesis) is not new and has been previously studied extensively in orthopedic surgery. It has demonstrated acceptable feasibility, efficacy, safety, and reproducibility of its treatment results. In its simplest form, distraction osteogenesis describes the generation of new bone in the stretched fracture callus. A screw-driven appliance that is firmly attached to the bone fragments slowly pulls apart the cut/or fractured bony edges, and new bone can fill in the stretched callus tissue. Distraction osteogenesis was first described by Alessandro Codvilla in 1905, who first reported the use of this technique in lengthening the long bone [4]. However, it is Ilizarov [8] who is credited with developing the current methods of distraction osteogenesis. Distraction osteogenesis in the maxillofacial region was first investigated by Snyder et al. [16] in the canine mandible. Karp et al. [10] demonstrated that bone formation during distraction osteogenesis in the maxillofacial region is similar to that of long bones, which is predominately by intra-membranous ossification. Surgical lengthening by distraction osteogenesis in the sagittal plane was first described by McCarthy at al. [13], who reported on the application of distraction osteogenesis of the human mandible in pediatric patients in 1992. The surgical expansion of the maxilla and that of the mandible by distraction osteogenesis were reported by Bell and Epker [1] and Guerrero [6]. Distraction osteogenesis is less invasive than the traditional technique. It requires less tissue manipulation, less blood loss, and has less skeletal relapse potential.

Preoperative Evaluation

Preoperative evaluation consists of a thorough head and neck evaluation combined with radiography (lateral and posteroanterior cephalometric as well as panoramic radiographs). Patients with significant maxillomandibular narrowing and/or the presence of cross bite are candidates for the procedure (Fig. 42.1). Fiberoptic airway assessment is helpful to assess the extent of airway obstruction in adults. The posteroanterior cephalometric radiograph provides information on the skeletal and airway dimension. The panoramic radiograph is essential to evaluate the maxillary and mandibular anatomy and the dentition. The space between the maxillary as well as the mandibular central incisor teeth is assessed to determine whether there is sufficient space to allow for the osteotomies in adults. A thorough understanding of the anatomy will minimize the potential of injury to the dentition as well as vital structures.

Patient Selection

Both adults and children with significant maxillomandibular narrowing and/or the presence of cross bite are candidates for the procedure (Fig. 42.1). Patients with soft-tissue redundancy should have the soft tissue addressed by conventional surgery first (such as tonsillectomy or palatopharyngoplasty).

Tips and Pearls

■ In general, ideal candidates are children or young adults with mild or moderate OSA and who are willing to undergo mandatory orthodontic intervention associated with the operation.

Maxillomadibular Widening

Maxillomandibular widening can be performed in the adult as well as in the pediatric population. In the pediatric population, maxillary widening usually does not require surgical intervention since the midpalatal suture is not yet ossified. However, with fusion of the midpalatal suture after adolescence, osteotomy is required to facilitate the expansion.

42

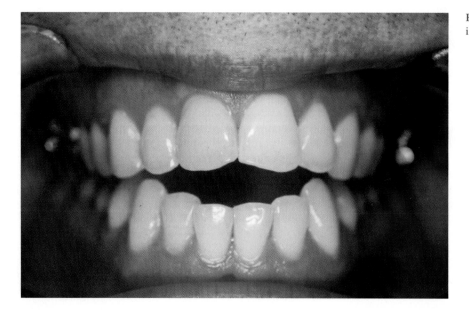

Fig. 42.1. Narrowed maxilla and mandible

The surgical technique is as follows. The procedure is performed in the operating room under general anesthesia technique. Maxillary widening is achieved by a limited osteotomy in the Le Fort I level without downfracturing. A limited osteotomy in the midline of the maxilla is also performed (Fig. 42.2). The distraction device is usually placed by the orthodontist before surgery, and it is activated for 0.5 mm at the completion of the operation (Fig. 42.3). In the mandible, a midline osteotomy is made, followed by application of the intraoral distraction device (Fig. 42.4). Following a latency period of 5–7 days, the device is activated two to four times per day to achieve 1 mm of bone lengthening per day.

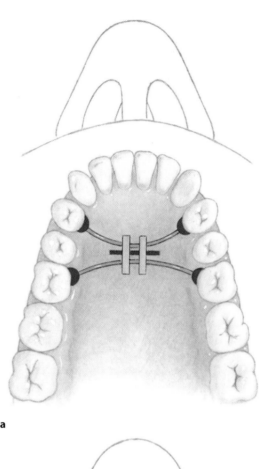

a

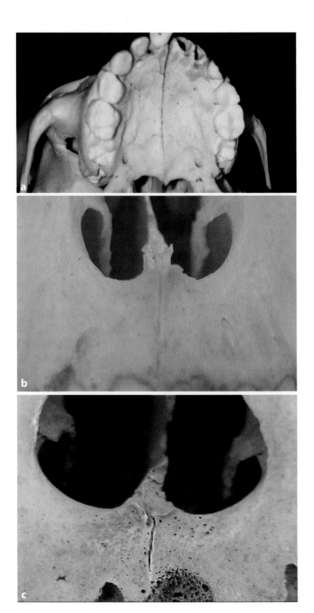

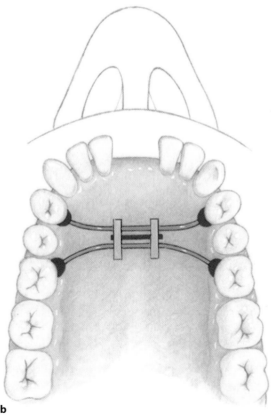

b

Fig. 42.2. Maxillary osteotomy to facilitate widening of the maxilla.

Fig. 42.3. Before (**a**) and after (**b**) maxillary widening

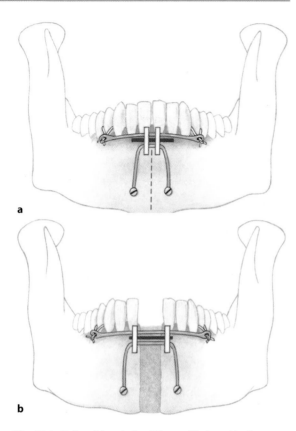

Fig. 42.4. Before (**a**) and after (**b**) mandibular widening

The total widening is determined preoperatively based on the patient's anatomy, dentition, facial appearance, and the severity of OSA. Typically, a widening of 5–10 mm can be achieved. After the completion of distraction (approximately 1–3 weeks), the distraction device is maintained for 2–3 months to facilitate ossification (Fig. 42.5, 42.6). The maxillary distraction device is removed by the orthodontist, and the mandibular distraction device is removed under general anesthesia.

Perioperative Management

Since patients who undergo maxillomandibular widening usually do not have severe OSA, the majority of the patients do not require observation in the intensive care unit setting. Patients are admitted to the recovery room following surgery and are transferred to the regular ward. All patients are encouraged to ambulate and begin a liquid diet. The majority of the patients are discharged on the first postoperative day. Discharge criteria include a stable airway, adequate

oral intake of fluids, and satisfactory pain control. A soft diet begins on day 10 and is continued until sufficient ossification occurs following distraction osteogenesis, which is usually 2–3 months postoperatively.

Surgical Outcomes

Tips and Pearls

- Distraction osteogenesis offers several advantages over the conventional techniques by eliminating the need for bone grafting, and it involves less surgical dissection because bone lengthening is the result of natural bone healing in a gap created by a simple osteotomy.

The incremental skeletal movement allows accommodation of the soft tissue, thus enabling large skeletal movement that usually cannot be achieved by conventional techniques. The gradual soft-tissue accommodation also improves the stability of the new skeletal position.

The major advantage in the application of distraction osteogenesis for maxillofacial skeletal expansion is in the pediatric population where the access for the conventional procedure is limited, the volume of bone is insufficient for the conventional procedure, there is need for much greater skeletal expansion than the conventional technique can achieve, and there is potential for surgical scarring by the conventional procedure, which can negatively impact future facial growth. Both advancement and widening of the maxilla and mandible were shown to improve OSA. Maxillary widening improves nasal airway resistance [18, 19], although the beneficial effect of maxillary expansion on nasal resistance may not be uniformly achieved in all patients, and it appears that patients with greater degrees of nasal resistance tend to have greater improvement after maxillary expansion [7, 20]. Nocturnal enuresis is improved in children [11, 17]. Cistulli et al. [2] performed maxillary expansion on ten OSA patients with maxillary constriction and improvement was achieved in nine of the ten patients. The mean apnea–hypopnea index (AHI) was reduced from 19 events per hour to seven events per hour, and the mean maxillary expansion achieved was 12.1 mm. It is unknown whether mandibular expansion can be performed with maxillary expansion, and if simultaneous maxillary and mandibular expansion can improve sleep-disordered breathing. Pirelli et al. [14] treated 31 children with orthodontic maxillary expansion. Nasal resistance was improved in all patients. The AHI was reduced from 12.2 events per hour to less than one event per hour. The mean expansion was 4.32 mm.

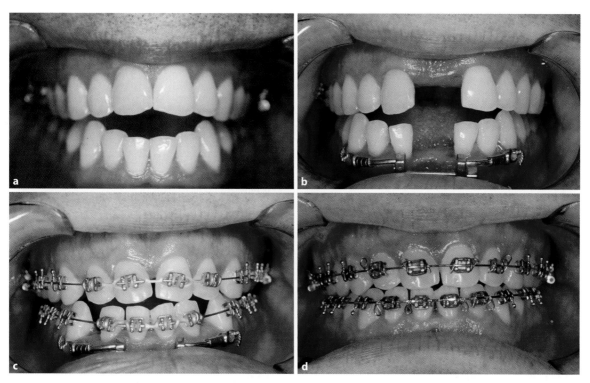

Fig. 42.5. Clinical and radiographic images showing the maxillomandibular widening. Note the expansion of the intraoral volume and the airway space

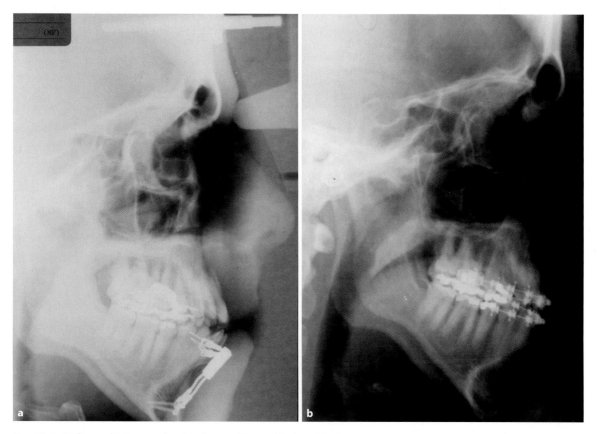

Fig. 42.6. Radiographic images showing the maxillomandibular widening

Conclusion

Distraction osteogenesis is a safe surgical technique in the management of children or young adults with mild or moderate OSA. The incremental skeletal movement allows accommodation of the soft tissue, thus enabling large skeletal movement that usually cannot be achieved by conventional techniques.

References

1. Bell WH, Epker BN. (1976) Surgical-orthodontic expansion of the maxilla. Am J Orthod;70:517–528.
2. Cistulli PA, Palmisano RG, Poole MD. (1998) Treatment of obstructive sleep apnea syndrome by rapid maxillary expansion. Sleep;21:831–835.
3. Cistulli PA, Richards GN, Palmisano RG, Unger G, Berthon-Jones M, Sullivan CE. (1996) Influence of maxillary constriction on nasal resistance and sleep apnea severity in patients with Marfan's syndrome. Chest;110:1184–1188.
4. Codvilla A. (1905) On the means of lengthening, in lower limbs, the muscles and tissues which are shortened through deformity. Am J Orthop Surg;2:353–369.
5. DeBerry-Borowiecki B, Kukwa A, Blanks R. (1988) Cephalometric analysis for diagnosis and treatment of obstructive sleep apnea. Laryngoscope;98:226–234.
6. Guerrero CA, Bell WH, Contasti GI, Rodriguez AM. (1997) Mandibular widening by intraoral distraction Osteogenesis. Br. J Oral Maxillofac Surg;35:383–392.
7. Hartgerink DV, Vig PS, Abbott DW. (1987) The effect of rapid maxillary expansion on nasal airway resistance. Am J Orthod Dentofac Orthop;92:381–9.
8. Ilizarov GA. (1988) The principles of the Ilizarov method. Bull Hosp Joint Dis Orthop Inst;48:1–11.
9. Jamieson A, Guilleminault C, Partinen M, Quera-Salva MA. (1986) Obstructive sleep apneic patients have craniomandibular abnormalities. Sleep;9:469–477.
10. Karp NS, McCarthy JG, Schreiber JS, Sissons HA, Thorne CHM. (1992) Membranous bone lengthening: a serial histological study. Ann Plast Surg;29:2–7.
11. Kurol J, Modin H, Bjerkhoel A. (1998) Orthodontic maxillary expansion and its effect on nocturnal enuresis. Angle Orthod;68:225–232.
12. Kushida C, Efron B, Guilleminault C. (1997) A predictive morphometric model for the obstructive sleep apnea syndrome. Ann Intern Med;127:581–587.
13. McCarthy JG, Schreiber J, Karp N, Thorne CHM, Grayson BH. (1992) Lengthening the human mandible by gradual distraction. Plast Reconstr Surg;89:1–10.
14. Pirelli P, Saponara M, Guilleminault C. (2004) Rapid maxillary expansion in children with obstructive sleep apnea syndrome. Sleep;15:761–766.
15. Seto BH, Gotsopaulos H, Sims MR, Cistulli PA. (2001) Maxillary morphology in obstructive sleep apnea syndrome. Eur J Orthod;23:703–714.
16. Snyder CC, Levine GA, Swanson HM, Browne EZ. (1973) Mandibular lengthening by gradual distraction: preliminary report. Plast Reconstr Surg;51:506–508.
17. Timms DJ. (1990) Rapid maxillary expansion in the treatment of nocturnal enuresis. Angle Orthod;60:229–233.
18. Timms DJ. (1986) The effect of rapid maxillary expansion on nasal airway resistance. Br J Orthod;13:221–228.
19. Timms DJ. (1984) The reduction of nasal airway resistance by rapid maxillary expansion and its effect on respiratory disease. J Laryngol Otol;98:357–362.
20. White BC, Woodside DG, Cole P. (1989) The effect of rapid maxillary expansion on nasal airway resistance. J Otolaryngol;18:137–143.

Chapter 43

Surgical Treatment of Children with Obstructive Sleep Apnea

43

Elisabeth Hultcrantz

Core Messages

- For children every apnea of obstructive origin is pathological.

- Snoring and apneas for an infant always require special investigations including polysomnography.

- Habitual snoring occurs in 6–10% of preschool children and obstructive sleep apnea in 1–2.5%.

- The purpose of surgery is to increase the diameter of upper airways and if necessary stabilize hypotonic muscles, thereby allowing for nasal breathing, which is the prerequisite for future normal growth and development.

- The most prominent symptom of obstructive sleep apnea is snoring in combination with oral breathing.

- The open mouth posture may cause underdevelopment of the maxilla with bite abnormalities.

- Increased daytime sleepiness is often noticed as hyperactivity and/or restlessness.

- Primary and secondary enuresis is common among children with sleep-disordered breathing. For very small children, "failure to thrive" is seen.

- Consider pulmonary hypertension in patients with organic heart disease.

- Adenoidectomy solely or in combination with partial reduction of the tonsil is in most cases the first surgical choice.

- Full tonsillectomy is only indicated if a history of multiple infections exists together with obstructive apneas.

- Avoid electrocoagulation in the tonsillar fossae, which causes unnecessary pain and an increased risk for delayed bleeding.

- Conservative uvulopalatopharyngoplasty with closing of the fossa supratonsillaris and partial resection of an elongated uvula are effective in children with a narrow nasopharynx, or in patients with muscular hypotonia.

- Primary or secondary orofacial skeletal deviations are treated in collaboration with orthodontics and/or maxillofacial surgeons if oral breathing and/or apneas continue after adenotonsillectomy. Distraction treatment of the mandible and/or expansion of the maxilla are effective in these patients.

- Long-term tracheostomy is rarely indicated, but may be preferred to extensive surgery in early childhood.

Contents

What Is Obstructive Sleep Apnea in Children?

Definition

All obstructive apneas in children are pathological. The definition of obstructive sleep apnea (OSA) in adults is not valid for children. Instead of speaking about children with sleep apnea, we should instead use the term sleep-related breathing disorder.

Etiology

Children snore when their upper airways are too narrow with lower than usual negative pressures secondary to a Bernoulli effect. When these patients have sleep-related muscular hypotonia, the breathing will cause audible vibrations. As in adults, the most common anatomy that contributes to the snoring sound is the soft palate and uvula. The level of obstruction in patients with apneas is usually at the level of the base of the tongue.

Children who snore at birth or before the age of 1 year usually have some congenital anatomical obstruction as a part of a congenital syndrome such as Pierre Robin syndrome, or are abnormally muscular hypotonic as in Down syndrome. When the snoring sound and apneas are produced in the laryngeal entrance, laryngomalacia is included in the differential diagnosis. Snoring and apneas in an infant always requires special investigation including polysomnography.

Epidemiology

Waldeyer's ring is poorly developed at birth, but then starts to grow, as a consequence of a normal immunological development. At the age of 2 years, the adenoid is usually well developed and can create breathing problems for children with a narrow face. At the age of 4 years, many children also have a relative hyperplasia of the pharyngeal tonsils. These organs are necessary as a first line of defense both for the breathing and eating functions and for the development of B and T cells. In spite of the relative narrowing of the airway, not all children snore; they maintain airway patency during sleep because of increased upper-airway neuromotor tone and an increased central ventilatory drive compared with adults [19].

Differences in muscular tone during sleep and in genetically influenced dimensions of the airway can make a difference such that one child develops OSA and another does not. All obstruction which increases the breathing effort in children should be evaluated for treatment. Between 6 and 10% of preschool children are habitual snorers and 1–2.5% develop OSA [5, 10].

Symptoms

Snoring in infants does not necessarily cause loud noise: small children do not have the volume of muscles and size of the lungs which are necessary for strong sounds. The most prominent symptom is, however, snoring in combination with oral breathing. The open mouth posture may in the long run cause abnormal development of the maxilla and mandible owing to the muscular influence and bite aberrations, since the tongue in the closed mouth normally acts like a mold for facial development [20].

When snoring becomes an effort, the child usually also develops increased daytime sleepiness, which is very often noticed as an increased difficulty in concentration and hyperactivity. Primary and secondary enuresis is common, and for very small children, a noticeable failure to thrive (which means low increase of length and weight irrespective of eating habits) because of influenced output of growth hormone during the disturbed sleep. The children are usually also slow eaters and have a poor appetite. Most often these symptoms momentarily vanish after treatment [1, 2]. As the condition continues to slowly develop, the parents do not always notice the problems as do visitors/grandparents or day care personnel. In severe long-lasting OSA, funnel chest or other deformities of the thorax may develop (Fig. 43.1c, Video 43.1).

How to Examine a Child with Suspected OSA

- Listen to the parents' spontaneous story about the child's sleep and their concerns.
- If possible, ask the parents to bring a video tape of their sleeping child.
- At the physical examination notice the child's general behavior: sleepy, alert or restless?
- Look at general physical development. Breathing with open mouth? Audible breathing? Running nose? Any deformities of the rib cage, such as "funnel" chest? Overweight? Failure to thrive?

- Examine the oral cavity with respect to bite and teeth. Open mouth posture, open bite, overbite and cross bite? Narrow/high or normal hard palate? Small mandible? These signs often confirm the case history of a long period

43

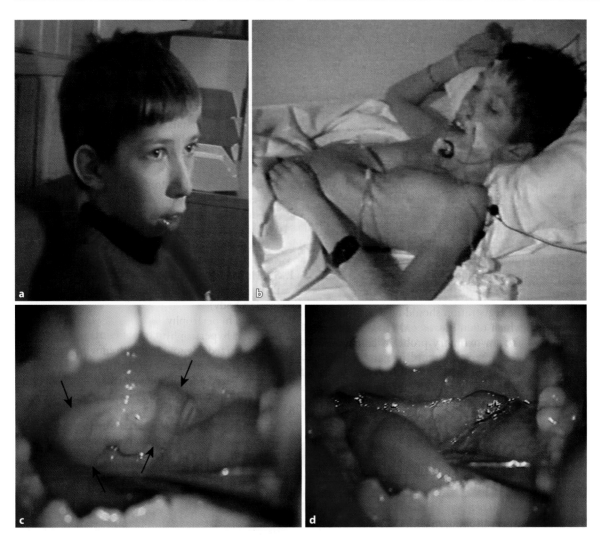

Fig. 43.1. A 12-year-old boy with sleep apnea. **a** Severe obstructive sleep apnea due to mandibular hypoplasia. Primary enuresis, hypersomnia. **b** Pronounced funnel chest which had developed postnatally. **c** Throat preoperatively. Notice the web-like edge of the soft palate. **d** Throat after uvulopalatopharyngoplasty (*UPPP*). Good passage to the nasopharynx. No snoring, no enuresis, alert and considerable weight gain

of breathing obstruction, although a genetic-component most often also exists. Look at the accompanying parents and ask about their snoring history in childhood and later.

■ What is the size of the tonsils in relation to the diameter of the throat during rest with a limp tongue and at provocation when the impact of the lower pole of the tonsils is evaluated?

■ If possible, examine the nasopharynx with a mirror or optics but never palpate the nasopharynx either with a mirror or with a finger in a nonanesthetized child. If examination with a mirror is not possible, a lateral X-ray may be necessary in children from 7 years and older. Younger children can always be expected to have an adenoid pad, which at least adds to the obstruction of large tonsils

When the history and clinical examination both suggest sleep-disordered breathing in an otherwise healthy, normally developing child, it is not always necessary to perform polysomnography before making a decision about whether or not to perform surgery.

However, if the history suggests severe disease or you do not find large tonsils or an occluding adenoid pad, partial polysomnography is necessary to verify the condition. In some cases, the sleep study is "therapeutic" as you can calm the parents that the child's breathing is normal despite some snoring. In all cases where preoperative polysomnography has demonstrated apneas/hypopneas and/or oxygen desaturation, a control postoperative polysomnography should be performed.

All parents should also be informed that during further growth and development of the child, snoring and apnea may reoccur and in that case the

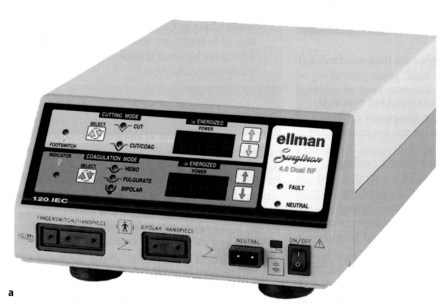

Fig 43.3. Surgitron®
dual-frequency 4.0-MHz
device (Ellman, New York,
USA). a Device console. b
Electrodes used for tonsillotomy and conservative
UPPP

a

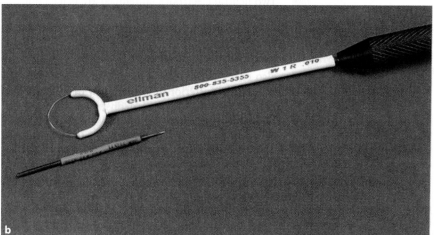

b

sion line. If there is bleeding, put a new swab in place and do the other side after changing to the other antenna. Remaining bleeding small vessels are coagulated using a needle or the ball electrode (Fig. 43.4e).

Conservative UPPP

The indication is narrow maxilla with a sharp angle between the tonsils and in cases where muscular hypotonia during sleep is the major problem. Children with Down syndrome are always candidates.

Perform a tonsillectomy or if there is a fossa supratonsillaris a partial intracapsular tonsillectomy (Fig. 43.5). Remove the mucus membrane in the fossa supratonsillaris all the way to the root of the uvula. Ex-

tirpate a half-moon-shaped piece of the mucus membrane above the uvula (Fig. 43.5c).

Remove redundant tissue from around the uvula. Do not damage the posterior pillars or the membranous lining of the uvula. Suture the upper part of the pillars (fossa supratonsillaris) together, thereby pulling the posterior pillar forward. Be careful to get the sutures through muscle. Use 00 Vicryl. Close the incision above the uvula, let the suture go into the muscle layer. Use 000 Vicryl (Fig. 43.5d).

Figure 43.5e shows the result 6 weeks after surgery. Notice the widening of the entrance to the nasopharynx and the fibrosis where the sutures were.

43

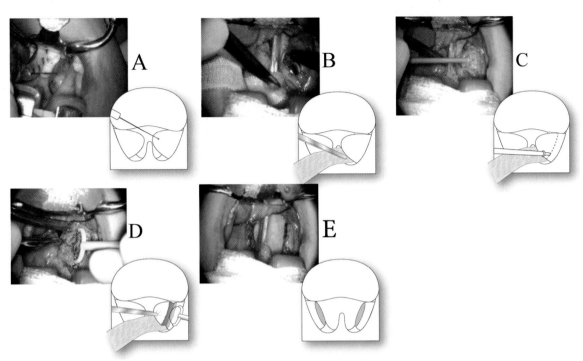

Fig. 43.4. Partial intracapsular tonsillectomy (tonsillotomy) with the Surgitron® dual-frequency 4.0-MHz device. **A** Injection of local anesthetics into the tonsils, to increase fluid content. **B** Application of a gauze strip through the fossa supratonsillaris to protect the posterior pillars. **C** Incision of the tonsil surface parallel to the anterior pillar **D** Cutting through the tonsil with the HTZ electrode **E** End result: small, normal-sized tonsils

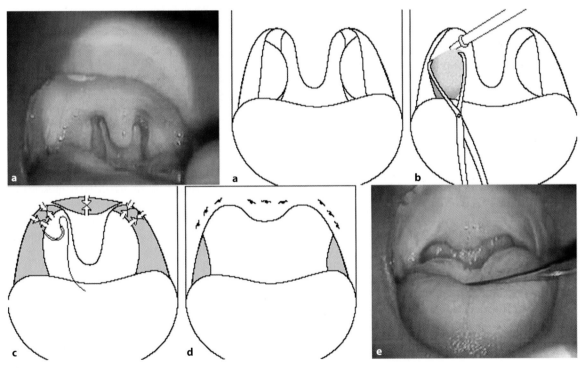

Fig. 43.5. Conservative UPPP. **a** Preoperative status in a 12-year-old boy with severe obstructive sleep apnea due to muscular hypotonia during sleep. Hypersomnia, hyperactive, loss of concentration, poor school performance. **b** Full tonsillectomy. **c** Removal of mucosa in fossa supratonsillaris and an oval incision of mucosa over the uvula. **d** Deep sutures in fossa supratonsillaris as well as over the uvula. **e** *End result:* Note the fibrosis where the sutures were placed – normal sleep and alertness, improved grades in school

Tonsillectomy: Blunt Dissection

The child should be under full anesthesia, intubated or using a laryngeal mask. Sufficient premedication is used to reduce postoperative pain, but intravenous morphine is usually necessary.

Local anesthesia including epinephrine is applied under the mucus membrane of the tonsil medially of the anterior pillar. The tonsil is grabbed with tonsil forceps and pulled medially so that the mucous membrane can be incised at the bottom of the fossa supratonsillaris and the tonsil be freed outside of its capsule without damage to the anterior pillar.

Continue to dissect inferiorly in the plane between the tonsillar capsule and the tonsillar fossa. Clamp visible blood vessels successively in advance with fine arterial forceps if needed, but as you dissect along the tonsillar capsule you rarely have to ligate them. Leave as much as possible of the mucus membrane intact also on the posterior pillar, thereby minimizing the extracapsular wound. At the lower pole dissect the tonsil free. If the pharyngeal tonsil continues into the lingual tonsil, arterial forceps can secure the end and a suture ligature may be needed.

If there is bleeding, find the vessels and use fine arterial forceps and ordinary ligatures. Do not use diathermy in the tonsillar fossae because there is a higher risk for late postoperative bleeding [25] and pain.

Postoperative Care

Most children operated on for OSA can be sent home after a few hours of observation (6–8 h). The breathing obstruction will be immediately relieved after adenoidectomy and tonsil surgery. The risk for postoperative bleeding is decreased if partial tonsil reduction is performed and the time for the child to return to normal activity is shortened [12, 16].

Pain relief is the most important part of care responsibility for the parents, who should be given a written schedule for medication. Diclophenac in combination with paracetamol is usually sufficient initially [18]. The parents and children are instructed to evaluate the pain using a pain scale before meals and to withdraw the medication successively while keeping pain "below 3" on the 7-graded scale, where 0 is no pain and 6 the worst possible. Antibiotics or steroids are only indicated in selected cases.

No restrictions concerning food or activity are necessary.

Complications

As for all tonsil surgery, the risk for primary and secondary bleeding has to be considered [25].

The risk for bleeding is less in a calm and pain-free child:

- Minor bleeding can be stopped by the child sucking on ice cubes.
- Desmopressin given intravenously or as a nasal spray will often be sufficient, both in normal children and in ones with unsuspected coagulation abnormality.
- If fresh blood is oozing out of the mouth, a small child usually has to be taken back to the operating theatre for bleeding control.
- An older child can be treated locally by injection of local anesthetics containing epinephrine and coagulation of bleeding vessels can be done with silver nitrate sticks.
- If it is necessary to reoperate, identify bleeding vessels and ligate them. Do not use electrocoagulation.
- If the bleeding has stopped when the patient is anesthetized, try to estimate from which area the blood originated and apply hemostatic material in that location. Avoid placing sutures deep in the muscles to avoid injury to neighboring large blood vessels.
- If major bleeding occurs in a child, manually compress the vessels before attempting definitive treatment.
- If there is a secondary bleeding, an infection is often part of the cause and antibiotics should be prescribed

In children with an undiagnosed submucous cleft or genetic underfunction of the palatal muscles or short soft palate, an adenotonsillectomy may cause speech problems with air leakage through the nose. This complication can be avoided by preoperatively identifying the anomaly. Always suspect the condition if there is a bifid uvula. In such cases, a "high adenoidectomy" can be performed, which means that only the part of the adenoid covering the choanae and the ceiling of the nasopharynx is removed. The portion of the adenoidal tissue on the posterior wall of the nasopharynx is left intact, since it participates in the closing at phonation. In the child who has developed speech problems, speech therapy may be beneficial, but in the worst cases pharyngeal reconstruction may be necessary.

Recurrence

Although the symptoms are resolved after surgery, the parents should be informed that there is a risk that the snoring, apneas and other symptoms may recur and if this occurs they should again contact a physician.

The reasons for recurrence can vary:

- If the original surgery has not accomplished transition to nasal breathing, there is risk that negative maxillofacial development continues with recurrence of symptoms, either in the teens or in adulthood. The child who continues to have predominantly oral breathing should be evaluated with respect to additional treatment of rhinological problems (allergy) or be referred to an orthodontist, even if the snoring and apneas have improved after primary surgery.
- After isolated adenoidectomy, hypertrophied tonsils may contribute to worsening snoring and disturbed sleep. This problem can partly be avoided if partial resection of the tonsils is performed routinely with adenoidectomy.
- If both adenoidectomy and a full tonsillectomy have been performed, later development of lingual tonsils may create new breathing problems. This problem is avoided by never doing an adenotonsillectomy in infants.

Conclusion

Sleep apnea in adults is a chronic disease which can be treated symptomatically, but seldom cured permanently. If sleep apnea is diagnosed and treated adequately in early childhood most children will be cured. Some will experience a return of symptoms during their physical development [6], but there will still be an opportunity for improvement once again and for normal development if sufficient treatment is given early enough [8].

References

1. Ahlquist, J., Hultcrantz, E., Svanholm, H. (1988). Children with tonsillary obstruction. Symptoms and efficacy of zonsillectomy. Acta Ped. Scand. 77:831–835.
2. Ahlquist-Rastad, J., Hultcrantz, E., Melander, H., Svanholm, H. (1992). Body growth in relation to tonsillar enlargement & tonsillectomy. Int. J. Pediatr. Otolaryngol. 24:55–61.
3. Cohen, S.R., Simms, C., Burstein, F.D., Thomsen, J. (1999). Alternatives to tracheostomy in infants and children with obstructive sleep apnea. J. Pediatr. Surg. 34(1):182–187
4. Friedman, M., Ibrahim H. (2001). Radiofrequency tonsil and adenoid ablation Operative Techn Otolaryngol Head Neck Surg 12:196–198.
5. Gislason, T., Benediktsdottir, B. (1995).Snoring, apneic episodes, and nocturnal hypoxemia among children 6 months to 6 years old: An epidemiologic study of lower limit of prevalence.Chest 107(4):963–966.
6. Guilleminault, C., Partinen, M., Praud, JP, Quera-Salva, MA., Powell N, Riley, R. (1989). Morphometric facial changes and obstructive sleep apnea in adolescents. J. Pediatr.114: 997-9
7. Hultcrantz, E., Svanholm, H., Ahlquist, J. (1988). Sleep apnea in children without tonsillary hypertrophy. Clin. Pediatr. 27:350–354.
8. Hultcrantz, E., Larson, M., Hellquist, R., Ahlquist-Rastad, J., Svanholm, H., Jacobsson, O.P. (1991). The influence of tonsillary obstruction and tonsillectomy on facial growth and dental arch morphology. Int. J. Pediatr. Otorhinolaryngol. 22:125–134.
9. Hultcrantz, E., Sunnegårdh, J., Svanholm, H. Riesenfeld, T. (1993). Uvulopalatopharyngoplasty in children with Down's syndrome. In: Sleep Apnea and Rhonchopathy, Basel, Karger, pp 8–12.
10. Hultcrantz, E., Löfstrand-Tideström, B., Ahlquist-Rastad, J. (1995). The epidemiology of sleep related breathing disorder in children. Int. J. Pediatr. Otorhinolaryngol. 32(Suppl):63–66.
11. Hultcrantz, E., Linder, A., Markström, A. (1999). Tonsillectomy or tonsillotomy?–a randomized study comparing postoperative pain and long-term effects. Int. J. Pediatr. Otorhinolaryngol. 51:171–176
12. Hultcrantz, E., Ericsson, E. (2004). Pediatric tonsillotomy with RF-technique-less pain and morbidity. Laryngoscope 114:871–877.
13. Hultcrantz, E., Ericsson, E., Graf, J. (2004). Intracapsular tonsillectomy with RF-surgery versus regular tonsillectomy. One year results. Otolaryngol. Head Neck Surg. 131(2):108
14. Hultcrantz, E., Linder, A. Markström, A. (2005). Long-term effects of intracapsular partial tonsillectomy (tonsillotomy) compared with full tonsillectomy. Int. J. Pediatr. Otorhinolaryngol. 69:463–469.
15. Johansson, E., Hultcrantz, E. (2003). Clinical consequences twenty years after tonsillectomy? Int. J. Pediatr. Otorhinolaryngol. 67:981–988.
16. Koltai, P.J., Solares, C.A., Mascha, E.J., Xu, M. (2002). Intracapsular partial tonsillectomy for tonsillar hypertrophy in children. Laryngoscope 112(8 II):17–19.
17. Löfstrand-Tideström, B., Thilander, B., Ahlqvist-Rastad, J., Jakobsson, O., Hultcrantz, E. (1999). Breathing obstruction in relation to craniofacial and dental arch morphology in four year-old children Eur. J. Orthod. 21:323–332.
18. Lundeberg, S., Lönnqvist, PA. (2004). Update on systematic postoperative analgesia in children. Pediatr. Anesth. 14:394–397.
19. Marcus, C.L. (2000).Pathophysiology of childhood obstructive sleep apnea: Curr. Concepts Respir. Physiol. 119(2–3):143–154.

20. Moss, M.L., Salentijn, L. (1969). The primary role of functional matrices in facial growth. Am. J. Orthod. 5(6):566–577.
21. Nord, P-G. (2001). Jaw bone elongation with distraction technique. Läkartidningen 98:2708–2712.
22. Shehata, E.M., Ragab, S.M., Behiry, A.B., Efran F., Gamea, A.M. (2005). Telescopic-assisted Radiofrequency adenoidectomy: a prospective randomized controlled trial. Laryngoscope 115:162–166.
23. Stanislaw, P. Jr., Koltai, P.J., Fuestel, P.J. (2000). Comparison of power-assisted adenoidectomy vs adenoid curette adenoidectomy. Arch. Otolaryngol. Head Neck Surg. 126:845–849.
24. Temple R.H., Timms M.S. (2001). Paediatric coblation tonsillectomy. Int. J. Pediatr. Otorhinolaryngol. 61:195–198.
25. National Audit UK. (2004). Tonsillectomy technique as a risk factor for postoperative haemorrhage. Lancet 364(9435):697–702.

43

Chapter 44

Complications of Palatal Approaches

44

Bridget Hathaway, Jonas Johnson

Core Messages

- Careful patient selection minimizes the risk of postoperative respiratory complications following palate surgery for obstructive sleep apnea.

- Excision of the soft palate in a rectangular fashion with preservation of the posterior tonsillar pillars may prevent scar contracture and nasopharyngeal stenosis after uvulopalatopharyngoplasty.

Contents

Early Complications

Respiratory Compromise

The most common and potentially severe complication of palate surgery in the early postoperative period is respiratory compromise. The severity of respiratory compromise is variable and may involve mild oxygen desaturation, airway obstruction, or postobstructive pulmonary edema (POPE). Patient selection is important in minimizing the risk of postoperative respiratory compromise. In general, patients with se-vere comorbidities or apnea-related cardiac events are not good candidates for palate surgery for obstructive sleep apnea (OSA) treatment. When positive pressure therapy fails, such patients should be offered tracheostomy.

Multiple authors have examined rates of respiratory complications following uvulopalatopharyngoplasty (UPPP) [3, 7, 10, 11, 14, 15]. Unfortunately, definitions of respiratory complications vary widely in these studies, with some authors only including major respiratory complications such as reintubation, emergent tracheotomy, pneumonia, and pulmonary edema.

Tips and Pearls

- Mild oxygen desaturation is the most commonly observed respiratory complication in the early postoperative period.

Since upper-airway surgical procedures are not immediately curative, the oxygen desaturation that OSA patients experience preoperatively is not expected to immediately resolve. In certain patients, postoperative edema and narcotic use may potentiate obstructive tendencies, causing worsening of symptoms in the short term. In general, postoperative oxygen desaturation is comparable to that observed during preoperative polysomnography [2, 15]. Riley et al. [14] reviewed 182 patients having surgery for OSA and found that six patients desaturated to the upper 80% range in the first two postoperative days. Hathaway and Johnson [7] recently reviewed 110 patients undergoing UPPP with or without concomitant septoplasty. Three percent of patients had oxygen desaturation in the recovery room.

Postobstructive Pulmonary Edema

Tips and Pearls

- POPE may occur after sudden relief of chronic upper-airway obstruction.

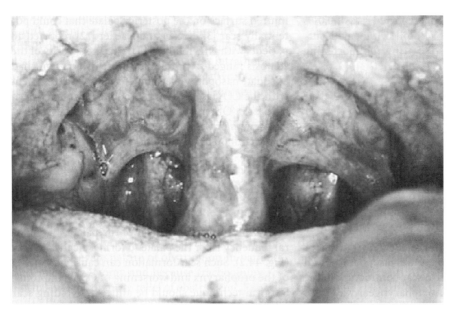

Fig. 44.2. Preoperative and postoperative intraoral photographs of a patient who underwent type 1 laser-assisted uvulopalatoplasty. **a** Preoperative view. **b** Immediate postoperative view. **c** Late postoperative view; note severe medial scar contracture of the posterior pillars (*white arrows*). (From [1], copyright 2001, American Medical Association)

the RDI in 60% of patients at follow-up polysomnography 5–48 months after LAUP. They attribute these results to progressive fibrosis of the soft palate initiated by thermal damage from the laser beam [2, 7].

Surgical Failure

Failure to improve the symptoms of OSA is perhaps the most common complication of palate surgery. The efficacy of individual surgical procedures is well described in other chapters. However, there are general considerations that apply to all surgical procedures for OSA.

Tips and Pearls

■ Patient selection is possibly the most important factor in determining success for a given procedure.

Patients with severe comorbidities or apnea-related cardiac events are generally not appropriate candidates for palate surgery. When these patients are unable to be effectively managed with positive pressure, they should be offered tracheostomy as the minimal procedure.

Recognition of other sites of upper-airway obstruction is also important in effectively treating the OSA patient. The tongue base, lateral pharyngeal walls, and epiglottis may all contribute to obstruction. Careful preoperative flexible endoscopic examination should provide useful information in developing a plan of treatment.

Finally, in the overweight or obese patient, the importance of weight control in treating OSA cannot be overemphasized.

Oropharyngeal and Voice Complaints

Hypogeusia has been reported as a complication of palate surgery but is seemingly rare. Possible mechanisms include direct or thermal injury to the glossopharyngeal nerve or its lingual branch [9]. Patients may also experience pharyngeal dryness or globus sensation following palate surgery. These symptoms are rarely permanent.

Finally, patients may report voice changes following palate surgery. While some investigators have not found any persistent changes in vocal function after UPPP [5], Tewary and Cable [17] prospectively studied patients undergoing UPPP for voice and speech changes and found that the fundamental frequency was significantly lower in patients undergoing UPPP compared with those undergoing tonsillectomy.

Tips and Pearls

■ While many patients may not be affected by or even notice such voice changes, professional voice users should be counseled preoperatively as to this potential outcome.

Conclusion

▼

Careful patient selection and meticulous surgical technique may reduce the risk for complications associated with UPPP. To avoid airway complications following surgery, the patient should not be extubated until fully awake, following commands, and breathing adequate tidal volumes.

References

1. Berger G, Finkelstein Y, Stein G, Ophir D. (2001) Laser-assisted uvulopalatoplasty for snoring: medium- to long-term subjective and objective analysis. Arch Otolaryngol Head Neck Surg; 127:415

2. Burgess LP, Derderian SS, Morin GV, Gonzalez C, Zajtchuk JT. (1992) Postoperative risk following uvulopalatopharyngoplasty for obstructive sleep apnea. Otolaryngol Head Neck Surg;106(1):81–6.

3. Fairbanks DF. (1990) Uvulopalatopharyngoplasty complications and avoidance strategies. Otolaryngol Head Neck Surg;102(3):239–45.

4. Fujita S, Conway W, Zorick F, Roth T. (1981) Surgical correction of anatomic abnormalities in obstructive sleep apnea syndrome: uvulopalatopharyngoplasty. Otolaryngol Head Neck Surg; 89:923–34.

5. Greene JS, Zipfel TE, Harlor M. (2004) The effect of uvulopalatopharyngoplasty on the nasality of voice. J Voice;18(3):423–30.

6. Guffin TN, Har-El G, Sanders A, Lucente FE, Nash M. (1995) Acute postobstructive pulmonary edema. Otolaryngol Head Neck Surg;112(2):235–7.

7. Hathaway B, Johnson JT. (2006) Safety of uvulopalatopharyngoplasty as outpatient surgery. Otolaryngol Head Neck Surg;134(4):542–4.

8. Jackson IT, Kennedy D. (1997) Surgical management of velopharyngeal insufficiency following uvulopalatopharyngoplasty: report of three cases. Plastic Recon Surg;99(4);1151–3.

9. Kamel UF. (2004) Hypogeusia as a complication of uvulopalatopharyngoplasty and use of taste strips as a practical tool for quantifying hypogeusia. Acta Otolaryngol;124(10):1235–6.

10. Kezirian EJ, Weaver EM, Yueh B, Deyo RA, Khuri SF, Daley J, Henderson W. (2004) Incidence of serious complications after uvulopalatopharyngoplasty. Laryngoscope;114:450–3.

11. Kieff DA, Busaba NY. (2004) Same-day discharge for selected patients undergoing combined nasal and palatal surgery for obstructive sleep apnea. Ann Otol Rhninol Laryngol;114:128–31.

12. Krespi YF, Kacker A. (2000) Management of nasopharyngeal stenosis after uvulopalatoplasty. Otolaryngol Head Neck Surg;123(6):692–5.

13. Madani M. (2004) Complications of laser-assisted uvulopalatopharyngoplasty and radiofrequency treatments of snoring and chronic nasal congestion: a 10-year review of 5,600 patients. J Oral Maxillofac Surg;62:1351–62.

14. Riley RW, Powell NB, Guilleminault C, Pelayo R, Troell RJ, Li KK. (1997) Obstructive sleep apnea surgery: risk management and complications. Otolaryngol Head Neck Surg;117(6):648–52.

15. Spiegel JH, Raval TH. (2005) Overnight hospital stay is not always necessary after uvulopalatopharyngoplasty. Laryngoscope;115:167–71.

16. Stevenson EW. (1969) Cicatricial stenosis of the nasopharynx: a comprehensive review. Laryngoscope;79:2035–67.

17. Tewary AK, Cable HR. (1993) Speech changes following uvulopalatopharyngoplasty. Clin Otolaryngol Allied Sci;18(5):390–1.

Chapter 45

Reasons for Failure in Surgery of Obstructive Sleep Apnea Syndrome

45

Metin Önerci, Oguz Ögretmenoglu, Taskın Yücel

Core Messages

- Systematic approach in preoperative evaluation and postoperative management is mandatory to avoid failure in obstructive sleep apnea syndrome (OSAS) surgery.

- Pathologic factors leading to airway obstruction such as alcohol consumption and drug use, and the predisposing systemic diseases such as hypothyroidism must be eliminated preoperatively.

- The relationship between obesity and OSAS should be explained to the patient. Postoperative weight gain must be prevented.

- The apnea–hypopnea index is not a summary of polysomnographic evaluation. To study obstructive sleep apnea treatment outcomes, all parameters of polysomnography must be determined, and bias of the test must be considered.

- Definition of success is not standardized as of yet. Because of this, study results cannot be compared without confusion.

Contents

Introduction

Surgical treatment of obstructive sleep apnea syndrome (OSAS) started with tracheotomy as it bypasses the whole upper airway and eliminates all possible obstruction. However, maintaining a tracheostomy in obese patients is difficult and patients in general resist accepting the procedure.

In 1981, Fujita [14] introduced the uvulopalatopharyngoplasty (UPPP) procedure, which targets only the obstructed velopharyngeal site during sleep, and during the same period, continuous positive airway pressure (CPAP) was developed as a noninvasive treatment of obstructive sleep apnea (OSA). Even though UPPP was commonly utilized, polysomnographic evaluation showed that it failed to improve OSAS in more than half of the patients. As the concept of multilevel airway obstruction in OSA was popularized, efforts to achieve a better cure rate led to development of multiple surgical techniques addressing multiple anatomic sites suspected for obstruction.

Successful surgical outcomes depend on the systematic preoperative evaluation and postoperative management along with the choice of surgical technique. The following list summarizes the parameters that influence treatment outcomes:

1. Preoperative evaluation
   (a) Risk factors
   Predisposing pathologic conditions
   – Endocrine diseases
   – Diseases affecting the neuromuscular system
   – Brainstem abnormalities
   – Obstruction of airway with the patient awake
      (A) Anatomic factors
      (B) Space-occupying lesions
   Medications
   – Iatrogenic
   – Alcoholism
   Obesity and age
   Other
   (c) Severity of disease
   (d) Determination of level of obstruction
   (e) Determinants in polysomnography

2. Surgical method
   (a) Indication and selection of method
   (b) Technical considerations
   (c) Tolerance to therapy in staged treatment

3. Postoperative management
   (a) Weight gain
   (b) Drugs and alcohol
   (c) Long-term effectiveness of therapy
   (d) Determinants in polysomnography
   (e) Determination of the surgical success

Preoperative Evaluation

Preoperative evaluation is an important step to assist in the selection of patients for surgery. Complicating factors such as systemic diseases, obstructed airway, drugs, and obesity can be easily recognized by a proper evaluation.

Systemic Disease

Daytime sleepiness and sleep apneas can be observed in various endocrine, neuromuscular and other types of disorders [2, 29, 42, 44, 52]. Examples are hypothyroidism, acromegaly, diabetic neuropathy with autonomic dysfunction, Parkinsonism, Alzheimer's disease, stroke, epilepsy, metabolic abnormalities such as hyponatremia and hypoglycemia due to adrenal insufficiency, Cushing's syndrome, brainstem abnormalities due to inflammation, hemorrhage, trauma, encephalitis, acute bulbar poliomyelitis, and rarely neoplasm. Neuromuscular disorders affecting the spinal conducting pathways, the anterior horn cells, the nerves to respiratory muscles, and the respiratory muscles themselves, such as compression of the cervical cord, muscular dystrophies, poliomyelitis, Guilliain–Barré syndrome, and myasthenia gravis, can cause hypoventilation. Clinical expression is quite obvious in most of the diseases mentioned above. Management includes treatment of the primary disease, and simultaneous addition of adjunctive therapy for sleep apnea. Acromegaly and hypothyroidism are exceptions as hormone therapy may improve sleep apnea [16, 18, 47, 48]. Surgery for OSAS without treatment of the underlying disease may result in failure. Conversely, Winkelman et al. [51] suggested that screening for hypothyroidism was not recommended in OSAS, since they discovered similar prevalence in OSAS patients as in individuals without OSAS. We recommend screening for these disorders since misdiagnosis will compromise the results of treatment.

Pathologic Conditions Causing Airway Obstruction

Obstruction of the airway during sleep is a dynamic process, and causes OSAS in patients who have a patent airway when awake. Disorders leading to permanent airway obstruction unrelated to sleep can cause OSAS. These include deviation of the nasal septum, chronic rhinitis, rhinolithiasis, turbinate abnormalities, nasal polyps, choanal atresia, a foreign body, cysts, hypertrophied lymphoid tissue (palatine and lingual tonsils, adenoid tissue), craniofacial anomalies, floppy epiglottis, laryngeal abnormalities, and neoplasms [3, 8, 33]. Although increased nasal resistance was reported as an aggravating factor for OSAS, correction of obstruction by performing septal surgery did not guarantee relief from apnea [12, 25, 49]. We recommend elimination of nasal obstruction and reduction of the hypertrophied adenoid tissue since it helps patients with or without sleep apnea.

It is also clear that removal of hypertrophied tonsils and adenoid tissue can cure symptoms of OSA in the majority of children [30]. In adults, the presence of hypertrophied tonsils significantly increases the success rate of surgery, when tonsillectomy is added to other OSA surgery [24].

To avoid missing any abnormality in the rest of the upper airway, nasopharyngolaryngeal endoscopic examination should be performed, which is well tolerated by patients.

Craniofacial Anomalies

Craniofacial anomalies involving the midface and mandible in syndromes such as Pierre Robin, Apert, Treacher Collins, Saethre–Chotzen, CHARGE, Nager, Stickler, Goldenhar, and Pfeiffer can cause airway obstruction and sleep apnea [4, 7, 37]. Lateral cephalometric radiography certainly provides reliable and objective information about these anomalies, and treatment should be individualized according to the clinical presentation of each patient.

Medications

Many medications with central nervous system effects can contribute to sleep difficulties. Different medication classes may have different effects on polysomnography. For example, barbiturates and benzodiazepines cause decreased sleep onset latency, increased sleep continuity and total sleep amount, and mild suppression of REM sleep. Morphine and heroin cause decreased and disturbed sleep with suppression of REM sleep. Antipsychotic drugs with sedative effects can cause decreased sleep latency, increased total sleep time, and improved sleep continuity. First-generation antihistamines (H1 antagonists) might produce daytime sleepiness and worsen OSA symptoms. This effect can be avoided by replacing them with second-generation antihistamines. Some antidepressant drugs have sedative effects. Sedative and hypnotic drugs can worsen sleep apnea, as does alcohol consumption. β-adrenergic blockers may cause daytime sleepiness owing to fragmentation of sleep, while α-adrenergic agonists, such as methyldopa and clonidine, may cause sedation. All stimulants, such as caffeine, theophylline, amphetamine, and cocaine, increase wakefulness and withdrawal of these agents may produce severe hypersomnia in chronic use. Alcohol consumption can increase snoring and worsen sleep apnea. It is also a major cause of sleep disruption. Always consider alcohol withdrawal prior to performing surgery for OSA. However, in chronic alcoholism, alcohol withdrawal may cause decreased total sleep time and poor sleep continuity for a significant length of time [32].

Obesity

It is well recognized that obesity is an important risk factor of OSA [6], and its severity is measured by the body mass index (BMI). Fat distribution is a more accurate evaluation of obesity than BMI, but both of them correlate with the severity of OSA [11, 34, 54]. It was reported that gross obesity (BMI more than 30 kg/m^2) can decrease the success rate of surgery [17, 19, 27]. In another study, a cutoff BMI of less than 40 kg/m^2 was suggested as one of the selection criteria for OSA surgery [10]. Although, the BMI was not found to correlate with surgical outcome in some studies, problems with the small number of patients, selection bias, or limited available raw data (meta-analysis) were stressed by the authors [20, 43, 45]. It is well known that weight loss in obese patients may improve or cure the disease; however, postoperative weight gain is an important problem in patients treated with surgery. Weight gain after UPPP might lead to worsening of OSAS [27, 40]. All patients must be informed of the importance of obesity in the etiology of OSA and the effect obesity has on the progression of the disease.

Severity of OSAS

The severity of OSAS as indicated by the apnea–hypopnea index (AHI) was found to correlate with the results of surgery in some studies: a higher AHI prior to surgery suggested higher failure rates [15, 20, 38, 41]. Millman et al. [31], found that an AHI less than 38 events per hour of sleep was a predictor of improvement after UPPP in 46 patients (success rate 50% for AHI < 38 versus 18% for AHI > 38). In all these studies only one surgical method was performed to address only one anatomic site of obstruction. Combined or staged procedures addressing multilevel obstruction in selected patients increased success rates dramatically, and this was unrelated to the AHI [41].

Determination of Obstruction Level

Determining the level of obstruction is the most important key factor in the success of the surgical treatment of OSA. UPPP and more aggressive modifications cured snoring in most patients, but polysomnographic data showed that a few of them still had higher apnea scores. Studies aimed at defining factors that influence the outcome of palatal surgery in order to eliminate the nonresponder group preoperatively. These studies showed that the main reason for failure after UPPP is the presence of obstructive anatomy other than at the retropalatal level, mainly the tongue base. Fujita [13] introduced a classification of the preoperative physical examination according to the level of obstruction and proposed that patients with type III (hypopharyngeal only) obstruction were poor responders to UPPP. Müller's maneuver was proposed as a more reliable method of evaluation by simulating the collapse of the upper airway, but later results showed lower sensitivity and specificity [23].

Imaging studies, including lateral cephalometric radiographs, CT scans, and MRI, are used to evaluate patients with OSAS. These imaging methods and physical findings evaluate the airway in the awaken state and not during sleep, when OSA occurs, and thus have limited specificity and sensitivity; however, these techniques can assist in the evaluation of the patient with OSA. Friedman et al. [10] correlated physical findings such as tonsillar size and Mallampati index (Figs. 45.1, 45.2) with BMI and developed a staging system that can assist in the selection of patients for surgery. They reported significantly higher success rates of UPPP with stage 1 OSA patients. It is clear that identifying an obstructed or narrowed airway segment can assist in the planning of surgery. The inability to do this leads surgeons to perform multi-

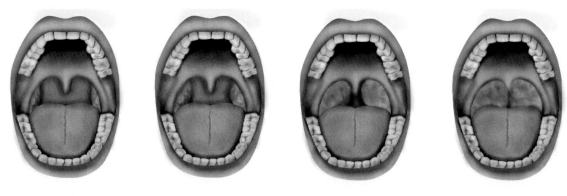

Fig. 45.1. Tonsil size, grades 1, 2, 3, and 4 *from left to right* (modified Mallampati score by Friedman et al. [31])

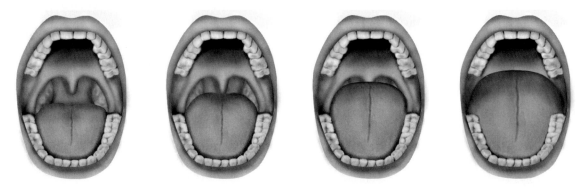

Fig. 45.2. Palate position, grades 1, 2, 3, and 4 *from left to right* (modified Mallampati score by Friedman et al. [31])

level or staged OSA surgery to avoid unsuccessful results [10, 41].

Evaluation of Polysomnography

Polysomnography cannot be summarized by the AHI only. Sleep architecture, body position, and oxygen saturation should be considered. Decreased total sleep time, REM sleep, and sleep position may result in decreased AHI values. The first-night effect can also underestimate the severity of disease. Apneas are seen more frequently during stages 3 and 4 and REM sleep. In some patients apneas are strictly position related and seen mainly when the patient is in the supine sleeping position [35]. It is also very important to compare preoperative and postoperative results of polysomnography in relation to sleep position in order to avoid artificial changes. For example, a preoperative AHI of 20 in a position-dependent apnea patient is not improved when a postoperative AHI of 10 is obtained, if the postoperative sleep time in the supine position is less than half of the preoperative supine sleep time period.

Surgical Techniques for OSA

Surgical techniques for OSA aim to correct airway obstruction in two main sites: retropalatal and/or retrolingual. Success rates of UPPP alone in all patients are significantly lower than those of tracheotomy or CPAP. Early modifications of UPPP with aggressive tissue resection were suggested to achieve better results, but these were associated with increased complication rates instead of success [53]. Electrosurgery, laser-assisted uvulopalatoplasty, radiofrequency and use of chemical agents were suggested for palate operations, as consequences of advanced technology [5, 21, 28, 39]. Instead of providing better results than UPPP, most of them tried to attain the success of UPPP, and have been recommended for snoring and mild OSAS only. It appears that multilevel and staged surgery provides the best surgical results in patients with OSA [40].

45

Careful dissection with respect to tissue and proper hemostasis is helpful to prevent edema, hematoma, and abscess formation. Nasopharyngeal stenosis is a rare complication of UPPP that can usually be related to the surgical technique.

Factors that might lead nasopharyngeal stenosis [9, 22] are:

- Injury to the posterior mucosal surface of the soft palate and posterior pharyngeal mucosa
- Excessive mucosa destruction
- Aggressive posterior pillar resection
- Excessive use of electrocautery
- Infection and necrosis

Suture dehiscence is another problem that can cause unpredictable healing. In most descriptions of UPPP, suture approximation of tonsillar pillars to eliminate redundant mucosa is included in the surgical technique. Breakdown of sutures after UPPP has a potential negative effect on eliminating redundant mucosa. The incision technique, suture material, and tension at the wound edges may contribute to this complication. Electrocautery is commonly used to incise the mucosa, but the tensile strength of the mucosal wounds created by a scalpel is superior to electrocautery [46]. In one study, the incidence of tonsillar pillar dehiscence was reported as 44.4% with electrocautery versus 33.3% with cold dissection (p=0.41) [1]. Resection of only redundant mucosa instead of aggressive tissue resection prevents the tension at the closure line. Suture materials which provide tensile strength for longer periods such as polyglactin should be used. Mattress sutures that include not only mucosa but also submucosal tissue and muscle provide for higher tensile strength.

One of the causes of persistent symptoms after UPPP is failure to obtain an enlarged lumen at the retropalatal level. Postoperative endoscopy and measurement of cross-sectional area in CT scans are helpful to confirm the pathology findings [26]. Langin et al, [26] reported that patients who failed to respond or who got worse after UPPP had persistent retropalatal narrowing. We feel that the complex relationship between the tongue and the soft palate in the pharynx might explain the reasons for failure (Fig. 45.3). In the absence of an enlarged tongue, reduction of soft-palate length by UPPP would achieve a wide lumen (Fig. 45.4). The extent of palate resection may be limited retropositioned maxilla and hard palate in some patients who are at risk for velopharyngeal insufficiency. We recommend transpalatal advancement pharyngoplasty in these patients.

Decreasing the length of the soft palate may not be enough to widen the lumen in the presence of an

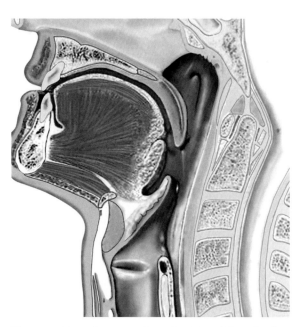

Fig. 45.3. Normal tongue volume. Excision of the soft palate will provide significant airway space

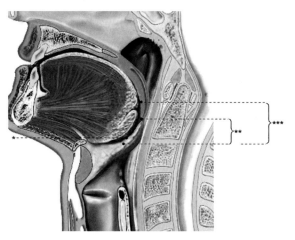

Fig. 45.4. An enenlarged tongue is present. Space superior to the vallecula narrowed (*one asterisk*). Long soft palate and uvula placed posteriorly to the enlarged tongue and occupied a part of the retrolingual space (*three asterisks*). Additionally, a more inferior segment is obstructed by an enlarged tongue (*two asterisks*)

enlarged tongue that pushes the soft palate against posterior pharyngeal wall (Fig. 45.3, 45.5). Langin et al. [26] also remarked that if the palate tended to have its long axis parallel to the posterior pharyngeal wall instead of there being a soft palate bulging into the pharyngeal lumen, surgical techniques to enlarge the pharyngeal lumen instead of excessive palatal resection were successful. This finding

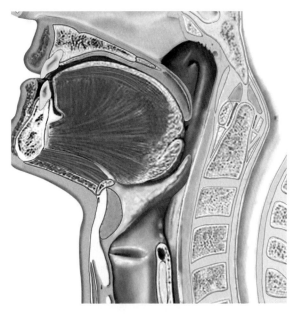

Fig. 45.5. Soft palate partially excised and retrolingual segment inferiorly obstructed by an enlarged tongue

supports our conclusion on the complex relation between an enlarged tongue and the soft palate. Narrowing of the lumen more inferiorly at the tongue base would clearly add to the list of different levels of anatomic obstruction (Fig. 45.5) and in these cases, surgical techniques to enlarge the retrolingual space are needed. A solution to prevent failure in such cases would include sufficient decrease in the length of the soft palate without compromising velopharyngeal insufficiency, transpalatal advancement pharyngoplasty, tongue-base reduction, or maxillomandibular advancement.

Tips and Pearls

Reasons for failure in UPPP:

- Nasopharyngeal stenosis
- Suture dehiscence
- Unable to obtain a wide velopharyngeal space
- Enlarged tongue

In genioglossus advancement, detachment of genioglossus muscle from the tubercule can be repaired with wire sutures to prevent further narrowing of the retrolingual space.

Suture suspension of the tongue base to the mandible also aims to enlarge the airway at the level of the tongue base. Although rare, breakdown of sutures could occur and require revision surgery [36]. Radiofrequency reduction of the tongue base requires sequential treatment sessions until the desired reduction is achieved. When the procedure is performed

aggressively, it may occasionally result in an abscess of the tongue base, which can drain spontaneously or with surgery, without permanent narrowing of the airway. However, the requirement of multisession treatment was not tolerated by all patients, many of whom withdrew from the study after only symptomatic relief and before a possible cure [10]. This is an interesting cause of failure to cure, which is similar to that of CPAP.

Conclusion

Preoperative evaluation, choice of procedure, proper application of technique, and postoperative management influence the outcome of surgery for OSA. Predisposing factors such as endocrine disease, extrinsic abnormalities causing airway obstruction such as neoplasms, and sedating-narcotic medications must be eliminated before surgery. Patients with OSA must be educated about the relationship between weight gain and sleep apnea, and advised to avoid weight gain after surgery. CPAP is an effective and noninvasive treatment for OSA, but the long-term compliance rate is reported as 76% [50]. Choosing the appropriate surgical technique and using proper dissection and hemostasis will reduce the risk for complications and increase the chance for successful surgical outcomes. All patients treated with surgery for OSA should undergo postoperative polysomnography to determine the long-term effectiveness of therapy.

References

1. Altman JS, Senior B, Ransom E: The effect of electrocautery versus cold scalpel technique on the incidence of early postoperative tonsillar pillar dehiscence after uvulopalatopharyngoplasty with tonsillectomy. Laryngoscope. 2004 Feb;114(2):294–6.
2. Arnulf I: Excessive daytime sleepiness in parkinsonism. Sleep Med Rev. 2005;9:185–200.
3. Aziz L, Ejnell H: Obstructive sleep apnea caused by bilateral vocal fold paralysis. Ear Nose Throat J. 2003 Apr;82(4):326–7.
4. Bravo G, Ysunza A, Arrieta J, Pamplona MC: Videonasopharyngoscopy is useful for identifying children with Pierre Robin sequence and severe obstructive sleep apnea. Int J Pediatr Otorhinolaryngol. 2005 Jan;69(1):27–33.
5. Brietzke SE, Mair EA: Injection snoreplasty: How to treat snoring without all the pain and expense. Otolaryngol Head Neck Surg 2001;124:503–10.
6. Brownman CP, Sampson MG, Yolles SF, et al: Obstructive sleep apnoea and body weight. Chest. 1984;85:435–46.

45

7. Cistulli PA, Gotsopoulos H, Sullivan CE: Relationship between craniofacial abnormalities and sleep-disordered breathing in Marfan's syndrome.Chest. 2001 Nov;120(5):1455–60.

8. Dahm MC, Panning B, Lenarz T: Acute apnea caused by an epiglottic cyst. Int J Pediatr Otorhinolaryngol. 1998 Jan;42(3):271–6.

9. Fairbanks DN: Uvulopalatopharyngoplasty complications and avoidance strategies. Otolaryngol Head Neck Surg. 1990 Mar;102(3):239–45.

10. Friedman M, Ibrahim H, Lee G, Joseph N: Combined uvulopalatopharyngoplasty and radiofrequency tongue base reduction for treatment of obstructive sleep apnea/ hypopnea syndrome. Otolaryngol Head Neck Surg. 2003 Dec;129(6):611–21.

11. Friedman M, Tanyeri H, La Rosa M, et al: Clinical predictors of obstructive sleep apnea. Laryngoscope. 1999;109:1901–7.

12. Friedman M, Tanyeri H, Lim JW, Landsberg R, Vaidyanathan K, Caldarelli D: Effect of improved nasal breathing on obstructive sleep apnea. Otolaryngol Head Neck Surg 2000;122:71–4.

13. Fujita S: Pharyngeal surgery for obstructive sleep apnea. In: Fairbanks DNF, Fujita S, editors, Snoring and Obstructive Sleep Apnea (2nd ed), Raven Press, New York, 1994, pp 77–96.

14. Fujita S, Conway WA, Zorick F, et al: Surgical correction of anatomic abnormalities in obstructive sleep apnea syndrome: uvulopalatopharyngoplasty. Otolaryngol Head Neck Surg. 1981;89:923–34

15. Gislason T, Lindholm CE, Almqvist M, Birring E, Boman G, Eriksson G, Larsson SG, Lidell C, Svanholm H: Uvulopalatopharyngoplasty in the sleep apnea syndrome. Predictors of results. Arch Otolaryngol Head Neck Surg. 1988 Jan;114(1):45–51.

16. Grunstein RR, Ho KK, Sullivan CE: Effect of octreotide, a somatostatin analog, on sleep apnea in patients with acromegaly. Ann Intern Med. 1994 Oct;121(7):478–83.

17. Hendler BH, Costello BJ, Silverstein K, Yen D, Goldberg A: A protocol for uvulopalatopharyngoplasty, mortised genioplasty, and maxillomandibular advancement in patients with obstructive sleep apnea: An analysis of 40 cases. J Oral Maxillofac Surg. 2001;59:892–897.

18. Ip MS, Tan KC, Peh WC, Lam KS: Effect of sandostatin LAR on sleep apnoea in acromegaly: correlation with computerized tomographic cephalometry and hormonal activity. Clin Endocrinol (Oxf). 2001 Oct;55(4):477–83.

19. Iwanaga K, Hasegawa K, Shibata N, Kawakatsu K, Akita Y, Suzuki K, Yagisawa M, Nishimura T: Endoscopic examination of obstructive sleep apnea syndrome patients during drug-induced sleep. Acta Otolaryngol 2003;Suppl 550:36–40.

20. Janson C, Gislason T, Bengtsson H, Eriksson G, Lindberg E, Lindholm CE, Hultcrantz E, Hetta J, Boman G: Long-term follow-up of patients with obstructive sleep apnea treated with uvulopalatopharyngoplasty. Arch Otolaryngol Head Neck Surg. 1997 Mar;123(3):257–62.

21. Kamami YV: Laser CO2 for snoring. Preliminary results. Acta Otorhinolaryngol Belg. 1990;44(4):451–6.

22. Katsantonis GP: Limitations, pitfalls, and risk management in uvulopalatopharyngoplasty. In: Fairbanks DNF, Fujita S, editors, Snoring and Obstructive Sleep Apnea (2nd ed), Raven Press, New York, 1994, pp 147–62.

23. Katsantonis GP, Maas CS, Walsh JK: The predictive efficacy of the Müller maneuver in uvulopalatopharyngoplasty. Laryngoscope. 1989;99:677–80.

24. Kern CR, Kutler DI, Reid KJ, Conley BD, Herzon GD, Zee P: Laser-assisted uvulopalatoplasty and tonsillectomy for the management of obstructive sleep apnea syndrome. Laryngoscope. 2003;113:1175–81.

25. Kim ST, Choi JH, Jeon HG, Cha HE, Kim DY, Chung YS: Polysomnographic effects of nasal surgery for snoring and obstructive sleep apnea. Acta Otolaryngol. 2004 Apr;124(3):297–300.

26. Langin T, Pepin JL, Pendlebury S, Baranton-Cantin H, Ferretti G, Reyt E, Levy P: Upper airway changes in snorers and mild sleep apnea sufferers after uvulopalatopharyngoplasty (UPPP). Chest. 1998 Jun;113(6):1595–603.

27. Larsson LH, Carlsson-Nordlander B, Svanborg E: Four year follow-up after uvulopalatopharyngoplaty in 50 unselected patients with obstructive sleep apnea syndrome. Laryngoscope. 1994 Nov;104(11 Pt 1):1362–8.

28. Mair EA, Day RH: Cautery-assisted palatal stiffening operation. Otolaryngol Head Neck Surg 2000;122:547–55.

29. Malow BA, Weatherwax K, Chervin R, et al: Identification and treatment of obstructive sleep apnea in adults and children with epilepsy: A prospective pilot study. Sleep Med. 2003;4:509–15.

30. Messner AH: Treating pediatric patients with obstructive sleep disorders: an update. Otolaryngol Clin North Am. 2003 Jun;36(3):519–30.

31. Millman RP, Carlisle CC, Rosenberg C, Kahn D, McRae R, Kramer NR: Simple predictors of uvulopalatopharyngoplasty outcome in the treatment of obstructive sleep apnea. Chest. 2000 Oct;118(4):1025–30.

32. Obermeyer WH, Benca RM: Effects of drugs on sleep. Otolaryngol Clin North Am. 1999; Apr;32(2):289–302.

33. Ogretmenoglu O: The value of endoscopy in the diagnosis of rhinolithiasis: a case report. Kulak Burun Bogaz Ihtis Derg. 2003 Sep;11(3):89–92.

34. Ogretmenoglu O, Suslu AE, Yucel OT, Onerci TM, Sahin A: Body fat composition: a predictive factor for obstructive sleep apnea. Laryngoscope. 2005 Aug;115(8):1493–8.

35. Oksenberg A., Silverberg D., Arons E. et al: Positional vs. non positional obstructive sleep apnea patients: Anthropomorphic, nocturnal Polysomnographic and multiple sleep latency test data. Chest. 1997;112, 629–639.

36. Omur M, Ozturan D, Elez F, Unver C, Derman S: Tongue base suspension combined with UPPP in severe OSA patients. Otolaryngol Head Neck Surg. 2005 Aug;133(2):218–23.

37. Perkins JA, Sie KC, Milczuk H, Richardson MA: Airway management in children with craniofacial anomalies.Cleft Palate Craniofac J. 1997 Mar;34(2):135–40.

38. Petri N, Suadicani P, Wildschiodtz G, Bjorn-Jorgensen J: Predictive value of Muller maneuver, cephalometry and clinical features for the outcome of uvulopalatopharyngoplasty. Evaluation of predictive factors using discriminant analysis in 30 sleep apnea patients. Acta Otolaryngol. 1994 Sep;114(5):565–71.

39. Powel NB, Riley RW, Troell RJ, et al: Radiofrequency volumetric tissue reduction of the palate in subjects with sleep-disordered breathing Chest 1998;113:1163–74.

40. Riley, RW, Powell NB, Guilleminault C: Maxillofacial surgery and nasal CPAP: a comparison of treatment for obstructive sleep apnea syndrome. Chest, 1990 Dec 98(6):1421–5.

41. Riley RW, Powell NB, Guilleminault C: Obstructive sleep apnea syndrome: a review of 306 consecutively treated

surgical patients. Otolaryngol Head Neck Surg. 1993 Feb;108(2):117–25.

42. Rosenow F, McCarthy V, Caruso AC: Sleep apnoea in endocrine diseases. J Sleep Res. 1998 Mar;7(1):3–11.

43. Sasse SA, Mahutte CK, Dickel M, Berry RB. The characteristics of five patients with obstructive sleep apnea whose apnea-hypopnea index deteriorated after uvulopalatopharyngoplasty. Sleep Breath. 2002 Jun;6(2):77–83

44. SeddonPC, Khan Y: Respiratory problems in children with neurological impairment. Arch Dis Child. 2003; 88(1);75–8.

45. Sher AE, Schechtman KB, Piccirillo JF: The efficacy of surgical modifications of the upper airway in adults with obstructive sleep apnea syndrome. Sleep. 1996 Feb;19(2):156–77.

46. Sinha UK, Gallagher LA: Effects of steel scalpel, ultrasonic scalpel, CO2 laser, and monopolar and bipolar electrosurgery on wound healing in guinea pig oral mucosa. Laryngoscope. 2003 Feb; 113(2):228–36.

47. Skatrud J, Iber C, Ewart R, Thomas G, Rasmussen H, Schultze B: Disordered breathing during sleep in hypothyroidism. Am Rev Respir Dis. 1981;Sep;124(3):325–9.

48. Skjodt NM, Atkar R, Easton PA: Screening for hypothyroidism in sleep apnea. Am J Respir Crit Care Med. 1999 Aug;160(2):732–5.

49. Verse T, Maurer JT, Pirsig W: Effect of nasal surgery on sleep disordered breathing disorders. Laryngoscope 2002;112:64–8.

50. Waldhorn RE, Herrick TW, Nguyen MC, O'Donnell AE, Sodero J, Potolicchio SJ: Long-term compliance with nasal continuous positive airway pressure therapy of obstructive sleep apnea Chest. 1990 Jan;97(1):33–8.

51. Winkelman JW, Goldman H, Piscatelli N, Lukas SE, Dorsey CM, Cunningham S: Are thyroid function tests necessary in patients with suspected sleep apnea? Sleep. 1996;Dec;19(10):790–3.

52. Yantis MA, Neatherlin J: Obstructive sleep apnea in neurological patients. J Neurosci Nurs. 2005;37(3):150–155.

53. Zohar Y, Finkelstein Y, Strauss M, Shvilli Y: Surgical treatment of obstructive sleep apnea. Technical variations. Arch Otolaryngol Head Neck Surg. 1993 Sep;119(9):1023–9.

54. Zonato AI, Bittencourt LR, Martinho FL, Junior JF, Gregorio LC, Tufik S: Association of systematic head and neck physical examination with severity of obstructive sleep apnea-hypopnea syndrome. Laryngoscope. 2003 Jun;113(6):973–80.

Chapter 46

Sedated Endoscopy and Management of Palatal Surgery Failure

46

B. Tucker Woodson

Core Messages

- There is no single cause of uvulopalatopharyngoplasty failure. A stepwise and systematic evaluation allows for identification of the cause of failure and allows for improved clinical, surgical, and medical outcomes.

- Surgical failure may result from medical, technical, or structural causes. Managing failure requires identifying these causes, including reassessing the diagnosis, critically identifying the previous surgical techniques, and reevaluating the structure of the airway.

- Medical failure includes both missed and inaccurate initial diagnosis.

- Technical failure may occur by applying the wrong procedure for a given anatomy, poor surgical techniques, or poor wound healing.

- Structural failure may occur from inadequate treatment of multiple interacting sites of abnormal resistance or obstruction in the upper airway.

- Failure of a surgical procedure is not a failure of patient selection but a failure of accurate diagnosis and appropriate reconstruction.

- Sedated endoscopy independently assessing collapse during inspiration and expiration may provide a means of assessing causes of failure.

Contents

Introduction

Sleep-disordered breathing defined by an apnea–hypopnea index (AHI) of greater than five events per hour is a prevalent disorder estimated to affect 9–24% of middle-aged adults [15]. Obstructive sleep apnea syndrome (OSAS) with both abnormal sleep-disordered breathing and excessive daytime somnolence affects 2–4% of adults. OSAS is strongly associated with significant medical and social morbidity, including increased risk of hypertension, decreased functional quality of life and performance, and increased frequency of accidents [6]. Most risks are elevated with moderate or severe OSAS. However, morbidity and symptoms of OSAS occur with milder forms of the disease and risks are associated with an AHI at both the mild and the severe end of disease spectrum without threshold effects.

Multiple surgical procedures have been advocated as treatment for OSAS. The most commonly performed procedure for OSAS remains uvulopalatopharyngoplasty (UPPP). For many surgeons, UPPP is the primary procedure used alone or in combination with nasal or other surgeries. Outcomes are variable [13]. Failure to adequately treat OSAS or snoring is not uncommon after isolated palatal surgery in adults. In addition, UPPP was associated with severe postoperative pain, increased sensation of phlegm, throat dryness, mild swallowing dysfunction, and continuous positive airway pressure (CPAP) intolerance [3, 11].

Rarely, UPPP is associated with more serious postoperative speech or swallowing changes and medical morbidity, or mortality.

When failure occurs following palatal surgery, no universal treatment protocol exists. Patients must be reevaluated for additional treatment. However, assessment and treatment of palatal surgery failure is not standardized. Few controlled or noncontrolled studies exist to provide recommendations, and so current recommendations are based on uncontrolled or poorly controlled case series and expert opinion. Treatment goals of primary palatal surgery for OSAS include:

- Elimination of symptoms
- Reduction of disease morbidity
- Reduction of mortality

When these goals are not met, additional treatment is indicated. Consensus of evaluating surgical outcomes is to compare results to a successful treatment threshold such as nasal CPAP.

Surgical outcomes are not only technical but also clinical. Palatal procedures may be technically successful in altering some of the characteristics of the palate, but clinically unsuccessful owing to obstruction at nonpalatal sites or other medical or sleep disorders. Conversely, failure of treatment after palatal surgery does not necessarily indicate that obstruction is occurring at other airway sites. Persistent palatal obstruction after palatal surgery is common [7].

Successful treatment of sleep apnea cannot be defined by fixed criteria. A 50% reduction in any currently used sleep study index (apnea index, AHI, or other arbitrary measure) may be an important research measure but rarely defines clinical success. Arbitrary disease thresholds defining sleep apnea as having 20 apneas or hypopneas per hour (or 15 or 10 events per hour) do not correlate to specific disease outcomes [5]. Ultimately, it is these disease outcomes that determine success. Disease outcomes for OSAS include snoring, sleepiness, neurocognitive functioning, risk of accidents, cardiovascular morbidity, and mortality. Lacking data on these, one uses polysomnographic metrics. It is important to understand that these measures define a test, not a patient. None of the measures or outcomes currently define a "cure." Obstructive sleep apnea is a chronic disease where outcomes may best be viewed as disease management rather than "cure."

Age, gender, race, and preexisting health problems alter outcomes and this variability complicates the disease assessment.

Outcomes must be interpreted in the context of other risk factors, but benchmarks for adults may include snoring elimination or reduction to mild intermittent levels, elimination of moderate sleepiness not explained by other conditions, an AHI reduction (using 4% desaturation) to less than 15 events per hour, and lowest oxygen desaturation to be rarely lower than 90%. At this level of disease, therapy with the "gold standard" of treatment (i.e., nasal CPAP) has not shown consistent evidence-based improvement above use of a placebo.

Tips and Pearls

Multiple causes of UPPP failure exist:

- Clinical failure may occur from inadequate medical diagnosis, including insomnia, narcolepsy, limb movement disorders, and idiopathic hypersomnolence.
- Clinical failure may occur owing to obstruction and increased airway resistance at other upper-airway sites, including the nose, hypopharynx, or larynx.
- Technical failure at the palate may occur owing to stenosis or narrowing of the airway.
- No consensus exists about methods of structural airway evaluation. Evaluation should identify the sites of collapse and, if possible, identify the structural cause.
- Revision surgery may be performed if clear abnormalities are identified. The best technical procedure to treat any given structural abnormality is not established.
- Alternatives to surgical correction exist and may include but are not limited to weight loss, oral appliances, and retrials of nasal CPAP.
- Individuals with severe structural upper-airway abnormalities, morbid obesity, and severe sleep apnea may best be treated by maxillofacial surgery or tracheotomy following failure of medical therapy.
- Following failed palatal surgery, the concept of additional surgery or treatment is unpleasant. An important initial treatment step is appropriate education and expectations for palatal surgery.

Indications and Patient Selection

Failure of UPPP may be multidimensional. Diagnostic reevaluation confirms the systems with which the patient presents. Prior testing should be reviewed and, if inadequate, testing should be repeated. A comprehensive head and neck examination focusing on the upper airway should be performed. This includes sitting and supine endoscopy. Additional special testing may include cephalometry, pharyngoesophagram (swallow study), sinus imaging studies, other head and neck imaging, sedated endoscopy, and further sleep tests such as multiple sleep latency or maintenance of wakefulness testing. Confounding medical disorders are identified and treated and retrial of medical therapy is warranted, which may include nasal CPAP, with or without expiratory pressure release, autonasal CPAP, bilevel pressure, and heated humidification. Problems with nasal or face masks should be discussed and addressed and the use of an oral appliance or mandibular repositioning splint may be considered. Oral appliances successfully salvage the surgical failure.

Tips and Pearls

Medical evaluation of disorders that may include symptoms of snoring, excessive sleepiness, or nocturnal choking:

1. Sleep disorders
   (a) Insufficient sleep syndrome
   (b) Drugs/alcohol
   (c) Insomnia
   (d) Idiopathic hypersomnolence
   (e) Periodic limb movement disorder
   (f) Restless leg syndrome
   (g) Narcolepsy
   (h) Increased upper-airway resistance
2. Medical disorders
   (a) Congestive heart failure
   (b) Thyroid disease
   (c) Acromegally
   (d) Depression
   (e) Gerd
   (f) Allergy

Nasal disease is diagnosed and treated with the goal of maximally reducing nasal resistance. Sinus disease should be treated when present, but no evidence supports sinus surgery alone for the treatment of apnea. During the pharyngeal evaluation, findings of overt stenosis or residual lymphoid hyperplasia may be identified. Other abnormalities may only be identified using the sitting and supine office fiberoptic examination or under general anesthesia.

To better treat current and future patients, prior surgical techniques should be evaluated. Errors may be in diagnostic assessment or in surgical technique. Procedures that create a scar will improve snoring but may do so at the expense of narrowing the airway and worsening sleep apnea. Stenosis is an almost certain result of excessive removal of pharyngeal mucosa. Current experience indicates a larger more open airway requires more mucosa not less to remain patent. Technical failure may also be intrinsic to the proce-

dure initially selected. Tonsillectomy without removal of obstructive adenoids (or vice versa) is an example. Unfortunately, failure to adequately enlarge the average OSAS patient's airway is more subtle. Simply identifying the level of obstruction may not provide the required information. Palatal collapse may occur in the proximal or distal pharyngeal isthmus or may occur from collapse of the lateral wall. Hypopharyngeal collapse may also occur in the proximal or distal tongue base, retroepiglottic segment, and larynx or hypopharyngeal lateral wall.

Surgical correction of persistent airway obstruction may include surgery at nonpalatal sites or additional palatal surgery. In the "Stanford algorithm," UPPP failure is usually followed by maxillofacial surgery [10]. Outcomes with this approach demonstrate very high objective success rates (greater than 90%). Unfortunately, the procedures are often poorly accepted by patients with mild or moderate disease.

An alternative approach is additional site-specific surgery. This method lacks a clear algorithm to guide the patient or the surgeon in making decisions about which interventions are appropriate. In a patient who has already undergone a major pharyngeal procedure, the concept of additional unplanned surgery is unpleasant. The need for multiple steps to achieve success is best addressed prior to any surgery. A partial list of available surgical procedures is as follows:

1. Palatal
   (a) Z-plasty pharyngoplasty
   (b) Palatal advancement
   (c) Palatal implants
   (d) Radiofrequency
2. Hypopharyngeal
   (a) Genioglossus advancement
   (b) Hyoid suspension
   (c) Partial glossectomy
   (d) Tongue-base ablation
   (e) Tongue suspension
   (d) Mandibular advancement
   (e) Lingual tonsillectomy
3. Combined
   (a) Maxillofacial advancement
   (b) Tracheotomy

Accurate diagnosis is important in selecting additional surgery. Endoscopy during nonsedated sleep, sedated sleep, and quantitative sedated sleep has been used as both clinical and research tools [8]. Improved surgical success rates have not been associated with many of the subjective methods described to predict success of palatal surgery for sleep apnea. Success in predicting outcomes for snoring surgery outcomes is also questioned with assessment of an audio "snore tape" potentially providing similar information [9].

In contrast, qualitative sedated sleep endoscopy for sleep apnea surgical technique and patient selection using quantitative methods was demonstrated successfully [4]. Differences in outcomes using these tests indicate that interpretation of the test is critical for the examination to be useful. Airway collapse is the result of an interaction of a structurally small airway, ventilatory drive, arousal thresholds, neuromuscular reflexes, lung volume, surface-adhesion forces, body and head position, and level of sleep. To accurately interpret sleep endoscopy, it is necessary to appreciate that the upper airway is a highly variable structure during sleep that is affected by these other physiologic factors. Identification of vibratory tissues or collapse alone is inadequate.

As part of the preoperative evaluation the surgeon should do the following:

■ Reconfirm diagnosis, review sleep study, repeat office upper airway evaluation
■ Understand the structures, mechanisms and physiologic factors that cause collapse and obstruction

Indications and contraindications for sedated endoscopy are as follows:

1. Indications
   (a) Unsuccessful office examination due to anxiety or failure to observe a relaxed airway
   (b) Unexplained surgical failure
   (c) Part of routine presurgical evaluation
2. Contraindications
   (a) Lack of adequate monitoring and airway equipment
   (b) Allergy or contraindications to medications used
   (c) Profound apnea or major medical risk (ASA class IV)
   (d) Lack of proper instrumentation

Technique of Sedated Endoscopy

Intravenous sedation uses a combination of midazolam and propofol in a monitored setting. It is critical to obtain a sedated steady state to mimic sleep. The concept is to maintain a constant brain level of the drugs and avoid undersedation or oversedation, which will alter results. Midazolam (a benzodiazepine) relaxes muscles and depresses respiratory reflexes mimicking rapid eye movement (REM) sleep. Propofol maintains respiratory reflexes and better mimics non-REM sleep. A continuous gradual infusion of medi-

cations is critical. This allows CO_2 levels to rise and to stimulate and maintain ventilation. A rapid induction of sedation causes an acute shift in the ventilatory threshold of CO_2 without time for a compensatory increase in $PaCO_2$. The result is a marked loss in muscle tone to the entire upper airway that does not recapitulate sleep. Sedation should mimic normal sleep and progression should be from snoring to apnea. It is preferable to have too little sedation and to observe snoring mechanisms and sites of primary airflow limitation than to have excess sedation.

Monitoring should include measures of ventilation, oxygen saturation, blood pressure, and heart rate.

The technical steps of sedated endoscopy include:

■ Nasal topical anesthesia
■ Induction of steady-state anesthesia
■ Nonmanipulated view of the airway in both the retropalatal and the hypopharyngeal/laryngeal segments
■ Observation with gentle jaw thrust
■ Observation with a nasopharyngeal airway
■ Oral observation

Equipment required for the procedure includes a rhino-laryngoscope, endoscopic video recording apparatus, a small adult-sized nasopharyngeal airway, topical 4% lidocaine anesthesia, and appropriate equipment for monitoring and handling the difficult airway. The patient should be supine with the head in a neutral position. The room should be quiet and excessive should be light avoided just as with normal sleep.

Step 1. Topical anesthesia (topical 4% lidocaine) and decongestant (oxymetazoline) should be applied with pledgets to the floor of the nose. Excessive topical anesthesia may increase the risk of aspiration and result in pharyngeal and/or laryngeal anesthesia eliminating ventilatory reflexes which confound results. Inadequate local anesthesia and failure to use gentle technique may result in arousal, rhinorrhea, and increased pharyngeal secretions which confound the examination.

Step 2. Sedation is gradually initiated. With the onset of snoring, the rhinolaryngoscope is inserted. This usually results in mild arousal which quickly reverts back to a sleep state. At this point mechanisms and locations of snoring may be observed. Placement of the endoscope is best in the smaller nostril if possible to allow the placement of the nasal airway into the larger nostril in step 5.

Step 3. Patterns, location, and structures associated with airway collapse and airway obstruction are noted.

46

Step 4. Jaw-thrust maneuver assesses both the retroglossal retropalatal area. If tolerated, a graded level of jaw advancement may allow the defining of a critical airway size that is a threshold for obstruction. Failure to observe changes in the retropalatal area may predict a higher risk of poor response to oral appliances.

Step 5. A small nasopharyngeal airway may be placed just beyond the free margin of the palate to eliminate upstream forces affecting the hypopharyngeal airway. This not only eliminates the affects of upstream obstruction in creating increased negative airway pressures, but also eliminates the effects of mechanoreceptor stimulation which augments muscle tone to the tongue and other airway muscles.

Tips and Pearls

The major criteria to evaluate are (1) site(s) of possible airflow limitation/snoring, (2) site(s) of primary (expiratory) obstruction or narrowing, and (3) sites of secondary obstruction:

- Collapse due to structure and anatomy is observed during expiration with loss of phasic ventilatory drive to upper-airway muscles.
- Inspiratory collapse occurs owing to both structure and physiologic factors, such as airflow, muscle tone, and negative inspiratory pressures.
- Inspiratory collapse (increased negative pressure) in an airway patent during the prior expiratory ventalatory cycle suggests a proximal level of obstruction.
- At a primary site of obstruction, progressive expiratory narrowing occurs until a critical calliber occurs and precedes collapse during inspiration .
- Starling resistor and Bernoulli forces result in inspiratory flutter (snoring) which is pathopneumonic for airflow limitation.
- Hypopharyngeal obstruction during vigorous inspiration with reopening during expiration is common and does not indicated lower pharyngeal obstruction.
- The goal is to measure the size and structure of the airway at levels of estimated muscle tone during sleep.
- Insertion of a nasopharyngeal airway reduces airway upstream resistance and decreases stimulation of airway mechanoreceptors. This may paradoxically worsen hypopharyngeal collapse.

Postoperative Assessment and Treatment Plan

Results of a comprehensive evaluation guide further treatment recommendations. Failure of medical therapy should not be accepted at "face value." Problems should be avoided if possible and causes identified and corrected if possible. Nasal CPAP adjustments should be made, including pressure changes, autoadjusting pressures, expiratory relief pressures, behavioral therapy, education, and mask changes. Oral appliances may salvage surgical-failure patients in some cases. Different mandibular splints are available and may be prefabricated or custom-made. These may be provided by the head and neck surgeon, who is familiar with dental and device issues, or may be performed by a dentist. Weight loss, treatment of allergy, and identifying other medical causes should also be addressed.

Decisions on additional surgery should incorporate both severity of disease and structural anatomy. Anatomy and structure guide selection of appropriate surgical procedures. Mild disease does not predict mildly abnormal anatomy and patients with mild or moderate sleep apnea may require major reconstruction for clinical success. Disease severity and patient motivation guide the aggressiveness of surgery. Generally, more morbid surgical procedures are reserved for more severe disease and more motivated patients.

Results and Complications

Limited data on medical or surgical treatment of palatal failures exist. Shepard, Metes, and Woodson used pharyngeal manometry to identify levels of airway obstruction following UPPP failures and found 80% of individuals continue to have obstruction in the retropalatal airway segment [6, 11]. More recently, studies suggested a higher rate of hypopharyngeal obstruction; however, these studies fail to document how such obstruction was defined. Computed tomography before and after UPPP demonstrate that the major difference is not narrowing at the level of the hypopharynx but failure to increase size in the retropalatal airway [1].

No studies have critically evaluated the management of UPPP failure. Woodson reported a high success rate following palatal advancement pharyngoplasty in a small group of patients many of whom had had prior UPPP. Similarly, Woodson and Robinson demonstrated a 70% success rate in reducing the AHI in patients with sleep apnea following palatal advancement and hypopharyngeal surgeries in a group where some had had prior UPPP [5, 6, 11]. Friedman (personal communication) reports surgical salvage of some individuals utilizing Z-plasty pharyngoplasty following failure of a conservative UPPP where excess soft tissue remained. Z-plasty pharyngoplasty has also been discussed as a method of addressing lateral pharyngeal stenosis.

In severe sleep apnea patients, multiple series report that maxillofacial surgery following UPPP failure resulted in very high success rates. Complications of velopharyngeal insufficiency are unusual, but may occur [2]. For this reason, individuals who are at high risk for UPPP failure should be considered for maxillofacial surgery as an initial procedure, with UPPP being reserved as a possible secondary procedure if needed. Hyoid advancement procedures have also been reported. In a subgroup of individuals who had undergone prior UPPP, hyoid advancement was markedly less successful than in a subgroup who had been selected to undergo a hyoid surgery alone [12]. Woodson et al. [14] in a multicenter study applied radiofrequency to the tongue base in a group of patients most of whom had failed prior UPPP. A small treatment effect was observed and subjective patient self-reports were significantly improved, but overall treatment success using this method was low. Nonetheless, a small subset of patients did note a significant improvement, and given the low morbidity of the procedure, it may be appropriate in some patients. Multiple authors have described midline glossectomy and lingual plasty in a group of patients most of whom had failed prior UPPP with variable success rates (20–80%) [12]. Finally, Isono et al. [5] reported on objective measures following UPPP over a 12-month period. For most patients, clinical and structural improvement was maintained; however, for a subset of patients, severe airway narrowing and stenosis occurred between 3 and 12 months after surgery. This indicates that not only may UPPP fail to adequately treat the retropalatal segment, but in some patients it may worsen retropalatal obstruction.

Conclusion

No single algorithm for the management of palatal failure exists. Management must include a comprehensive reassessment of the patient's complaint, underlying disease, medical conditions, and upper-airway structure. Successful salvage of those patients with persisting anatomic abnormalities can be achieved, but requires a thorough understanding of the underlying anatomy and the effects of given surgical procedures on this anatomy.

References

1. Caballero P, Alvarez-Sala R, Garcia-Rio F. CT in the evaluation of the upper airway in healthy subjects and in patients with obstructive sleep apnea syndrome. Chest 113:111–116, 1998.
2. Fairbanks DNF. Uvulopalatopharyngoplasty complications and avoidance strategies. Otolaryngol Head Neck Surg 102:239–245, 1990.
3. Farmer W, Giudici S. Site of airway collapse in obstructive sleep apnea after uvulopalatopharyngoplasty. Ann Otol Rhinol Laryngol 109:581–584, 2000.
4. Gotsopoulos H, Chen C, Qian J, Cistulli P. Oral appliance therapy improves symptoms in obstructive sleep apnea: A randomized, controlled trial. Am J Respir Crit Care Med 166:743–748, 2002.
5. Isono, I, Shimada, A, Tanaka, A, Ishikawa, T, Nishina T, Konno A. Effects of uvulopalatopharyngoplasty on collapsibility of the retropalatal airway in patients with obstructive sleep apnea. Laryngoscope 113:362–367, 2003.
6. Metes A, Hoffstein V, Mateika S, Cole P, Haight JS. Site of airway obstruction in patients with obstructive sleep apnea before and after uvulopalatopharyngoplasty. Laryngoscope 101:1102–1108, 1991.
7. Moore K, Phillips C. A practical method for describing patterns of tongue-base narrowing (modification of Fujita) in awake adult patients with obstructive sleep apnea. J Oral Maxillofac Surg 252–261, 2002.
8. Nieto F, Young T, Lind B, et al. Association of sleep-disordered breathing, sleep apnea, and hypertension in a large community-based study. JAMA 283(14):1829–1836, 2000.
9. Pringle MB, Croft CB. A comparison of sleep nasendoscopy and the Muller Manoeuvre. Clin Otolaryngol 16:559–562, 1991.
10. Riley RW, Powell NB, Guilleminault C. Obstructive sleep apnea syndrome: A review of 306 consecutively treated surgical patients. Otolaryngol Head Neck Surg 108:117–125, 1993
11. Shepard JW, Thawley SE. Localization of upper airway collapse during sleep in patients with obstructive sleep apnea. Am Rev Respir Dis 141:1350–1355, 1990.
12. Sher A, Piccarillo J, Schechtmank K. The efficacy of surgical modifications of the upper airway in adults with obstructive sleep apnea syndrome. Sleep 19:156–177, 1996.
13. Skatvedt O, Akre H, Godtlibsen OB. Continuous pressure measurements in the evaluation of patients for laser assisted uvulopalatoplasty. Eur Arch Otorhinolaryngol 253:1–5, 1996.
14. Woodson BT, Nelson L, Mickelson S, et al. A multi-institutional study of radiofrequency volumetric tissue reduction for OSAS. Otolaryngol Head Neck Surg 125(4):303–11, 2001.
15. Young T, et al. The occurrence of sleep-disordered breathing among middle-aged adults. N Engl J Med 328:1230–1235, 1993.

Permanent Tracheostomy as Treatment of Obstructive Sleep Apnea

Robert H. Maisel, Selena Heman-Ackah

Core Messages

■ Permanent tracheostomy is indicated for patients who have failed medical and surgical management and cannot tolerate continuous positive airway pressure or other devices.

■ Permanent tracheostomy is planned after discussion with the patient/caregivers and thorough preoperative planning involving the anesthesia and perioperative medical management services.

■ Permanent tracheostomy improves morbidity and mortality rates in patients with severe intractable obstructive sleep apnea who do not improve with more conservative medical and surgical techniques.

Contents

Introduction

Obstructive sleep apnea (OSA) is a disease that has been recognized for the last 40 years. With the recognition and evaluation of disease parameters, the medical literature began to recognize that an upper-airway obstruction was the mechanical cause of OSA. The first treatment available was tracheostomy and there was a time in the late 1960s and early 1970s when a permanent tracheostomy was the only recommended treatment for patients with severe behavioral or cardiopulmonary consequences of OSA. Tracheostomy remains the only uniformly totally effective surgical option to permanently relieve OSA. A full understanding of the physiology of OSA led to mechanical techniques and devices to treat the disease and resulted in patients with little need for a tracheostomy. There remain occasional patients with severe OSA who because of their anatomy or surgical complications of treatment are unable to tolerate other mechanical choices such as continuous positive airway pressure (CPAP) or have failed sequential upper-airway surgery, and these patients will benefit from a tracheostomy [4].

Indications and Contraindications of Tracheostomy for OSA

Indications are:

■ Severe OSA
■ Moderate OSA
■ Failure of CPAP or upper-airway expansion surgery
■ Temporary airway bypass during recovery from maxillary-mandibular surgery or bariatric surgery
■ Upper-airway obstruction in difficult intubation patients
■ Aggressive airway surgery requiring temporary airway control

47

Contraindications are:

- Refusal of the patient or family to accept the surgery
- Patient self-destructive behavior
- Medical or anesthesia contraindications

Preoperative Workup

Preoperative workup involves:

- General medical, cardiopulmonary, and coagulation workup and management
- Avoidance of coagulopathy-causing medications for 2 weeks before surgery
- Explaining and describing to the patient, family and all caregivers the appearance and care of tracheostomy
- In-hospital and posthospitalization management, including education about tracheostomy
- Communication with anesthesia and medical subspecialty services and coordination of anesthetic, surgical and postsurgical decisions and management
- Formal anesthesia preoperative consult for potential airway difficulties

Surgical Technique

Tracheostomy for planned permanent airway bypass is best performed in the operating room. The patient is intubated after techniques of airway control and management and stepwise plans to safely perform endotracheal translaryngeal intubation have been agreed. Patients who are anticipated to have a temporary tracheostomy are treated in the standard fashion through a transverse skin incision, retraction of the strap muscles and division of the thyroid isthmus with retraction of soft tissue to allow a direct tracheal puncture, either with extraction of an anterior tracheal window or with a transverse or vertical incision through the trachea.

Tips and Pearls

- When performing a permanent tracheostomy, skin incisions are planned to allow a cutaneous-tracheal mucosal anastomosis which aims to achieve a 360° skin-lined flap surrounding the stoma.
- The skin-lined stoma minimizes granulation tissue, thus avoiding bleeding, occlusion of the airway and crusting/low-grade infection with malodor.
- The stoma, when secured by mucocutaneous flaps, maintains its size and allows for easy stoma management by the patient and caregivers. When healed, the permanent tracheostomy prevents airway emergencies.
- Permanent tracheostomy permits more choices of stoma occlusion than a routine tracheostomy.

The originally described technique, a modification of which we have used for many years, required skin incisions drawn in the pattern of a horizontally directed H with extension of the superior flaps laterally (Fig. 47.1) [1, 7]. Once the flaps have been elevated and defatted as necessary, a cervical lipectomy is performed from the level of the hyoid bone to the level of the third or fifth tracheal ring, depending on the length of the trachea that is easily exposed in the neck (Fig. 47.2). Patients requiring flap tracheostomy are often obese and have retraction of the upper trachea below the level of the clavicle.

When indicated, a submental lipectomy is performed through this incision or even by standard liposuction technique. Removing this unnecessary fat allows the skin flaps to lie in better opposition to the strap muscles and makes the stoma more manageable. Partial removal of the redundant submental fat may prevent tracheostomy occlusion.

The anterior trachea is then fully exposed with retraction of the strap muscles. The thyroid gland is divided in the midline with suture ligation of each lobe to prevent bleeding from the free edges. Sharp and blunt dissection of the pretracheal fascia allows full exposure of the anterior trachea. The trachea is incised in the pattern of a vertical H (Fig. 47.3), creating superior and inferior tracheal flaps, which are then rotated to meet the skin and sutured with absorbable sutures between the skin of the neck and the tracheal wall (Figs. 47.4, 47.5). The inferior tracheal flap may be created slightly longer so it meets the inferior skin flap with less tension and thus creates a stable tracheocutaneous junction without granulation formation.

Nylon or silk sutures can be used to complement the previously placed absorbable suture and must be removed 7–10 days after surgery. At the completion of the operation, a double-cannulated cuffed tracheostomy tube with a balloon is placed. When the tracheostomy tract is long, as in very obese patients, an extended shaft or a customized tracheostomy tube is used. If the original tube placed at surgery is satisfactory, it is substituted with a noncuffed tube of similar size 5–14 days later.

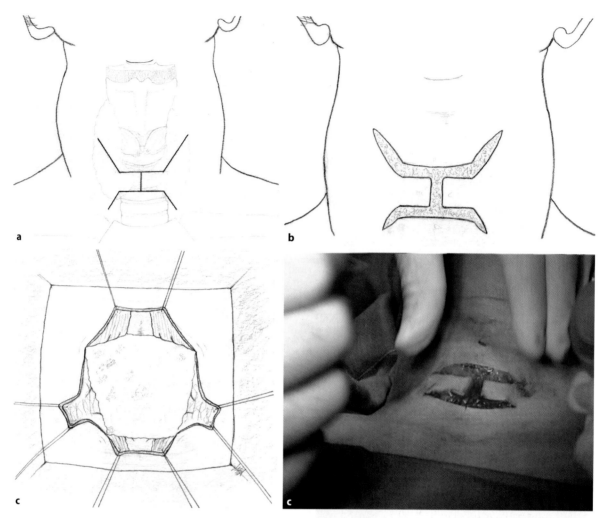

Fig. 47.1 Design and performing skin incisions drawn in the pattern of a horizontally directed H with extension of the superior flaps laterally

There are several variations from this standard technique that we often use, but we most frequently use a single transverse incision placed midway between the cricoid and the sternal notch. This incision allows for better cosmesis, minimizes dead space and reduces risk for seroma formation. The goal of sleep apnea tracheostomy is to keep the stoma occluded during the day so that patients can communicate, humidify their airway and function physiologically. The stoma button is removed at night in preparation for sleep to prevent the symptoms of OSA.

For those patients who still develop shortness of breath, we have been successful with the Montgomery tracheal cannula [5, 6]. This cannula (Fig. 47.6) permits drainage from the wound in the early healing phases and is less likely to dislodge owing to the multiple rings holding it in place. For the mature stoma, a softer and shorter Montgomery tube is used. Many patients become very adapt at recognizing the correct position of the stoma cannula and find it very easy to manage. The tube is designed to capture the inferior and superior tracheal wall anteriorly with flanges that compress during intubation and expand once they are in the open lumen of the trachea. This tube is used in patients without wound complications and is successful in minimizing future wound granulation as well as achieving a more open lumen for the patient. The Montgomery tube must be changed at least every 3–6 months.

Complications

Complications from permanent tracheostomy for OSA were reported [8] in a series of 79 patients, with